NURSING PROCESS AND NURSING DIAGNOSIS

THIRD EDITION

Nursing Process and Nursing Diagnosis

Patricia W. Iyer, RN, MSN, CNA

President, Patricia Iyer Associates
Med League Support Services
Stockton, New Jersey

Barbara J. Taptich, RN, MA

Program Director, Heart Institute
Saint Francis Medical Center
Trenton, New Jersey

Donna Bernocchi-Losey, RN, MA

Office Nurse
San Jose, California;
Formerly Faculty, School of Nursing
University of Nevada at Las Vegas
Las Vegas, Nevada

W.B. SAUNDERS COMPANY
A Division of Harcourt Brace & Company
Philadelphia London Toronto Montreal Sydney Tokyo

W.B. SAUNDERS COMPANY
A Division of Harcourt Brace & Company

The Curtis Center
Independence Square West
Philadelphia, Pennsylvania 19106

Library of Congress Cataloging-in-Publication Data

Iyer, Patricia W.
    Nursing process and nursing diagnosis / Patricia W. Iyer, Barbara J. Taptich,
Donna Bernocchi-Losey. — 3rd ed.
        p.   cm.
    Includes bibliographical references and index.
    ISBN 0-7216-5614-5
    1. Nursing.   2. Nursing diagnosis.   I. Taptich, Barbara J.   II. Bernocchi-Losey,
Donna.   III. Title.
    [DNLM: 1. Nursing Process.   2. Nursing Diagnosis.   WY 100 I97n 1995]
RT41.I94   1995
610.73—dc20
DNLM / DLC   94-17892

Nursing Process and Nursing Diagnosis   ISBN 0-7216-5614-5
Copyright © 1995, 1991, 1986 by W.B. Saunders Company.

Printed in the United States of America

Last digit is the print number: 9 8 7 6 5 4 3 2 1

*To Our Family Members
Who Supported Our Ability
to Complete this Edition:*

Raj, Raj Jr., and Nathan Iyer

Bob, Bobby, and Michael Taptich

Michael, David, Heather, Robert, and Bridgette Losey

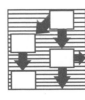

The Saunders Nursing Process Symbols depict the five steps of the nursing process through the use of shapes, arrows, and shading. In *Assessment*, the first step, the multidirectional arrows demonstrate the exploration that occurs during data collection. In *Diagnosis*, judgments are made about the assessment data, and a nursing diagnosis is derived based on these inferences. Each square in the symbol for *Planning* signifies a desired outcome of actions based on the nursing diagnosis. The directional arrows indicate that the plan is outcome-directed and client-oriented. *Intervention* involves the collaborative efforts of the nurse and client in the implementation of the nursing care plan. In this symbol, the changing tonality of the arrows connotes the client's health status as it progresses toward a high level of wellness. The arrow in the last symbol represents *Evaluation* as a flexible and ongoing process. Thus, it indicates that the nurse and client must evaluate each step of the nursing process to determine correct assessment data, an accurate nursing diagnosis, an appropriate nursing care plan, and effective nursing implementation.

Patricia W. Iyer, RN, MSN, CNA is president of two businesses: Patricia Iyer Associates, providing nursing consulting and educational services, and Med League Support Services, assisting attorneys with malpractice and personal injury cases. She has a diploma from Muhlenberg Hospital School of Nursing, a Bachelor of Science in Nursing, and a Master of Science in Nursing from the University of Pennsylvania, Philadelphia. She is certified in nursing administration. Correspondence may be directed to the author at 55 Britton Road, Suite 500, Stockton, NJ 08559.

Barbara J. Taptich, RN, MA, is Director for the Heart Institute at Saint Francis Medical Center, Trenton, New Jersey. She has a diploma from Saint Joseph's Hospital School of Nursing, Reading, Pennsylvania, a Bachelor of Arts in Health Education and School Nursing from Glassboro State College, Glassboro, New Jersey, and a Master of Arts in Health Care Administration from Rider College, Lawrenceville, New Jersey. Correspondence may be directed to the author at 20 Martin Lane, Mercerville, NJ 08619.

Donna Bernocchi-Losey, RN, MA, practices jointly with Michael C. Losey, an Internal Medicine Specialist in San Jose, California. She has a Bachelor of Science in Nursing from Seton Hall University, South Orange, New Jersey, and a Master of Arts in Nursing from New York University, New York, New York. Correspondence may be directed to the author's office at 2895 The Villages Parkway, San Jose, CA 95135.

PREFACE

The nursing process is the foundation on which nursing practice is based. *Nursing Process and Nursing Diagnosis* began as a self-learning module designed to introduce the concept of nursing diagnosis within the framework of the nursing process. We identified the need for a current, comprehensive presentation of the nursing process with an emphasis on the diagnostic phase. This text evolved from that need.

The book provides a comprehensive presentation of each of the five phases of the nursing process. The continuing emphasis on nursing diagnosis within the nursing community has been reinforced by professional standards, regulatory agencies, reimbursement systems, and the desire for a nomenclature specific to the profession. The text is particularly strong in its comprehensive discussion and utilization of the concept of nursing diagnosis.

Nursing Process and Nursing Diagnosis is designed for nursing students and nursing practitioners wishing to learn or review nursing process theory. The material is presented in a clear, understandable manner and provides guidelines for the development of nursing diagnoses, outcomes, and interventions. Exercises and case studies in a self-test format provide the learner with an opportunity to apply these concepts. The appendices include additional information that expands upon the theory contained in the text and also provide additional exercises to reinforce the theory.

This third edition reflects the changes that have occurred within nursing and the health care environment since the first edition was published in 1986. All the chapters have been reviewed, revised, and rewritten. Many of the examples have been altered to reflect the decreasing length of stay and increasing acuity of hospitalized clients. Our examples include additional issues of concern to nurses in a variety of settings. The nursing diagnoses used throughout the text have been updated to include the most current diagnoses available at the time of publication, and include the new Diagnoses in Progress submitted to the 1994 North American Nursing Diagnosis Association conference. In order to clearly relate the nursing process to professional standards, the most recent American Nurses' Association standards are discussed in the text. Content on critical thinking has been added to draw attention to this important aspect of care which is a key component of the nursing process. Critical thinking exercises are included in almost all of the chapters. Patient-focused care and the use of critical pathways is described in the discussion of nursing care delivery systems in Chapter 8. The chapter on evaluation has been rewritten to further clarify the steps in evaluation.

Reflecting the multicultural aspect of our society, the examples use names of patients from many different ethnic groups and reflect social issues such as domestic violence, homosexuality and AIDS. The examples also illustrate the varied roles of nurses and include nurses working in outpatient areas, nursing homes, schools, homes and hospitals. This edition also makes extensive use of the margins to provide a running outline of the chapter, highlight key definitions, and relate the content to the American Nurses' Association standards. This feature has been added to enhance the usefulness of the book. The appendices have been revised to include a section that lists the definition, defining characteristics and related/risk factors for each of the NANDA nursing diagnoses. We hope this section will be particularly useful for developing nursing diagnoses for the exercises, care plans and as a reference throughout the curriculum.

We would like to thank Thomas Eoyang, Editor-in-Chief, W.B. Saunders Company, for his ongoing support, patience and encouragement.

CONTENTS

3 THE DIAGNOSTIC PROCESS   92

4 Writing a Nursing Diagnosis   120

5   PLANNING: PRIORITY-SETTING AND DEVELOPING OUTCOMES   156

7 IMPLEMENTATION   222

8 IMPLEMENTATION: NURSING CARE DELIVERY SYSTEMS   268

9 EVALUATION   286

10 LEGAL AND ETHICAL ISSUES AND THE NURSING PROCESS   314

ONE

THE NURSING PROCESS

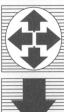

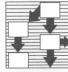

OBJECTIVES

After completing this chapter, you will be able to:

1. Define nursing according to nursing leaders, professional organizations, and nursing functions.
2. Define the nursing process and list six properties.
3. List three prerequisites for the use of the nursing process.
4. Define critical thinking and describe five dimensions of critical thinkers.
5. Explain the implications of the nursing process for the profession of nursing, the client, and the nurse.

INTRODUCTION

Early nursing practice encompassed many roles. The nurse focused on comfort measures and maintaining a sanitary environment. In addition, the roles of pharmacist, dietitian, physical therapist, and social worker were part of nursing practice. The nurse as a health care provider met the total needs of the client. Since that time, there have been a number of factors that have altered the dimensions of nursing practice. These include social, scientific/technological, educational, economic, and political changes. During the evolutionary process, the common thread that has remained is the nurse's focus on the total needs of the client. However, the previously identified factors have also changed the complexion of health care in general. A variety of disciplines—physical therapy, social services, and dietetics—have evolved to assist in meeting client needs. The role of the nurse in the delivery of these ancillary services has shifted from provider to coordinator. This allows the nurse to concentrate on the body of knowledge unique to nursing in the resolution of client problems. The method by which this is accomplished is

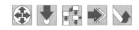
the *nursing process*. It may be helpful to explore some definitions of nursing prior to examining the nursing process in detail.

DEFINITIONS OF NURSING

The profession of nursing has been defined by nursing leaders, by professional organizations, and according to functions. These definitions help to describe the framework upon which the nursing process is based.

Nursing Leaders

The earliest definition of nursing was provided by Florence Nightingale in 1859. Nightingale's *Notes on Nursing—What It Is, What It Is Not* defined nursing as having "charge of the personal health of somebody . . . and what nursing has to do . . . is to put the patient in the best condition for nature to act upon him." The nature of nursing is complex, and efforts to define it have continued to the present day.

Nursing theorists are nurses who develop specific and concrete concepts and propositions that attempt to account for or characterize phenomena of interest to nursing (Fawcett, 1989). Nursing theorists frequently derive theories from models that reflect the profession's goals and philosophies. These models are based on the principles, values, and beliefs that guide the practice of nursing. Nursing theorists develop definitions of nursing based on the model and describe the nursing activities required to achieve the goals of nursing. Table 1-1 summarizes nursing definitions developed by major theorists.

These definitions are just a sample of the many descriptions of nursing. Nursing is both a science and an art. It has its own body of knowledge based on *scientific* theory and focuses on the health and well being of the client. Nursing is concerned with the psychological, spiritual, social, and physical aspects of the person, rather than only the client's diagnosed medical condition. In other words, the focus is on the responses of the total person interacting with the environment. These responses may be influenced by past experiences, the physical environment, the social situation, and family dynamics. Nursing is an *art* that involves caring for the client during times of illness and assisting the client to achieve maximum health potential throughout the life cycle. Nursing strives to adapt to the needs of people in a variety of settings—home, work, ambulatory care centers, and hospitals—through personal interaction with individuals, families, and communities.

INTRODUCTION
DEFINITIONS OF
NURSING
Nursing Leaders
Professional
Organizations

Professional Organizations

The mission of defining nursing has been undertaken by others in addition to nurse leaders. In 1979, the American Nurses' Association (ANA), the profes-

TABLE 1-1   Definitions of Nursing by Major Theorists

THEORIST	MODEL	DEFINITION OF NURSING
Virginia Henderson	Basic Needs	Assisting the individual, sick or well, in the performance of those activities contributing to health or its recovery (or to peaceful death) that s/he would perform unaided if s/he had the necessary strength, will or knowledge
Myra Levine	Conservation	A human interaction whose goal is the promotion of wholeness for all people, well or sick
Dorothy Johnson	Behavioral System	An external regulatory force that acts to preserve the organization and integration of the patient's behavior at an optimal level under those conditions in which the behavior constitutes a threat to physical or social health, or in which illness is found
Martha Rogers	Unitary Human Beings	A science with an organized body of abstract knowledge arrived at by scientific research and logical analysis; it is an art in the imaginative and creative use of the body of knowledge in human service
Dorothea Orem	Self-care	A special concern for the individual's need for self-care action and the provision and management of it on a continuous basis in order to sustain life and health, recover from disease or injury, and cope with their effects
Imogene King	Interacting Systems	A process of action, reaction, and interaction whereby nurse and client share information about their perceptions in the nursing situation; it includes promotion of health, maintenance and restoration of health, care of the sick and injured, and care of the dying
Betty Newman	Systems	Concerned with keeping the client system stable through accuracy in both assessment of effects and possible effects of environmental stressors and assisting client adjustments required for an optimal wellness level
Sister Callista Roy	Adaptation	A theoretical system of knowledge that prescribes a process of analysis and action related to the care of the ill or potentially ill person; it is needed when unusual stresses or weakened coping mechanisms make the person's usual attempts to cope ineffective

Adapted with permission from Fawcett, J: Analysis and Evaluation of Conceptual Models of Nursing. Philadelphia: FA Davis, 1989.

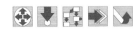

Nursing is the diagnosis and treatment of human responses to actual or potential health problems.

sional organization for nursing in the United States, defined nursing and established the scope of nursing practice. The end result of the ANA's efforts was the publication of "Nursing: A Social Policy Statement (1980)." The definition of nursing presented in this document reflected the historical evolution of the profession and its theoretical base: *"Nursing is the diagnosis and treatment of human responses to actual or potential health problems."*

Human responses are the phenomena of concern to nurses. They have been described as the response of individuals, families, or communities to interaction with their environment. The nurse focuses on two types of responses: "(1) reactions of individuals and groups to actual health problems (health-restoring responses), such as the impact of illness—effects upon the self and family—and self care needs; and (2) concerns of individuals and groups about potential health problems (health-supporting responses), such as monitoring and teaching in populations or communities at risk in which educative needs for information, skill development, health-oriented attitudes, and related behavioral changes arise" (ANA, 1980). More simply, this means that the scope of nursing practice includes the activities of assessing, diagnosing, planning, treating, and evaluating the responses observed in both sick and well persons. Nursing interventions can be directed to the management of the response to an actual problem, such as an illness or disease, or to the prevention of a health problem in a client at risk. Additionally, nursing interventions may focus on reinforcing and supporting health-seeking behaviors. In short, the nurse deals with the client's response to health problems or wellness behaviors. Nurses are concerned with the effect of the disease or health problem on the client's life. These human responses are dynamic in nature and change as the client and/or family progresses along the continuum between health and illness. The client usually has one or more human responses to an acute illness or long-term disease. The human responses are diverse and vary in nature because each client is a unique individual, and the response to the health problem or potential health problem will be a reflection of the individual's interaction with the environment. Consider the following situation.

Example. Mr. Vegas is a 52-year-old cross-country truck driver. While driving his truck 1000 miles from home, he began to develop some tightness in his chest. At first, he passed it off as indigestion. When the discomfort failed to dissipate, he drove to the nearest hospital. Mr. Vegas is admitted to the cardiac care unit with severe chest pain. He is restless and withdrawn. Later, he says that this is his first time in the hospital and he is afraid he might die. Feeling isolated in a hospital so far from home, he asks the nurse to call his wife to ask her to come as quickly as possible. Fortunately, Mr. Vegas had an uncomplicated heart attack. After a few days, he is transferred to another floor. While the nurse is transferring him, Mr. Vegas expresses his concern over the fact that he is going to a new unit. Once on the unit, the physician informs him that it would be in his best interest to change his lifestyle and perhaps retire from truck driving. Mr. Vegas states

TABLE 1-2 Human Responses

1. Self-care limitations such as feeding and dressing
2. Impaired functioning in areas such as rest, sleep, ventilation, circulation, activity, nutrition, elimination, skin care and sexuality
3. Pain and discomfort
4. Emotional problems related to illness and treatment, life-threatening events, or daily experiences, such as anxiety, loss, loneliness and grief
5. Distortion of thought processes, reflected in interpersonal and intellectual dysfunction, such as hallucinations
6. Deficiencies in decision-making and ability to make personal choices
7. Self-image changes created by altered health status
8. Dysfunctional health practices
9. Stress related to life processes, such as birth, growth and development, and death
10. Problems with affiliative relationships

Modified from the American Nurses' Association: Nursing: A Social Policy Statement. Washington, DC, 1980

that this is impossible for he has no other way to support his wife and four children.

This example demonstrates some of the human responses Mr. Vegas had to the health problem of a heart attack. During his hospitalization, the medical diagnosis remained the same from the time of admission to discharge. However, the human responses were multiple in nature and varied on the basis of his progress along the health care continuum. Upon admission, the responses exhibited were those of pain, fear of death, and loneliness. As his health status improved, he exhibited fear about his transfer and had difficulty in accepting the major change in lifestyle suggested by the physician. The nurse's role was to identify the responses of pain, fear, and anxiety and to assist the client in managing them. These are the types of human responses that are within the realm of nursing practice.

Table 1-2 is a list of some of the human responses that are the focus for nursing intervention.

Nursing Functions

Nursing has also been defined in terms of functions or roles. In nursing practice, roles can be divided into two areas: independent and interdependent functions.

Independent Functions

Independent functions are those activities that are considered to be within nursing's scope of diagnosis and treatment. These actions do not require a physician's order. Some examples are shown in Box 1-1.

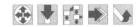

BOX 1-1

Examples of Independent Functions

---

1. *Assessment* of the client/family through health history and physical examination to ascertain health status

2. *Diagnosis* of responses requiring nursing interventions

3. *Identification* of nursing interventions that are likely to maintain or restore health

4. *Implementation* of measures designed to motivate, guide, support, counsel, or teach the client/family

5. *Referral* to other members of the health care team when indicated and allowed by individual state nurse practice acts

6. *Evaluation* of the client's response to nurse and medical interventions

7. *Participation* with consumers or other health care providers in the improvement of health care systems

---

Interdependent Functions

Interdependent functions of the nurse are those that are carried out in conjunction with other health team members. For example, in the case of a pregnant woman with diabetes in a high-risk clinic, the nurse and dietitian collaborate to develop a plan for meeting the nutritional needs of the expectant mother and developing fetus. The dietitian contributes in meal planning and teaching, while the nurse reinforces the teaching and monitors the client's ability to incorporate the diet into daily food selection. Another example of interdependent functions might be seen in the physician's office. The physician diagnoses the medical problem of hypertension and orders medications and dietary modifications in an elderly client. In response to the physician's findings, the office nurse evaluates the client's reaction to the diagnosis and initiates teaching about the disease, drugs, and diet. These are examples of interdependent functions of the nurse.

It is important to note that each state has legally defined the practice of nursing in its nurse practice act. Once licensed, the nurse is responsible and accountable for practicing nursing within the state's legal definition. For example, the practice of nursing, as described in the New Jersey Nurse Practice Act (1993), is clearly defined in terms of its independent and interdependent roles. It states:

Independent
Function

"The practice of nursing as a registered professional nurse is defined as diagnosing and treating human responses to actual or potential physical and emotional health problems through such services as casefinding, health teaching, health counseling, and provision of care supportive to or restorative of life and well being. . .

Interdependent Function   . . . and executing medical regimens as prescribed by a licensed or otherwise legally authorized physician or dentist."

1-1   TEST YOURSELF
Human Responses

After reading the situation below, identify four human responses to actual or potential health problems.

  Mrs. Hart is a 32-year-old white woman admitted to the acute care facility for removal of her right breast. Mrs. Hart informs the nurse that her husband had noticed the lump in her breast approximately six months ago. She had put off going to the doctor because she was afraid that it might be cancer. She explains that she has a 2-year-old child at home and is hoping to become pregnant in the near future, but now that the lump had been discovered, her own future is in doubt. She had delayed childbirth because of her career as an accountant. During the conversation she becomes teary-eyed. After questioning her, the nurse determines that she is anxious about receiving anesthesia.

  Mrs. Hart undergoes a right modified mastectomy. On her first day after surgery, she experiences pain, and because of the nature of the surgery her ability to move her right arm is impaired. This is disturbing to her because she is right-handed. She is not accustomed to being so dependent. On the fourth day after surgery, the physician informs Mrs. Hart that because the disease had spread to two lymph nodes she will require chemotherapy, radiation therapy, or both. After the physician left, Mrs. Hart starts to cry. She tells the nurse that she is afraid she will never be able to have another child or see her little girl grow up. She also refuses to look at her incision when the dressing is changed and expresses that she is scarred for life and will never be attractive to her husband again.

  Human Responses Displayed by Mrs. Hart:

1.

2.

3.

4.

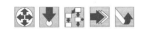

1-1 TEST YOURSELF

Human Responses: Answers

1. Self-care limitations
2. Pain
3. Fear of anesthesia
4. Fear of death
5. Change in self-image
6. Change in relationship with husband
7. Impaired sexuality
8. Grief

The following example illustrates the independent and interdependent functions of the nurse. As you read it, see if you can identify these two different types of functions.

Example. Mr. Rubin Paul, age 64, had surgery five days ago for cancer. While caring for Mr. Paul, the nurse notes he is withdrawn and noncommunicative. The client's wife verbalizes her concern about this dramatic change in her husband's behavior. The nurse discusses this information with the surgeon, and they reach a mutual agreement that a psychiatric evaluation would benefit Mr. Paul. The client and his wife agree, and the physician orders a psychiatric consultation. The nurse notifies the consultant and shares information pertinent to Mr. Paul's physical and psychological status. The psychiatrist evaluates the client, confirms the diagnosis of postoperative depression, and orders medications. The nurse incorporates the administration of this medication along with the use of therapeutic communication into the client's plan of care. In addition, the nurse monitors Mr. Paul's response to both of these modalities.

The lists on the next page identify the independent and interdependent functions that the nurse performed in this example.

In conclusion, the practice of nursing has been defined by nursing leaders, by professional organizations, and according to function to include independent and interdependent components. This definition will evolve in response to nursing research and theory building as well as to the increasing complexity of

INDEPENDENT	INTERDEPENDENT
1. Assessment of psychological status (withdrawn and noncommunicative)	1. Discussion with surgeon regarding psychiatric evaluation
2. Therapeutic communication	2. Administration of medications
3. Evaluation for response to medication and therapeutic communication	3. Communication with psychiatrist about physical and psychological status

health care. However, meeting the total needs of the client will continue to be the focus of nursing practice.

THE NURSING PROCESS

The science of nursing is based on a broad theoretical framework. The nursing process is the method by which this framework is applied to the practice of nursing. It is a deliberative problem-solving approach that requires cognitive, technical, and interpersonal skills and is directed to meeting the needs of the client/family system. The nursing process consists of five sequential and interrelated phases: assessment, diagnosis, planning, implementation, and evaluation. These phases integrate the intellectual functions of problem solving in an effort to define nursing actions.

History

The nursing process has evolved into a five-phase process consistent with the developing nature of the profession. It was first described as a distinct process by Hall (1955). Johnson (1959), Orlando (1961), and Wiedenbach (1963). Each developed a different three-phase process that contained rudimentary elements of the existing five-phase process. In 1967, Yura and Walsh authored the first text that described a four-phase process: assessment, planning, implementation, and evaluation. In the mid 1970s, Bloch (1974), Roy (1975), Mundinger and Jauron (1975), and Aspinall (1976) added the diagnostic phase, resulting in a five-phase process.

Since that time, the nursing process has been legitimized as the framework of nursing practice. The ANA used the nursing process as a guideline in developing standards of care. The nursing process has been incorporated into the conceptual framework of most nursing curricula. It has also been included in the definition of nursing in the majority of nurse practice acts. More recently, the state board licensing examinations were revised to test the ability of the aspiring registered nurse to utilize the steps of the nursing process.

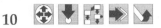
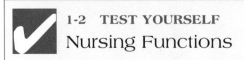

1-2 TEST YOURSELF
Nursing Functions

The following example will give you a chance to practice identifying the independent and interdependent functions of the registered nurse. After reading the example, determine whether the nursing functions identified are independent or interdependent.

Example.   Mr. Ease is an 84-year-old white man admitted to your unit at 6 AM. The night charge nurse reports that Mr. Ease has a history of urinary incontinence at home. His skin is intact, but she noted a reddened area approximately 2 inches in diameter at the base of his spine. He has limited range of motion in all his extremities and is unable to reposition himself in bed.

On first rounds, you find Mrs. Ease, his 80-year-old wife, outside the room crying. She states that she is worried about what is going to happen to her husband because they had no children and she could no longer care for him.

Based on the physician's physical examination and information obtained from the nurse's assessment, the physician's orders include intravenous therapy, vital signs every four hours, two acetaminophen (Tylenol) by mouth every four hours for a temperature elevation above 102°F, insertion of a Foley urinary catheter, and consultation with a physical therapist.

During the course of the day, Mr. Ease's temperature rises to 103°F (rectally). You administer Tylenol and decide to monitor the client's vital signs every hour for the next three hours. You insert the Foley catheter and establish a turning schedule. You also initiate intravenous therapy and record intake and output. You notify the physical therapy department and make a social service referral. After consultation with a physical therapist, you develop a regimen for range of motion exercises. This includes bedside physical therapy twice a day on the day shift by the therapist and specific active and passive exercises on the evening shift by the nursing staff.

Identify the following functions performed by the nurse in this example as independent (IND) or interdependent (INT):

Continued

1-2 TEST YOURSELF
Nursing Functions—cont'd.

FUNCTION	IND	INT
1. Administration of Tylenol		
2. Increasing frequency of vital signs		
3. Insertion of Foley catheter		
4. Establishment of turning schedule		
5. Initiation of intravenous therapy		
6. Initiation of intake and output		
7. Social service referral		
8. Performing range of motion exercises		
9. Assessment of skin integrity		

Definition

The nursing process is the framework for nursing practice in that it provides the mechanism by which nurses use their beliefs, knowledge, and skills to diagnose and treat the client's response to actual or potential health problems. Yura and Walsh (1988) state that "the nursing process is the designated series of actions intended to fulfill the purpose of nursing—to maintain the client's optimal wellness—and, if this state changes, to provide the amount and quality of nursing care his situation demands to direct him back to wellness. If wellness cannot be achieved, the nursing process should contribute to the client's quality of life, maximizing his resources to achieve the highest quality of living possible for as long a time as possible."

Purpose

The major purpose of the nursing process is to provide a framework within which the individualized needs of the client, family, and community can be met. The nursing process involves an interactional relationship between the client and the nurse, with the client as the focus. The nurse validates observations with the client, and together they utilize the process. This assists the client to deal with changes in health status and results in individualized care.

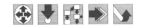

1-2 TEST YOURSELF
Nursing Functions: Answers

FUNCTION	IND	INT
1. Administration of Tylenol		✔
2. Increasing frequency of vital signs	✔	
3. Insertion of Foley catheter		✔
4. Establishment of turning schedule	✔	
5. Initiation of intravenous therapy		✔
6. Initiation of intake and output	✔	
7. Social service referral	✔	
8. Performing range of motion exercises		✔
9. Assessment of skin integrity	✔	

Organization

As previously noted, the nursing process is organized into five identifiable phases: assessment, diagnosis, planning, implementation, and evaluation. Each can be further described as follows.

Assessment

Assessment is the first phase of the nursing process. Its activities are focused on gathering information regarding the client, the client/family system, or the community for the purpose of identifying the client's needs, problems, concerns, or human responses. Data are collected in a systematic fashion, utilizing the interview or nursing history, physical examination, laboratory results, and other sources.

Diagnosis

During this phase, the data collected during assessment are critically analyzed and interpreted. Conclusions are drawn regarding the client's needs, problems, concerns, and human responses. Nursing diagnoses are identified and provide a central focus for the remainder of the phases. Based on the nursing diagnoses, the plan of care is designed, implemented, and evaluated. The nursing diagnoses supply an efficient method of communicating the client's problems.

Planning

In the planning phase, strategies are developed to prevent, minimize, or correct the problems identified in the nursing diagnosis. The planning phase consists of several steps:

1. Establishing priorities for the problems diagnosed.
2. Setting outcomes with the client to correct, minimize, or prevent the problems.
3. Writing nursing interventions that will lead to the achievement of the proposed outcomes.
4. Recording nursing diagnoses, outcomes, and nursing interventions in an organized fashion on the plan of care.

Implementation

Implementation is the initiation and completion of the actions necessary to achieve the outcomes defined in the planning stage. It involves communication of the plan to all those participating in the client's care. The interventions can be carried out by members of the health care team, the client, or the client's family. The plan of care is used as a guide. The nurse continues to collect data regarding the client's condition and interaction with the environment. Implementation also includes recording the patient's care on the proper documents. This documentation verifies that the plan of care has been carried out and can be used as a tool to evaluate the plan's effectiveness.

Evaluation

The last phase of the nursing process is evaluation. It is an ongoing process that determines the extent to which the goals of care have been achieved. The nurse evaluates the progress of the client, institutes corrective measures if required, and revises the nursing care plan.

This discussion has separated the nursing process into five distinct phases. In actual practice, you may not always complete one phase before moving to the next. For example, if your preliminary assessment data determine that the client is having difficulty breathing, you may give oxygen before completing the remainder of your assessment. The phases of the process are, however, interrelated and interdependent. The assessment data provide information for the diagnosis and planning phases. Similarly, the plan of care guides the implementation phase and determines the criteria for evaluation.

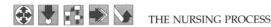
Properties

The nursing process has six properties: it is purposeful, systematic, dynamic, interactive, flexible, and theoretically based. The nursing process can be described as *purposeful* because it is goal directed. The nurse utilizes the phases of the process to provide quality client-centered care. The process is *systematic* because it involves the use of an organized approach to achieve its purpose. This deliberate method promotes the quality of nursing and avoids the problems associated with intuition or traditional care delivery.

The nursing process is *dynamic* because it involves continuous change. It is an ongoing process focused on the changing responses of the client that are identified throughout the nurse-client relationship. The *interactive* nature of the nursing process is based on the reciprocal relationships that occur between the nurse and the client, family, and other health professionals. This component ensures the individualization of client care.

The *flexibility* of the process may be demonstrated in two contexts: (1) it can be adapted to nursing practice in any setting or area of specialization dealing with individuals, groups, or communities; (2) its phases may be used sequentially and concurrently. The nursing process is most frequently utilized in sequence; however, the nurse may utilize more than one step at a time. For example, while implementing the plan of care, the nurse may evaluate its effectiveness.

Finally, the nursing process is *theoretically based*. The process is devised from a broad base of knowledge, including the sciences and humanities, and can be applied to any of the theoretical models of nursing.

Prerequisites

The use of the nursing process is influenced by the nurse's beliefs, knowledge, and skills. The nurse's beliefs and knowledge form the foundation for nurse-client interactions. Knowledge and skills are the tools that enable the nurse to (1) acquire data, (2) determine their significance, (3) develop interventions that promote individualized nursing care, (4) evaluate the effectiveness of the plan of care, and (5) initiate changes to assure that the client receives quality care.

Beliefs

The nurse's beliefs include philosophies about nursing, health, the client as an individual and as a health care consumer, and the interactions between these factors. These beliefs become part of the theoretical framework upon which the nurse's practice is based. This framework is reflected as the nurse implements each of the five phases of the nursing process.

Example. Steven Bodine, age 25, is admitted to the hospital with a medical diagnosis of metastatic cancer of the lung. His primary tumor, testicular cancer,

1-3   TEST YOURSELF
Nursing Process Phases

Match the nursing activities in Column I with the correct phase of the nursing process identified below:

  Assessment
  Diagnosis
  Planning
  Implementation
  Evaluation

NURSING ACTIVITY	PHASE
Analyzing and interpreting data	
Initiating nursing interventions	
Performing a physical examination	
Determining outcomes with the client	
Revising the plan of care	
Interviewing the client	
Writing a nursing diagnosis	
Determining if outcomes have been achieved	
Developing interventions to achieve outcomes	
Recording care on the proper documents	
Developing a plan of care	

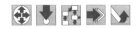

 1-3 TEST YOURSELF

Nursing Process Phases: Answers

NURSING ACTIVITY	PHASE
Analyzing and interpreting data	Diagnosis
Initiating nursing interventions	Implementation
Performing a physical examination	Assessment
Determining outcomes with the client	Planning
Revising the plan of care	Evaluation
Interviewing the client	Assessment
Writing a nursing diagnosis	Diagnosis
Determining if outcomes have been achieved	Evaluation
Developing interventions to achieve outcomes	Planning
Recording care on the proper documents	Implementation
Developing a plan of care	Planning

Purpose
Organization
Properties
Prerequisites
Beliefs

was diagnosed three years ago, and he has completed an extended series of both radiation and drug therapies. Steven and his wife have reached a mutual decision that his disease process and the need for continuing therapy have severely affected the quality of his life. Therefore, he has chosen to discontinue all therapy. This decision is supported by his physician.

You believe that Steven has the right to make an informed decision and to control the manner in which he spends the remainder of his life. Your role as a client advocate directs you to assist him in accomplishing these goals. You determine that Steven would like to be made comfortable and to die at home with the support of his family. Your interventions, in this case, would therefore focus on the implementation of a pain management regimen, client/family teaching, and referral to a hospice program.

INTRODUCTION
DEFINITIONS OF
NURSING
THE NURSING
PROCESS

Knowledge

The nursing process demands that you possess an extensive body of knowledge from a variety of disciplines. This knowledge base includes both physical and behavioral sciences. You are expected to master basic concepts of anatomy, physiology, chemistry, nutrition, microbiology, psychology, and sociology. The components of this scientific base allow you to assess the client's physiological and psychological state. You use this knowledge base to diagnose the client's human responses to health issues and identify the factors that contribute to their presence. Individualized nursing interventions are selected based on your understanding of those actions that are most likely to be effective. Subsequently, the effectiveness of the interventions is evaluated based on your knowledge of identified expected client outcomes.

Example. John Thomas is an obese 42-year-old salesman who is admitted to the hospital for a cholecystectomy. On the third postoperative day, Mr. Thomas calls you and indicates that he feels as though his "stitches are popping." You note that he is pale and diaphoretic, and further observation reveals four open sutures at the incisional area. A loop of bowel is protruding through the lower end of the opening. In addition, the client is hypotensive, with a BP of 100/68.

Based on this assessment, you instruct the client not to eat or drink, place a sterile saline soaked dressing over his abdomen, and contact Mr. Thomas's surgeon. Your knowledge base is used to anticipate the need for further surgery. Application of your knowledge about postoperative care resulted in prompt nursing actions that prevented more serious complications.

Skills

A variety of skills are necessary to implement the nursing process. These skills are related to the knowledge base and may be both technical and interpersonal in nature.

Technical skills associated with the nursing process involve specific techniques and procedures that allow you to collect the data and develop, implement, and evaluate a comprehensive plan of care. Some technical skills are associated with the use of equipment such as the stethoscope, sphygmomanometer, and thermometer for the measurement of vital signs. Others involve the performance of procedures such as administration of medications, turning and positioning clients, and changing dressings.

Interpersonal skills are important during all phases of the nursing process. Because this is a communicative, interactive process, you must have highly developed communication skills. These skills facilitate the development of positive relationships between you and the client or family. These positive relationships allow you to:

- determine what the client/family sees as priorities.
- identify additional nursing concerns.
- create a therapeutic environment in which mutual outcomes may be accomplished.

Development of the therapeutic environment begins with your first interaction with the client and requires you to possess verbal and nonverbal

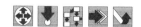
communication skills. Certainly, you must be able to share information by choosing language that accurately conveys the desired message at a level appropriate for the client. In addition, you must have highly developed listening skills, which contribute to the therapeutic environment by allowing the client/family to feel comfortable expressing thoughts, feelings, and concerns. The nonverbal component of communication is of particular importance in the development of nurse-client relationships.

Implications

The use of the nursing process in practice has implications for the profession of nursing, the client, and the individual nurse.

Implications for the Profession

Professionally, the nursing process concretely demonstrates the scope of nursing practice. Through the five phases, nursing continues to define its role to the consumer and other health care professionals. This clearly points out that the realm of nursing is more than just implementing the plan of care as prescribed by the physician.

In addition, the nursing process has been incorporated into Standards of Clinical Nursing Practice developed and published by the ANA (1991). Standards of Clinical Nursing Practice consists of Standards of Care and Standards of Professional Performance. Standards of Care define the care that should be provided to all clients requiring professional nursing services (Table 1-3). These standards are based on the nursing process, include significant interventions initiated by nurses to provide care to clients, and form the foundation for clinical decision-making by nurses. Standards of Care include the following components:

- Assessment
- Diagnosis
- Outcome identification
- Planning
- Implementation
- Evaluation

Nurses are held accountable for practicing according to these standards regardless of the setting or their area of specialization.

Standards of Professional Performance identify additional expectations of nurses in their roles as professionals. Nurses include these activities when appropriate based on their education, position, and practice setting.

TABLE 1-3   Standards of Clinical Nursing Practice

STANDARDS OF CARE	STANDARDS OF PROFESSIONAL PERFORMANCE
Standard I: *Assessment* The nurse collects client health data	**Standard I:** *Quality of Care* The nurse systematically evaluates the quality and effectiveness of nursing practice
Standard II: *Diagnosis* The nurse analyzes the assessment data in determining diagnoses	**Standard II:** *Performance Appraisal* The nurse evaluates his/her own nursing practice in relation to professional practice standards and relevant statutes and regulations
Standard III: *Outcome Identification* The nurse identifies expected outcomes individualized to the client	**Standard III:** *Education* The nurse acquires and maintains current knowledge in nursing practice
Standard IV: *Planning* The nurse develops a plan of care that prescribes interventions to attain expected outcomes	**Standard IV:** *Collegiality* The nurse contributes to the professional development of peers, colleagues, and others
Standard V: *Implementation* The nurse implements the interventions identified in the plan of care	**Standard V:** *Ethics* The nurse's decisions and actions on behalf of clients are determined in an ethical manner
Standard VI: *Evaluation* The nurse evaluates the client's progress toward attainment of outcomes	**Standard VI:** *Collaboration* The nurse collaborates with the client, significant others, and health care providers in providing client care
	Standard VII: *Research* The nurse uses research findings in practice
	Standard VIII: *Resource Utilization* The nurse considers factors related to safety, effectiveness, and cost in planning and delivering client care

Reprinted with permission from *Standards of Clinical Nursing Practice,* © 1991, American Nurses Association, Washington, DC.

These standards include criteria related to:

- Quality of care
- Performance appraisal
- Education
- Collegiality
- Ethics
- Collaboration

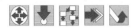
- Research
- Resource utilization

Both Standards of Care and Standards of Professional Performance include measurement criteria which define the activities that demonstrate that the standards have been achieved.

Implications for the Client

The use of the nursing process benefits the client and family. It encourages them to participate actively in care by involving them in all five phases of the process. The client provides assessment data, validates the nursing diagnosis, confirms outcomes and interventions, assists with implementation, and provides feedback for evaluation. In addition, the written plan of care promotes **continuity of care**, which results in a safe, therapeutic environment. The absence of this continuity may cause problems similar to those described in the following situation.

Example. Verna MacCarthy was a nursing supervisor of a medical surgical unit. On rounds, she encountered Mrs. Martin, the wife of one of the clients, who stated that she had some complaints concerning the care of her husband. She explained that her husband developed an infection of his incision following bowel surgery. The doctor told her the dressing had to be changed and the wound irrigated three times daily. She indicated that this procedure was being done but that each nurse did it differently. Some even asked her or her husband how to do the procedure. "How come the nurses don't all do it the same? Who is doing it right? Shouldn't it be written somewhere? How will my husband ever get better?"

This situation demonstrates that when nursing care is uncoordinated, the family loses confidence in the staff's ability to meet the client's needs. An anxiety-producing environment is created rather than a therapeutic one.

The use of a systematic method of providing nursing care also improves the **quality** of that care.

Example. Rosalind Brosier, a 30-year-old teacher, delivered her second child a week ago. Usually the public health nurse's first visit includes teaching about growth and development and contraception. However, the nurse's assessment of this client's learning needs reveals adequate understanding in both of these areas. Therefore teaching focuses on providing information about infant nutrition—a topic of concern to the client.

The use of the nursing process in this situation ensured a thorough assessment of the client's learning needs and involved her in planning approaches to meet them. The absence of this type of approach can lead to error, omissions, and duplications in care. Failure to use a systematic method of providing care might result in a frustrating experience for the client, which could also compromise the quality of care delivered.

Individualized care is also promoted by the use of the nursing process. For example, the priorities of care for a client with pneumonia frequently focus on temperature monitoring, hydration, and antibiotic therapy.

Example. When Bonnie O'Malley is admitted for pneumonia, her three preschool children are left with a 15-year-old baby sitter. The physician's plan of care includes temperature control, intravenous therapy, and antibiotics. In the assessment phase, you identify Bonnie's concern about her children. Because of her child-care problem, Bonnie feels that she has no choice but to leave the hospital against medical advice. You initiate a social service consultation that resolves Bonnie's dilemma. This allows Bonnie to remain in the hospital and to participate in those measures designed to restore her health. By addressing Bonnie's special needs, you are able to provide quality individualized care.

Implications for the Nurse

The nursing process increases **job satisfaction** and **enhances professional growth**. The development of meaningful nurse-client relationships is facilitated by the nursing process. The rewards obtained from nursing practice are frequently derived from the nurse's ability to assist the client to meet identified needs. The genuine "thank you," regardless of the manner in which it is expressed by clients and their families, often outweighs any other type of recognition.

Job satisfaction may also be increased through the use of the plan of care developed from the nursing process. Well-written plans save time and energy and prevent the frustration that is generated by trial and error nursing. Consider this situation.

Example. Walter Lodge was a 300-lb man who had a right total hip replacement three days ago. Today you are caring for him and must get him out of bed. The nurse giving change of shift report states that yesterday was his first time out of bed. You are concerned about how you will accomplish this task. You know that Mr. Lodge is overweight, cannot bear weight on the right leg, and is at risk for dislocating his hip. You are familiar with several recommended procedures for getting the client out of bed safely; however, the chart and care plan give no indication of which method was successfully used on the previous day. Mr. Lodge is unable to describe the method used, and the nurses who assisted him yesterday are not available. You finally select a strategy, choose a chair, and estimate the amount of assistance you will need to move Mr. Lodge.

This situation illustrates how the nursing process can save time and decrease frustration. In this instance, if the plan of care had specific directions on how to get Mr. Lodge out of bed, you would not have experienced frustration and anger. You would have been able to get Mr. Lodge out of bed more efficiently. As demonstrated here, coordinating a client's nursing care through the use of the nursing process greatly increases the chances of achieving the desired outcome.

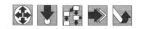
The nursing process enhances **professional growth**. The application of the nursing process encourages the development of cognitive, technical, and interpersonal skills. As you proceed through your nursing curriculum, you will accumulate additional knowledge through interaction with colleagues, clients, and other health care providers. Interaction with a variety of clients and other health care professionals encourages refinement of your verbal and nonverbal communication skills. The effectiveness of the nurse in daily practice is therefore enhanced. The nursing process provides the framework for implementation of the nurse's professional role behaviors identified in the Standards of Professional Performance developed by the ANA (Table 1-3).

CRITICAL THINKING AND THE NURSING PROCESS

Nurses make purposeful, goal-directed decisions in their professional practice. Critical thinking involves questioning assumptions, determining conclusions, and identifying the justifications to support them. Critical-thinking skills are necessary for you as an individual and a professional—you must be able to make informed personal decisions as well as those necessary to provide safe, competent, and skilled nursing care. You entered your nursing program with at least basic critical-thinking skills. For example, when preparing to rent an apartment, you might use critical thinking to identify and analyze the factors that will influence your decision. You gather information about cost, location, condition, size, furnishings, and the availability of security systems. After analyzing each of your options, you conclude that the most effective solution is to rent a two-bedroom apartment with one of your classmates. In this situation you have utilized the elements of critical thinking to make a personal decision.

In your nursing practice, you use similar thinking processes to make professional decisions. You will be required to collect data, define actual and potential problems accurately, make the best choices among alternatives, safely implement a plan of care, and evaluate the effectiveness of nursing interventions. Thus, the nursing process becomes the framework within which you can apply critical-thinking skills. This approach is based on the scientific method and reduces the limitations imposed when your beliefs, values or feelings influence your thinking process. The consistent use of well-developed critical-thinking skills increases the potential for success in your nursing practice and positive outcomes for your clients.

Definition

There are a variety of definitions for critical thinking. Kurfiss (1988) defines critical thinking as "... *an investigation whose purpose is to explore a situation, phenomenon, question or problem to arrive at a hypothesis or conclusion about it that*

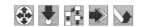

integrates all available information and that therefore can be convincingly justified." Ennis (1985) defines critical thinking as *"rational, reflective thinking concerned with what we do or believe."*

Watson and Glaser (1980) provide an explanation that is more easily adapted to nursing practice. They describe the following components of critical thinking:

1. Defining a problem
2. Selecting pertinent information for the solution
3. Recognizing stated and unstated assumptions
4. Formulating and selecting relevant hypotheses
5. Drawing conclusions
6. Judging the validity of inferences

Example. Nora Hafford is a 61-year-old woman admitted for elective knee joint replacement. You greet her, make her comfortable, and begin the nursing history. When you indicate that you would like to interview her, Mrs. Hafford states that she would like her daughter, a nurse-attorney, to be with her during the interview. She states that she expects her within the hour.

In this situation, you demonstrate your critical-thinking skills in selecting the timing of the health history. This sensitivity puts Mrs. Hafford at ease and strengthens your relationship with this client. Please refer to the table on the next page.

The outcomes of critical thinking are a conclusion and the justification to support it. These two components differentiate critical thinking from everyday thinking and characterize it as purposeful and goal directed.

Dimensions of Critical Thinkers

INTRODUCTION
DEFINITIONS OF
NURSING
THE NURSING
PROCESS
CRITICAL
THINKING
Definition
Dimensions
Logical

Nurses use the concepts described above as they apply the nursing process. This is particularly important as health care continues to be more complex, its knowledge base expands, and nurses seek to practice more autonomously. Professional nurses who are most successful in the use of critical thinking are logical, competent, flexible, and creative. They also use initiative and communicate effectively.

Logical

The use of logical, organized, and consistent approaches to critical thinking is key to its success and to positive outcomes. You must determine what the issue or problem is in each situation. You must also decide what information you need to make a judgment about the situation and how you can obtain it. You must be able to decide whether the data you have gathered are valid and determine what they mean. Next, you must develop an action plan based on the facts and

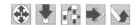
STEP	CRITICAL THINKING
1. Defining a problem **(What is the issue?)**	1. Client prefers to have her daughter present during the interview but you would prefer to collect the data now.
2. Selecting pertinent information for the solution **(What information do I need and where can I get it?)**	2. Client verbalized her preference. Waiting for her daughter will positively influence the interview and will not compromise the client's care. You have the time to wait for the client's daughter.
3. Recognizing differences between fact and assumptions **(Is my data valid?)**	3. You are unfamiliar to the client. The client may be anxious about hospitalization and the interview. The client may be more comfortable with her daughter present.
4. Formulating and selecting relevant hypotheses **(What do the data mean?)**	4. The client is typically anxious and will feel supported by her daughter.
5. Drawing conclusions **(Based on the facts, what should I do?)**	5. Waiting for the client's daughter is important to her and is in her best interest.
6. Judging the validity of inferences **(Is this the best way to deal with the issue?)**	6. When you indicate your intent to return when her daughter arrives, the client thanks you and restates how important her daughter's presence is to her.

question whether your plan is the *best* way to deal with the issue, considering the facts.*

Example.   You walk into Barbara Draper's hospital room and find her on her side in fetal position, clutching her lower abdomen, shaking and crying. You initiate a logical critical thinking approach to identifying what is happening with this client.

1. *What is the issue?*
   The issue in this case is that there has been a change in Barbara since your last observation.

2. *What information do I need and how do I get it?*
   You may want to talk to Barbara to determine her perception of what is happening. It will also be helpful to evaluate her physical condition by checking her vital signs and identifying whether she is having pain. When you last observed Barbara, she was walking in the hall and talking with

*Using Watson and Glaser's framework you can ask a series of questions. In this text we have varied the questions slightly as critical thinking is discussed in relation to each step of the nursing process. These variations illustrate how critical thinking is used throughout the nursing process.

her roommate. You may want to talk with the client and examine the medical record to determine what has changed since your last observation.

3. *Are my data valid?*
   When you talk with her, Barbara states that her doctor says that she needs an operation. Your review of the physician's progress notes supports that he is planning exploratory surgery. The past medical history component of the client's health assessment indicates that she has never had surgery. You note that the client's vital signs; B/P 140/78, P 92, R 24, are elevated compared to previous findings and note that Barbara is shaking and crying. This behavior is different from that observed before the physician's visit.

4. *What do the data mean?*
   The presence of shaking, crying, fetal posturing, and increased blood pressure, pulse rate, and respiratory rate following the physician's visit and discussion about impending surgery suggest that the client is fearful about the surgery.

5. *Based on the facts, what should I do?*
   In this case, it may be helpful to discuss strategies to decrease fear with the client and decide which will be most helpful to her. Barbara indicates that she would like to talk to her physician again about the surgery when her husband and sister can be with her. She also feels that she will do better if she can go home for about two weeks to prepare herself and make arrangements for her three young children. She does not want to speak to a social worker at this time but feels that her minister will be of assistance. You know that the surgery is not emergent, therefore you:

   - arrange to have her physician visit at a time when her husband and sister are present.
   - support her decision to go home.
   - call the minister and ask her to visit Barbara before she leaves the hospital.

6. *Are there other questions I should ask?*
   You may want to explore Barbara's fears about surgery. For example, has she known someone who had a complication after surgery?

7. *Is this the best way to deal with the issue?*
   In this situation, the strategies developed to deal with Barbara's fear are both scientifically sound and consistent with the client's needs at this time.

Competent

Nurses become competent by acquiring and updating the profession's rapidly expanding knowledge base and developing and maintaining required skills through experience. Your knowledge base must include the fundamentals of problem solving and decision making. You must be able to analyze data,

INTRODUCTION
DEFINITIONS OF NURSING
THE NURSING PROCESS
CRITICAL THINKING

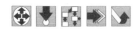
Definition
Dimensions
Logical
Competent

recognize significant relationships among data, develop valid conclusions, and subsequently make sound nursing judgments that contribute to the client's progress. Experiences from within and outside of nursing promote the development of appropriate alternatives for resolving client care and management issues. As you acquire more experience and develop more confidence in your abilities, you will be able to identify your strengths and recognize your limitations, particularly in the process of critical thinking. You may also feel more comfortable in questioning what is being done, why you are doing it, and what the implications of your actions might be.

Based on the work of Benner (1984), you can expect to enter the nursing profession as a novice and progress in your level of competence through advanced beginner, competence, proficiency, and expert. Box 1-2 describes each level of competency. Based on these principles, you will also identify that you are not expected to be perfect and that the errors you make as you develop professionally become the framework for continued learning.

Example. Pat Magovern is a new graduate nurse assigned to care for a client with a draining wound. Pat acknowledges her inexperience in caring for clients with this challenging problem. She works with the wound care specialist to learn specific nursing interventions commonly used in the effective management of draining wounds. Her observation of and participation in care provide

---

BOX 1-2
Levels of Competency

Novice	Nurse who has had no experience in the situations in which he/she is expected to perform and requires detailed analysis for problem-solving
Advanced Beginner	Nurse who can demonstrate marginally acceptable performance, has some experience but requires support in clinical decisions
Competent	Nurse who can master, cope with and manage the many contingencies of clinical nursing but may not have speed and flexibility
Proficient	Nurse who perceives a clinical situation as a whole, including its implications for long-term planning and modification
Expert	Nurse who has sufficient experience to possess an intuitive grasp of clinical situations rather than relying on analysis for routine problem-solving

Modified from the Dreyfus Model Applied to Nursing from *From Novice to Expert*, by Patricia Benner. Copyright (©) 1984 by Addison-Wesley Publishing Company. Reprinted by permission.

the experience that will allow her to recognize similarities and differences when applying this experience to future care of clients with draining wounds. It will also assist her to develop strategies for client care independently in the future. Her ability to be open-minded, consider the views of clients/peers, and persevere in finding the best solution for problems will provide the framework for the integration of critical thinking activities into her nursing practice.

Flexible

Traditionally, nursing systems have not encouraged flexibility in the resolution of client care issues. This is often influenced by: (1) the bureaucracy imposed by internal and external regulation, (2) rigid policies and procedures in health care settings that frown on change, and (3) the lack of teamwork within and between health care disciplines. In today's environment, the concepts of teamwork, client-focused care, recognition of constantly changing priorities, and ability to compromise and be comfortable with divergent thinking and ideas will promote flexibility in determining alternatives and solutions to client care issues.

Example.   Consider the case of Karen and Glenn Stanton, who are brought to the emergency department with multiple injuries after a car accident. You determine that Mr. and Mrs. Stanton were extremely apprehensive about being separated from each other. You know that there is no hospital policy prohibiting their sharing a room. You also recognize that the traditional approach of admitting them to separate rooms would add additional stress and interfere with their recuperation. Therefore, you intervene for the clients by requesting that the admitting department place the couple in the same room. Upon discharge, the couple expressed their appreciation.

In this example, your flexibility in placing the Stantons in the same room was an effective nursing action that probably hastened their recovery. Your success in this situation will encourage you to initiate similar interventions for the benefit of your clients in the future.

Creative

Historically, creativity has been stifled in both education and practice settings. Nurses were taught that there was one way to perform tasks/procedures and creativity was not rewarded. Today, in a competitive health care system, where resources are limited, creative solutions to client and management problems are both common and rewarded. As a creative thinker, you will be expected to be curious, and to question often and appropriately. You will be asked to contribute strategies to improve the way nursing is practiced in your work setting. You will use ingenuity and resourcefulness to acquire data, diagnose client responses, and develop innovative strategies to manage them. In addition, you will document and validate your success for subsequent use by clients and other professionals.

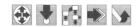
Example. Cindy is a 3-year-old who was brought to the university clinic by her mother. She is complaining of abdominal pain and is obviously frightened. Cindy screams when you attempt to examine her abdomen. You ask Cindy to show where it hurts on her doll or on mommy. This creative approach allows you to obtain important information in a manner that is much less threatening to Cindy.

Initiative

In the context of critical thinking, initiative requires a variety of strategies. In addition to the most obvious approach of assertively addressing problems or issues, initiative implies that you model positive behaviors, serve as a resource to clients, families and other professionals, identify multiple resources, and delegate effectively. This creates an environment where problems are anticipated, early intervention is encouraged, and risk-taking and creative thinking are rewarded.

Example. You are caring for Andrew Kochis, a client who is receiving outpatient chemotherapy for recurrent colon cancer. You know that during his last two treatments, the client experienced both nausea and vomiting after refusing pretreatment antiemetic medication. Based on this information, you initiate a conversation with the client sharing the benefits of the medication. He agrees to try it "just this time" and experiences only mild nausea. As he prepares to leave after the treatment he tells you that this is the best he has felt after a treatment and indicates that he wants that medicine before all of his treatments.

Your initiative in meeting with Andrew and informing him of the benefits of the medication significantly affected the client's treatment experience. Interventions of this nature often influence the quality of care provided as well as client outcomes.

Communication

Critical thinking requires effective communication including verbal, nonverbal, and written skills. These approaches, which are explored in detail in Chapter 2, create an environment that facilitates the exchange of information between the nurse, the client, and others to optimize successful outcomes. In a previous example, Pat Magovern used her resources, including the wound care specialist, to identify interventions for the management of a client's draining wound. Her communication of these strategies both verbally and in writing to the client, family, nurses, and other professionals is key to effective critical thinking and individualized care. For example, she *writes* instructions for wound care on the client's plan of care, and *tells* the nurses on the next shift what the wound looks like. This communication helps to ensure that each nurse who cares for the client will use the same procedure for wound care. This improves the continuity of care and promotes confidence in the client's caregivers. Your critical-thinking skills will enable you to continually evaluate the messages you receive as well as those you send in order to identify opportunities for improving communication with clients, families, and other caregivers.

Critical thinking is a complex skill that is integral to daily living as well as to professional nursing practice. The nurse uses critical thinking skills in all steps of the nursing process, reaches conclusions, justifies them based on the science of nursing, and initiates nursing activities to support them.

SUMMARY

The dimensions of nursing practice have evolved in response to the scientific/technological, educational, economic, and political changes in society. The practice of nursing has been defined by nursing leaders, by professional organizations, and by regulatory agencies.

The nursing process is the method by which the theoretical frameworks of nursing are applied to actual practice. It provides the framework to meet the individualized needs of the client, family, and community. It is organized into five phases: assessment, diagnosis, planning, implementation, and evaluation. The nursing process has been characterized as purposeful, systematic, dynamic, interactive, flexible, and theoretically based.

The nursing process requires prerequisite beliefs, knowledge, and skills. Beliefs form the theoretical framework upon which the nurse's practice is based. Knowledge and skills provide the tools for assessment, diagnosis, planning, implementation, and evaluation.

The use of the nursing process has implications for the profession of nursing, the client, and the individual nurse. Professionally the nursing process defines the scope of nursing practice and identifies standards of nursing care. The client benefits by the use of the nursing process, since it ensures quality care while encouraging the client to participate in care. Finally, the benefits for the individual nurse are increased job satisfaction and enhancement of professional growth.

Critical thinking facilitates purposeful, goal-directed definition of client care and management problems. It requires logic, competency, flexibility, creativity, initiative, and effective communication.

REFERENCES

American Nurses' Association: Nursing: A Social Policy Statement. Kansas City, MO: American Nurses' Association, 1980.

American Nurses' Association: Standards of Clinical Nursing Practice. Washington, DC: American Nurses' Association, 1991.

Aspinall MJ: Nursing diagnosis—the weak link. Nurs Outlook 1976; 24:433–437.

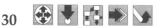
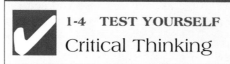

1-4 TEST YOURSELF

Critical Thinking

Apply your critical-thinking skills using the logical approach discussed in the chapter to resolve the following dilemma. There are no definitive answers because you have to make a personal decision, but some are suggested in the Test Yourself answers.

In review, the logical approach to critical thinking framework includes asking seven key questions:

1. What is the issue?
2. What information do I need and how can I obtain it?
3. Are my data valid?
4. What do the data mean?
5. Based on the facts, what should I do?
6. Are there other questions I should ask?
7. Is this the best way to deal with the issue?

You have been in a car accident. Your 1989 model car suffered a significant amount of damage. You need transportation to and from school. Public transportation is not available. Your insurance company wants to settle the claim. They inform you that the cost to repair the car would be very close to the Blue Book value. You are now faced with having to resolve this dilemma.

1. What is the issue?

2. What information do I need to know and how do I obtain it?

INFORMATION	SOURCE OF INFORMATION
a.	a.
b.	b.
c.	c.
d.	d.

Continued

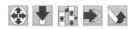

 1-4 TEST YOURSELF
Critical Thinking—cont'd.

3. Are my data valid?

4. What do the data mean?

5. Based on the facts, what should I do?

6. Are there other questions I should ask?

7. Is this the best way to deal with the issue?

Benner P: From Novice to Expert: Excellence and Power in Clinical Nursing Practice. Menlo Park, CA: Addison Wesley, 1984.

Bloch D: Some crucial terms in nursing—what do they really mean? Nurs Outlook 1974; 22:689–694.

Ennis RH: A logical basis for measuring critical thinking. Educational Leadership. October 1985; 43:44–48.

Fawcett J: Analysis and Evaluation of Conceptual Models of Nursing. Philadelphia: FA Davis, 1989.

Hall LE: Quality of Nursing Care. Public Health News, June 1955.

Johnson D: A philosophy for nursing diagnosis. Nurs Outlook 1959; 7:198–200.

Kurfiss JC: Critical thinking: Theory, research, practice and possibilities, Washington, DC: Association for the Study of Higher Education: 1988. Report No. 2.

Mundinger M and Jauron G: Developing a nursing diagnosis. Nurs Outlook 1975; 23:94–98.

Nightingale F: Notes on Nursing—What It Is, What It Is Not. New York: Dover Publications, 1969. (Originally published 1859.)

Orlando I: The Dynamic Nurse-Patient Relationship. New York: GP Putnam's Sons, 1961.

Roy C: The impact of nursing diagnosis. AORN 1975; 21:1023–1030.

State of New Jersey Nurse Practice Act. Newark, NJ: New Jersey Board of Nursing, 1993.

Watson G and Glaser EM: Watson-Glaser Critical Thinking Appraisal Manual. New York: Harcourt Brace Jovanovich, 1989.

Wiedenbach E: The helping art of nursing. Am J Nurs 1963; 63(11):544–557.

Yura H and Walsh M: The Nursing Process: Assessing, Planning, Implementing, Evaluation, 1st ed. New York: Appleton Century Crofts, 1967.

Yura H and Walsh M: The Nursing Process: Assessing, Planning, Implementing, Evaluation, 5th ed. New York: Appleton Century Crofts, 1988.

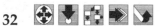

1-4 TEST YOURSELF

Critical Thinking: Answers

1. What is the issue?
   To repair present vehicle or to buy another one.

2. What information do I need and how can I obtain it?

INFORMATION	SOURCE OF INFORMATION
A. What is the exact amount of damage to the car?	**A.** Insurance adjuster Personal mechanic look at car for a second opinion
B. What is the difference between damage costs and Blue Book value?	**B.** Insurance adjuster Can get Blue Book value from a car dealer
C. Do I want a new car or do I like the old one enough to repair it?	**C.** Need to ask myself
D. Can I afford to buy a brand new car or a previously owned car?	**D.** Look at savings account Check car loan rates Determine how much insurance company would give me to settle the claim Check newspaper for advertisements for new and previously owned cars Phone car dealerships and owners selling their cars independently

3. Are my data valid?
   I believe so because I have confirmed it with documented sources and got several quotes from car dealers. I obtained a second opinion from my own mechanic, whom I trust, regarding cost of repairs.

4. What do the data mean?
   The data mean that the car is very close to being totaled. My mechanic feels that it's not worth fixing the car considering its age and possible problems with the car in the future.

Continued

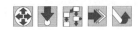

1-4 TEST YOURSELF
Critical Thinking: Answers—cont'd.

- I can get a fairly nice previously owned car with a warranty for about an additional $1000
- I can get a brand new car for an additional $5000
- I was getting tired of driving the car and was considering buying another

5. Based on the facts, what should I do?
   Buy previously owned car with the desired safety features and warranty.

6. Are there other questions I should ask myself?

- If I get the car repaired, how long will I be happy driving it?
- Will I be able to get my money out of it if I want to sell it at a later date?

7. Is this the best way to deal with the issue?
   Based on the insurance settlement and a low cost loan, I feel it is better to get a previously owned car with a warranty. My old car with high mileage is close to needing major repair work from wear and tear. I would also have a hard time selling it later on because a car that has been in a major accident has a lower resale appeal.

BIBLIOGRAPHY

Birx EC: Critical thinking and theory-based practice. Hol Nurs Pract 1993; 21–27.

Dean-Baer SL: Application of the new ANA framework for nursing practice standards and guidelines. J Nurs Care Qual 1993; 8(1):33–42.

Fitzpatrick JM et al: The role of the nurse in high quality patient care: A review of the literature. J Adv Nurs 1992; 17(10):1210–1219.

Jones SA and Brown LN: Alternative views on defining critical thinking through the nursing process. Hol Nurs Pract 1993; 7(3):71–76.

Schank MJ: Wanted: Nurses with critical thinking skills. J Cont Educ Nurs 1990; 21(2):86–89.

White NE: Promoting critical thinking skills. Nurse Educ 1990; 15(5):16–19.

Wright K: An overview of the nursing process. Gastroenterol Nurs 1992; 15(1):14–17.

TWO

ASSESSMENT

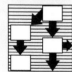

After reading this chapter, you will be able to:

1. Define assessment.
2. Describe four types of data.
3. Name two sources of data.
4. Set priorities for the collection of assessment data.
5. List three methods of data collection.
6. Describe two characteristics of data collection.
7. Discuss the importance of critical thinking in assessment.
8. Use seven guidelines to document assessment data.
9. Explain the role of computers in nursing assessment and documentation.

INTRODUCTION

ANA Standard I. THE NURSE COLLECTS CLIENT HEALTH DATA

Assessment is the first step of the nursing process and can be described as the organized and systematic process of collecting data from a variety of sources in order to analyze the health status of a client. It consists of two components: data collection and documentation. The importance of this phase of the nursing process has been addressed specifically in the Standards of Care published by the American Nurses' Association (ANA). The first standard defines the need for the collection of data that are (1) prioritized according to the client's needs, (2) collected using appropriate techniques, and (3) involve clients, significant others, and health care providers in collection when appropriate; (4) are the result of a systematic and ongoing process; and (5) are documented in a retrievable form (ANA, 1991). The fact that the assessment standard is the first of the six standards is significant in reinforcing its importance as the key to the remaining steps of the nursing process. This chapter is organized around the standard and the five criteria related to assessment described above and illustrated in Figure 2-1.

Assessment is the organized, systematic process of collecting data from a variety of sources to analyze the health status of a client.

The assessment phase provides a solid foundation that promotes the delivery of quality individualized care. Accurate, complete assessment is

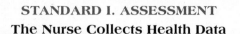

STANDARD I. ASSESSMENT
The Nurse Collects Health Data

Measurement Criteria

1. The priority of data collection is determined by the client's immediate condition or needs.
2. Pertinent data are collected using appropriate assessment techniques.
3. Data collection involves the client, significant others, and health care providers when appropriate.
4. The data collection process is systematic and ongoing.
5. Relevant data are documented in a retrievable form.

FIGURE 2-1. ANA standard I: Assessment.

(Reprinted with permission from *Standards of Clinical Nursing Practice,* © 1991, American Nurses' Association, Washington, DC.)

necessary to facilitate the diagnosis and treatment of human responses—the scope of nursing practice as defined by the ANA (1980). Assessment forms the basis for the identification of nursing diagnoses, development of outcomes, implementation of nursing interventions, and evaluation of nursing actions.

INTRODUCTION
DATA AND
ASSESSMENT

Data are specific information obtained about a client.

INTRODUCTION
DATA AND
ASSESSMENT
Types of Data
Subjective
Objective

DATA AND ASSESSMENT

In the context of the nursing assessment, data might be defined as specific information obtained about a client. You systematically accumulate the information required to diagnose the client's health responses and to identify contributing factors. This data base subsequently forms the foundation for the remaining phases of the nursing process: diagnosis, planning, implementation, and evaluation.

Types of Data

Four types of data are collected by the nurse during assessment: subjective, objective, historical, and current. A complete and accurate data base usually includes a combination of these types.

Subjective Data

Subjective data might be described as the individual's perspective of a situation or a series of events. This information cannot be determined by the nurse independent of interaction or communication with the individual. Subjective data are frequently obtained during the nursing history and include the client's perceptions, feelings, and ideas about self and personal health status. Examples include the client's descriptions of pain, weakness, frustration, nausea, or embarrassment. Information supplied by sources other than the client—e.g., family, consultants, and other members of the health care team—may also be subjective if based on the individual's opinion rather than substantiated by fact.

Subjective data are the individual's perspective of a situation or a series of events.

Objective Data

In contrast, objective data consist of observable and measurable information. This information is usually obtained through the senses—sight, smell, hearing, and touch—during the physical examination of the client. Examples of objective data include respiratory rate, blood pressure, presence of edema, and weight.

During the assessment of a client, you must consider both subjective and objective findings. Frequently, these findings substantiate each other, as in the case of John Thomas, the client whose incision opened three days after surgery. The subjective information provided by Mr. Thomas, "feels like my stitches are popping," was validated by the nurse's objective findings: pallor, diaphoresis, hypotension, and protrusion of the bowel through the incision.

Example. You observe Peggy Malletts crying as she stands in front of the nursery two days after the premature delivery of her first child. You suggest that Peggy seems "upset," and the client validates that she is "afraid that her baby might die."

Here, the objective data you observe (crying) is substantiated by subjective data obtained from the client (feelings of fear).

At times, subjective and objective data may be in conflict.

Objective data consist of observable and measurable information.

Example. Casey Smithson is a 15-year-old client in your eating disorders clinic. She is 5 ft, 5 in. tall and weighs 82 lb. Her blood pressure is 80/50, her pulse rate is 62, and her skin is dry with little turgor. Casey looks malnourished, however, when you ask her how she is feeling, she pinches a fold of skin and replies, "Fat! Look at this roll—I just have to lose weight."

Clearly, your objective data—height, weight, vital signs, and appearance—are in conflict with the client's subjective expression of feeling "fat." Therefore you must discuss your findings with the client in an effort to resolve the discrepancy.

Historical Data

Another consideration when describing data concerns the element of time. In this context, data may be either historical or current (Bellack and Bamford, 1984). Historical data consist of situations or events that have occurred in the past. These data are particularly important in identifying the client's normal health patterns and in determining past experiences that may impact on the client's current health status. Examples of historical data might include previous hospitalizations or surgery, ECG results, normal elimination patterns, or chronic diseases.

Historical data include situations or events that have occurred in the past.

Example. As a community health nurse, you visit John Kelly, age 62, at his home to teach him how to change a dressing on his abdominal burn. When you begin writing out the directions for him, the client says, "I can't read. I left school after the first grade to help my father on the farm."

In this case, John's educational background (historical data) influences your assessment of his ability to follow written instructions for changing his dressing.

Current data refer to events that are occurring now.

Current Data

In contrast, current data refer to events that are occurring now. Examples might include blood pressure, vomiting, or postoperative pain. These data are particularly important in your initial assessment and in reassessments to compare current information with previous data to determine the client's progress.

Example. Kelly O'Keefe, age 5, is admitted for tonsillectomy. In the immediate postoperative period, her pulse rate ranges from 90 to 108. Four hours later, the nurse observes that Kelly is swallowing frequently and her pulse rate is 124.

In this situation, current data (pulse rate 124) and frequent swallowing substantiate the existence of a problem (bleeding) when compared with historical data (pulse rate 90 to 108).

For the data base to be complete, you should collect all four types of data. Subjective and objective data provide specific information regarding the client's health status and help to identify problems. Additionally, current and historical data assist in this process by establishing time frames or usual behavioral patterns.

The test yourself exercise on the next page is designed to assist you to recognize subjective, objective, historical, and current data.

Sources of Data

During the assessment phase, data are collected from a variety of sources. These sources are classified as either **primary** or **secondary**. The client is the primary source and should be used to obtain pertinent subjective data. The client can most accurately (1) share personal perceptions and feelings about health and illness, (2) identify individual goals or problems, and (3) validate responses to diagnostic or treatment modalities.

Secondary sources are those other than the client. These are used in

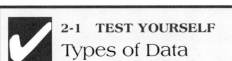

2-1   TEST YOURSELF
Types of Data

The following is a list of data. Indicate by checking (✔) whether each item is subjective or objective.

DATA	SUBJECTIVE	OBJECTIVE
1. "I feel tired today."		
2. Blood pressure 180/96.		
3. Speaks only when spoken to.		
4. "She seems nervous."		
5. "My leg hurts."		
6. Dirt under nails.		
7. Rash on flank.		
8. "I need help."		
9. Absent bowel sounds.		
10. Respirations 24.		

Now, identify each of the following as historical or current.

DATA	HISTORICAL	CURRENT
1. No prior surgery.		
2. "I used to eat when I was nervous."		
3. Temperature 97.8° F.		
4. "I'm allergic to sulfa."		
5. Weight 118 lb.		
6. Smoked three packs of cigarettes a day until last month.		
7. Warm, dry skin.		
8. Worked part time until one year ago.		
9. Two episodes of nocturia six months ago.		
10. Diminished breath sounds at base of right lung.		

2-1 TEST YOURSELF

Types of Data: Answers

The following is a list of data. Indicate by checking (✔) whether each item is subjective or objective.

DATA	SUBJECTIVE	OBJECTIVE
1. "I feel tired today."	✔	
2. Blood pressure 180/96.		✔
3. Speaks only when spoken to.		✔
4. "She seems nervous."	✔	
5. "My leg hurts."	✔	
6. Dirt under nails.		✔
7. Rash on flank.		✔
8. "I need help."	✔	
9. Absent bowel sounds.		✔
10. Respirations 24.		✔

Now, identify each of the following as historical or current.

DATA	HISTORICAL	CURRENT
1. No prior surgery.	✔	
2. "I used to eat when I was nervous."	✔	
3. Temperature 97.8° F.		✔
4. "I'm allergic to sulfa."		✔
5. Weight 118 lb.		✔
6. Smoked three packs of cigarettes a day until last month.	✔	
7. Warm, dry skin.		✔
8. Worked part-time until one year ago.	✔	
9. Two episodes of nocturia six months ago.	✔	
10. Diminished breath sounds at base of right lung.		✔

situations in which the client is unable to participate or when additional information is required to clarify or validate data supplied by the client. Secondary sources might include the client's family or significant other, individuals in the client's immediate environment, other members of the health care team, and the medical record. Family, friends, and coworkers may also provide pertinent historical data regarding the client's normal patterns in the home, at work, and in recreational environments.

Example. Cathy Johnson, age 24, is admitted to the ICU following an automobile accident. Because Cathy is comatose, you interview her father. During this conversation, Mr. Johnson indicates that Cathy was hit in the eye when she was 13 and has a permanently dilated right pupil.

In this situation, the information obtained from the client's family provides historical data that clarify your physical findings. These are significant in view of the client's history.

Other members of the health team may also contribute significant data.

- Other *nurses* who have cared for the client during hospitalization may provide information concerning that client's responses.
- The *physical therapist* may be able to assist the nurse to compare the motor skills demonstrated by the client during therapy with those observed on the nursing unit.
- The *physician* may be able to describe the client's emotional response to a previous heart attack.

Each of these secondary sources may add to your knowledge base and therefore expand the data available for comparing and evaluating client responses.

The individuals in the client's immediate hospital environment may also provide additional information. Visitors may substantiate your opinion that the client is less communicative today than on a previous day. Other clients may be able to offer current data about events that occur when you are not present. For example, the client in another bed may validate your impression that an elderly client climbed over the siderails and fell out of bed.

The medical record contains an abundance of demographic data: marital status, occupation, religion, insurance. This adds insight into the client's socioeconomic status. Additionally, the record contains current and historical data documented by personnel in other disciplines (physician, dietitian, respiratory therapist, social worker, discharge planner). Diagnostic data are also available, including laboratory and radiological findings.

Carefully consider the client's rights to privacy and confidentiality when obtaining information from secondary sources. Additionally, these client rights may outweigh the needs of others to obtain sensitive data.

Example. Mr. Turi's employer brings him to the emergency department after

ANA Measurement Criteria I-3. Data collection involves the client, significant others, and health care providers when appropriate.

Primary Sources: Data obtained from the client

Secondary Sources: Data obtained from sources other than the client

---

BOX 2-1

Types and Sources of Data

TYPES OF DATA

Subjective	The individual's perception of a situation or a series of events
Objective	Observable and measurable information
Historical	Situations or events that have occurred in the past
Current	Situations or events that are occurring now

SOURCES OF DATA

Primary	Information obtained directly from the client
Secondary	Information about a client obtained from other people, documents, or records

---

he vomits blood while at work. The client tells you that he has been drinking a fifth of Scotch a day for five years. While providing information to you, Mr. Turi's employer states, "He drinks, doesn't he? That's why he's bleeding again!"

In this situation, the client's employer is attempting to obtain confidential information about the client's drinking patterns. You must protect the client's privacy by tactfully focusing the conversation on other topics rather than confirm Mr. Turi's alcoholism without his approval. Box 2-1 summarizes the types and sources of data.

DATA COLLECTION

Systematic and ongoing data collection is the key to accurate assessment of your clients. This segment of the chapter will discuss determining priorities in data collection, methods of data collection, and methods of enhancing data collection.

Priorities in Data Collection

ANA Measurement Criteria I-1. The priority of data collection is determined by the client's immediate condition or needs.

A thorough nursing assessment may identify many actual or potential client responses that require nursing intervention. Assessment of each of these may be unrealistic or unmanageable. Therefore, a system must be established to determine which data will be collected first. One such mechanism is the human needs hierarchy.

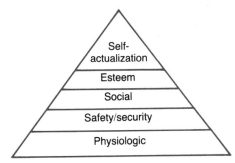

FIGURE 2-2.   Maslow's model.

(Reprinted with permission from Maslow A: A theory of human motivation. *Psychol Rev* 50:370, 1943.)

Maslow's Hierarchy

Abraham Maslow (1943) described human needs on five levels: physiological, safety or security, social, esteem, and self actualization (Fig. 2-2). He suggested that the client progresses up the hierarchy when attempting to satisfy needs. In other words, physiological needs are generally of greater priority to the client than the others. Therefore, when these basic needs are unsatisfied, the client may be unwilling or unable to deal with higher level needs.

Kalish's Hierarchy

Richard Kalish (1983) further refined Maslow's system by dividing physiological needs into survival needs and stimulation needs (Fig. 2-3). This division is particularly useful in assisting the nurse to prioritize data collection.

Physiological

SURVIVAL NEEDS

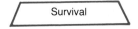

Kalish identified survival needs as those for food, air, water, manageable temperature, elimination, rest, and pain avoidance. When a deficit occurs in any of these areas, the client tends to utilize all available resources to satisfy that particular need. Only then is it possible to be concerned about higher-level needs, such as security or esteem.

For this reason, the confused client with an oxygen (air) deficit may continuously climb out of bed to open the window in a hospital room. The basic need for oxygen supersedes concerns about safety. Likewise, the individual who

2-2 TEST YOURSELF
Types and Sources of Data

CASE STUDY

Mr. Ted Alexander, a 50-year-old white divorced salesman from Las Vegas, was on a business trip to Atlantic City when he developed pain in the left upper abdominal quadrant. He took Alka-Seltzer with little relief, and the pain persisted for the next two days. He was busy with appointments during the day and evening and was able to ignore the pain. He ate very little and took two sleeping pills at night. On the afternoon of the third day, the pain became much more intense, and when it continued for several hours and he began to vomit bloody fluid, he went to the emergency department.

Physical examination and laboratory data at this time revealed an alert, well-groomed male with generalized abdominal tenderness, rigidity of the abdominal wall, absent bowel sounds, and a hemoglobin level of 11.6 (normal = 16 ± −2) with a hematocrit of 38 (normal = 47 ± −5). The diagnosis of bleeding gastric ulcer was made. He was admitted to the hospital for initial medical management, with surgery anticipated at a later date.

Your examination of the patient reveals the following: B/P 104/60, P 120, R 26, T 98.2. The patient indicates that he is 6 ft, 2 in. tall and weighs 196 lb. He is alert and oriented and states, "I've never had this bleeding before—it's serious isn't it?" His skin is cool to the touch and slightly diaphoretic. The patient states that he had been a heavy drinker for 15 years and was admitted to the hospital with cirrhosis two years ago by his family doctor, Dr. Martland, but has never had surgery. He denies drinking for the past two years but smokes two packs of cigarettes daily.

Mr. Alexander is tense throughout your conversation but shares a number of concerns with you, including his separation from his two teenage children who live with him. He is also anxious about being cared for by an unfamiliar physician. The Emergency Department nurse indicates that he wears contact lenses and is concerned because he has left his case and supplies as well as his glasses in his hotel. He gives you $750.00 in cash and traveler's checks to deposit in the hospital safe. He has a partial lower plate of dentures and caps on his four front teeth. Further inquiry reveals that the patient prefers a low-fat diet, occasionally uses laxatives, and has had several occurrences of urinary urgency and nocturia in the last six months.

Continued.

2-2 TEST YOURSELF
Types and Sources of Data–cont'd.

The physician states that his treatment plan includes gastric suction, antiulcer medications, and replacement therapy with IV fluid, blood, electrolytes, and vitamins until the patient is stabilized enough for exploratory surgery. Mr. Alexander agrees to this plan but is concerned about his job demands and wonders how he will deal with "getting back home when all of this is over."

Based on the case study, identify three examples of each subjective, objective, current, and historical data as well as three secondary sources of data.

SUBJECTIVE DATA

1.
2.
3.

OBJECTIVE DATA

1.
2.
3.

CURRENT DATA

1.
2.
3.

HISTORICAL DATA

1.
2.
3.

SECONDARY SOURCES

1.
2.
3.

2-2 TEST YOURSELF
Types and Sources of Data: Answers

SUBJECTIVE DATA

1. Abdominal pain
2. Height and weight; concerns about separation from children and private physician; concerns about condition
3. Low-fat diet preference; smoking

OBJECTIVE DATA

1. Abdominal rigidity, absent bowel sounds
2. B/P 104/60, P 120, R 26, T 98.2°, skin cool and diaphoretic, Hemoglobin 11.6, Hematocrit 38
3. Partial dentures, caps, well groomed, wears corrective lenses

CURRENT DATA

1. Vital signs
2. Skin cool, diaphoretic
3. Smokes two packs of cigarettes daily

HISTORICAL DATA

1. Drinking heavily for 15 years, no drinking past two years
2. No previous surgery; occasional use of laxatives
3. Urgency and nocturia in last six months; pain for two days

SECONDARY SOURCES

1. Laboratory data
2. Emergency department nurse
3. Physician

has not slept for three days because of anxiety may not be able to focus on preoperative teaching, even though such information is particularly important for safety in the postoperative period.

Examples of nursing assessment data reflecting survival needs include the following:

SURVIVAL NEED	ASSESSMENT DATA
Food	Anorexia, lack of interest in food, weight loss or gain, altered taste sensation
Air	Dyspnea, cyanosis, confusion, restlessness, abnormal blood gases, abnormal breath sounds, retained secretions
Water	Dry skin/mucous membranes, thirst, nausea, weakness, persistent vomiting, edema
Temperature	Increased or decreased body temperature, shivering, flushed, hot or cool skin, perspiration
Elimination	Diarrhea, constipation, dysuria, incontinence, abdominal distention, decreased or increased bowel sounds
Rest	Fatigue on awakening, dark circles under eyes, headache, irritability, difficulty in concentrating
Pain	Reports of pain, facial grimacing, clutching of painful area, changes in posture or gait

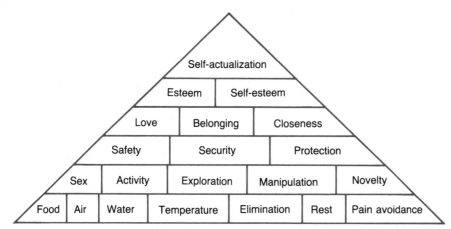

FIGURE 2-3. Kalish's refinement of Maslow's model.

(Reprinted by permission of Brooks/Cole, Monterey, CA, from Kalish R: The Psychology of Human Behavior, 5th ed. Wadsworth, Inc., 1983, 1977, 1973, 1970, 1966.)

STIMULATION NEEDS

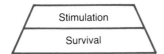

Kalish suggests that stimulation needs include those related to sex, activity, exploration, manipulation, and novelty. When survival needs are met, the client will attempt to satisfy stimulation needs before moving up the hierarchy. For this reason, the younger client who is hospitalized for a prolonged period of time in a psychiatric setting may be unable to focus on therapy when strong sexual urges remain unsatisfied. Similarly, the client who is required to maintain prolonged bedrest at home may require frequent diversionary activities to suppress the desire to get out of bed.

Examples of nursing assessment data reflecting stimulation needs include the following:

STIMULATION NEED	ASSESSMENT DATA
Sex	Decreased vaginal secretions, decreased or absent sexual desire, impotence
Activity	Complaints of boredom, restlessness, inability to participate in usual hobbies
Exploration	Limited range of motion, reluctance to attempt movement, falling or stumbling
Manipulation	Requests help in bathing, toileting, dressing, child reaching for a toy
Novelty	Inattentiveness, daydreaming, decreased sensitivity to smell, change in usual response to stimuli

In the example of Ted Alexander, who was described in Test Yourself 2-2, the primary physiological need is control of bleeding. The client who is bleeding is frequently unable to deal with higher-level concerns. Note that Ted verbalized this need in very concrete terms ("I've never had this bleeding before—it's serious, isn't it?") early in the interviewing process. This is frequently the case, because the physiological need is the most important reason for the client's visit to the physician's office or to the hospital.

KEY ASSESSMENT DATA: Bloody emesis, pain, decreased hemoglobin and hematocrit.

Safety

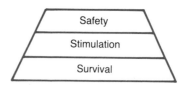

The next levels in the hierarchy are the needs for safety, security, and protection. These become of particular concern to the client when physiological needs have been satisfied. Safety needs are particularly evident in the elderly or very young when they are placed in an unfamiliar environment. Children frequently require the presence of a favorite toy or blanket for security. The elderly client may be at risk for falls, bruises, and the like while trying to adapt to the strangeness of a nursing home environment. Clients who undergo treatments or procedures such as chemotherapy or heart surgery are frequently at risk because of changes in the body's protective mechanisms.

Some examples of assessment data reflecting safety needs include the following:

SAFETY NEED	ASSESSMENT DATA
Security	Insufficient finances, lack of food, expressed fear of new environment
Safety	Falls at home, lack of safety education, decreased sensory or motor abilities
Protection	Low white blood-cell count, abuse of self or others, stated inability to protect self

Mr. Alexander's concern about being managed by an unfamiliar physician reflects a safety need. He has verbalized confidence in his family physician who is 3000 miles away but faces major surgery by a surgeon who is basically unknown to him. Additionally, Mr. Alexander has never had surgery and may be concerned about his safety during the surgical experience.

KEY ASSESSMENT DATA: Verbalized concern about unfamiliar physician, separation from usual support systems and lack of previous surgical experience.

Love and Belonging

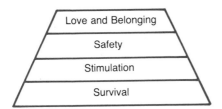

Maslow's social needs are described by Kalish as the necessity for love and a sense of belonging or closeness. These needs reflect a person's ability to affiliate or interact with others in the environment and are met through involvement with family, friends, and coworkers. The nurse frequently identifies social deficits in clients requiring prolonged hospitalization, those isolated for protection or because of infection, and those placed in such areas as critical care units, where visiting privileges may be restricted.

Examples of nursing assessment data reflecting love and belonging needs include the following:

LOVE/BELONGING NEED	ASSESSMENT DATA
Love	Lack of maternal infant bonding, depression after loss of significant other
Belonging	Separation from family, verbalized disparity between self and others, discomfort in interpersonal interactions
Closeness	Isolation because of disease process, recent separation or divorce, prolonged hospitalization

Mr. Alexander has verbalized his concern about being separated from his children during hospitalization. This reflects his parental role and the need for interaction with his children. Fulfillment of this need may be particularly difficult because of the children's location.

KEY ASSESSMENT DATA: Verbalized concern about separation from children, history of divorce, unfamiliar environment.

Esteem

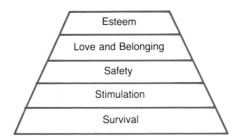

The need for the respect of oneself and others is reflected in this level of the hierarchy. The individual strives for recognition, usefulness, independence, dignity, and freedom. The client's position in the health care system frequently leads to deficits in these areas. Clients may unnecessarily surrender responsibility for elements of daily care to the nurse. Examples might include those who expect the nurse to pour their water, comb their hair, or shave them because they are in a hospital when, in fact, they are capable of self care.

Examples of nursing assessment data reflecting esteem needs include the following:

ESTEEM NEED	ASSESSMENT DATA
Esteem	Self-negating verbalization, expressions of shame or guilt, lack of eye contact, nonassertive or passive behavior, difficulty in making decisions, apathy, avoidance of conflict

In Mr. Alexander's case, the need for esteem is demonstrated by his concern about his job demands.

KEY ASSESSMENT DATA: Verbalized concern about job demands.

Self-Actualization

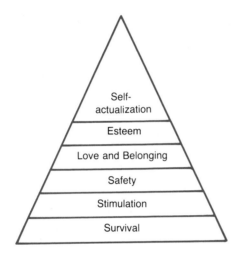

The highest level need is self-actualization, or the need "to make the most of your physical, mental, emotional and social competencies in order to feel that you are being the sort of person you wish to be" (Kalish, 1983). Clients wish to function according to a lifestyle that utilizes their individual knowledge, talents, and skills. Clients in a hospital setting are frequently not concerned with self-actualization needs, because they are preoccupied with fulfilling lower level needs. However, clients may demonstrate concerns about their ability to achieve self-actualization as a result of changes that may have occurred during hospitalization. Nurses who work with clients in other settings, such as in clients' homes, physicians' offices, and health maintenance organizations, may see clients who are focusing on self-fulfillment. This is possible because their needs for survival, stimulation, and safety are being satisfied. Therefore, they are able to focus on esteem and self-actualization.

Examples of nursing assessment data that relate to self-actualization include the following:

SELF-ACTUALIZATION NEED	ASSESSMENT DATA
Self-actualization	Verbalized concern regarding role conflicts, changes in self-perception, physical limitations affecting role functions, concerns regarding usual pattern of responsibility, disruption in caretaking routines, perceived loss of control, reluctance to participate in favored activities, extended period of denial or anger regarding health status changes

Mr. Alexander has verbalized concern about the effects of the impending surgery on his role as salesman. This reflects a need for self-actualization.

KEY ASSESSMENT DATA: Verbalized concern regarding ability to perform role.

Maslow's hierarchy provides a constructive resource for the nurse to utilize in setting priorities for data collection. Kalish's expansion of Maslow's model assists the nurse in differentiating more clearly between levels of physiological needs. Ordinarily, clients progress up the hierarchy of needs. For example, they attempt to satisfy survival needs before focusing on security or esteem. However, it is important to note that clients may have unsatisfied needs on more than one level at the same time. Lower level needs do not have to be completely resolved before the client begins to address higher-level needs.

Example. Victor Klein, a 48-year-old man, is admitted to the hospital with a diagnosis of pneumonia. He exhibits an elevated temperature and is dehydrated. He verbalizes concern about his disabled wife who is confined to bed at home. Additionally, he owns a home-based business with no employees to provide income while he is hospitalized.

In this example, the client has simultaneous survival, security, and love or belonging needs. Mr. Klein's immediate concerns relate to his temperature and fluid problems (survival needs). When collecting assessment data, you focus on temperature and fluid concerns (survival needs). Your next priority includes collection of data dealing with his anxieties about his job (security) and his disabled wife (love and belonging).

ANA Measurement Criteria I-2. Pertinent data are collected using appropriate assessment techniques.

Methods of Data Collection

Three major methods are utilized to gather information during a nursing assessment. These methods include interview, observation, and physical examination. These techniques provide the nurse with a logical, systematic, and ongoing approach to the collection of data required for subsequent nursing diagnosis and care planning.

2-3 TEST YOURSELF

Identification and Prioritization of Assessment Data

The following are statements made by Louisa Perez, a 28-year-old woman who had a cesarean section two days ago. She is married and has two other children, age 4 and 2. Utilizing the Kalish hierarchy of needs, identify the need being addressed in each of the following statements. Prioritize the assessment of needs by using a scale of 1 through 6, with 1 being the highest level of need. The first question is completed for you.

STATEMENT

- **A.** "I have not had a bowel movement since I had the baby."
- **B.** "When will I be getting out of bed?"
- **C.** "I have not had many visitors in the past two days."
- **D.** "I gained so much weight with this baby, I really feel ugly."
- **E.** "I'm afraid to walk to the bathroom myself; I feel dizzy when I get up."
- **F.** "My husband called and said he is losing his job in two weeks."
- **G.** "After this baby, I may not have time to work as a volunteer at the Hispanic Center."
- **H.** "My sister will not be able to come to help out when I get home."
- **I.** "I'm afraid I will not have enough breast milk to satisfy the baby."
- **J.** "My hair is a mess. When can I take a shower and wash my hair?"

	NEED		LEVEL OF NEED
A.	Survival (Physiological)	**A.**	1
B.		**B.**	
C.		**C.**	
D.		**D.**	
E.		**E.**	
F.		**F.**	
G.		**G.**	
H.		**H.**	
I.		**I.**	
J.		**J.**	

2-3 TEST YOURSELF

Identification and Prioritization of Assessment Data: Answers

NEED		LEVEL OF NEED
A. Survival (physiological)	**A.** 1	
B. Stimulation (physiological)	**B.** 2	
C. Love/belonging	**C.** 4	
D. Esteem	**D.** 5	
E. Safety/security	**E.** 3	
F. Safety/security	**F.** 3	
G. Self-actualization	**G.** 6	
H. Safety/security	**H.** 3	
I. Survival (physiological)	**I.** 1	
J. Esteem	**J.** 5	

Interview

Purposes. The interview serves four purposes in the context of a nursing assessment: (1) it allows you to acquire specific information required for diagnosis and planning; (2) it facilitates your relationship with the client by creating an opportunity for dialogue; (3) it enables the client to receive information and to participate in identification of problems and goal setting; and (4) it assists you in determining areas for specific investigation during the other components of the assessment process.

The nursing interview is a complex process that requires refined communication and interaction skills. It differs from the types of interviews performed by other members of the health care team since it focuses on identification of client responses that may be treated through nursing intervention. It is a purposeful process designed to allow both the nurse and the client to give and receive information. Figure 2-4 illustrates the interview process, including purposes, components, and factors affecting its success.

Segments of the Interview. The interview consists of three segments: introduction, body, and closure.

INTRODUCTION In the introductory phase, nurse and client begin to develop a therapeutic relationship. Your professional attitude is probably the most significant factor in creating an environment in which a positive relationship can

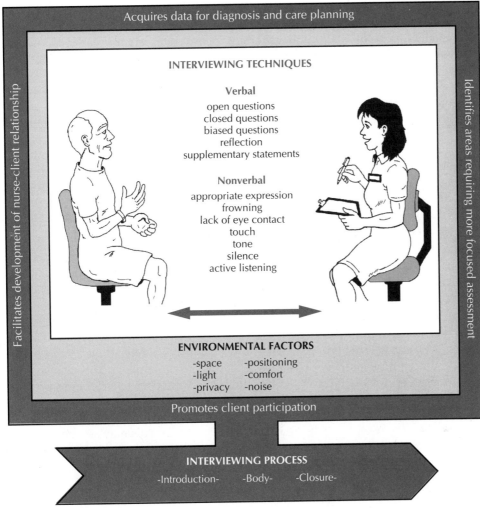

FIGURE 2-4. Interviewing process.

be developed. Your approach should convey respect for the client; therefore it is appropriate to share introductions. You should address the client by name—e.g., "Mr. Jones" rather than "Bill" or "Pop." You should also explain the purpose of the interview, estimate the time required, and assess for factors that may inhibit involvement (e.g., pain, lack of privacy). All questions should be directed to the client. Family and other sources should be utilized when the client is unable to respond. Assure the client that the information gathered is confidential. These approaches create an atmosphere of trust and sensitivity in which the client may feel comfortable sharing information of a personal nature.

BODY During this second part of the interview, focus the dialogue on specific areas designed to obtain the data required. This usually begins with the client's chief complaint and generally incorporates other areas such as past medical history, family history, and religious and cultural data. A more complete listing is seen in Table 2-1.

Interviews are done in a variety of settings, including the hospital, clinic, nursing home, physician's office, college infirmary, and client's home. The format for collecting assessment data is dependent on the type of setting and the purpose of the interview. Some nurses prefer to use a free-flow approach that begins with the client's chief complaint and extends to other areas based on individual client cues. Others prefer a more structured approach that utilizes a specific format. Content areas are defined, and the nurse utilizes a form as a checklist to ensure that all content areas have been addressed (Fig. 2-5). Use the format that is found to be most comfortable and that results in a logical, systematic accumulation of pertinent information about the client.

CLOSURE The final phase of the interview is closure. During this phase, you prepare the client for termination of the interview: "Mrs. Black, we'll be finishing in a few minutes." Do not introduce new material at this time; however, the client may want to discuss additional topics. If time allows, this may be accomplished, or you may suggest a second interview at another time. The most significant points discussed during the interview should be summarized. This allows the client to verify or negate the nurse's perceptions of major problems, client concerns, and other pertinent data. This also lays the foundation for clarification and mutual goal-setting in the planning process. Attempt to end the interview in a manner that conveys warmth and appreciation: "Mrs. Black, thanks for sharing this information about yourself; it will be very useful in helping us to plan your care." This may set the scene for future nurse-client interactions throughout the therapeutic relationship. Table 2-2 summarizes guidelines for interviewing.

Observation

The second method of data collection used during the assessment phase is observation. Systematic observation involves the use of the senses to acquire information about the client, significant other, the environment, and interactions among these three variables. Observation is a skill that requires discipline and practice on your part. It demands a broad knowledge base and conscious use of the senses: sight, smell, hearing, and feeling. Table 2-3 provides a list of the types of observations that can be obtained by the use of the senses.

The observations identified by the senses may be either positive or negative indices in the individual client. For example, crying may be viewed as a positive expression of grief in the parents of a terminally ill child, the odor of perfume may indicate progress in a woman after disfiguring breast surgery, or the presence of bowel sounds may signal the return of bowel function following abdominal surgery.

TABLE 2-1   Health History Content

CLIENT PROFILE

Brief statement about the client

CHIEF COMPLAINT

Client's statement about reason for seeking medical assistance

HISTORY OF PRESENT ILLNESS

Description of client's symptoms, including onset; location; duration; quality; intensity; aggravating, alleviating, and associated factors; course of illness; problem

PAST MEDICAL HISTORY

Summary of client's health, including major and minor adult illnesses, previous hospitalization and surgery, major injuries or accidents, drug or food allergies, usual response to illness

FAMILY HISTORY

Identification of family members and health trends, including age, sex, and health status of living family members; age, sex, and cause of death of deceased family members; familial history of cancer, heart disease, hypertension, stroke, epilepsy, renal disorders, diabetes, arthritis, tuberculosis

MEDICATION HISTORY

Listing of medications, including name, dosage, frequency of administration, duration of therapy, time of last dose (should include nonprescription drugs taken, including aspirin, laxatives, antihistamines, etc.)

ALCOHOL, TOBACCO, AND DRUG HISTORY

Description of usual patterns of usage, including alcohol type, average consumption; tobacco type, amount per day, age started, stopped; drug type, frequency of use

SOCIAL HISTORY

Summary of employment, occupation, education, hobbies, living environment, recreation, religion

PATTERNS OF DAILY LIVING

Identification of client's usual patterns, including sleep/rest, hygiene, activity, elimination, diet/fluids, health practices

PART II - PATIENT/ FAMILY HISTORY

PATIENT HISTORY (major illnesses/operations/major injuries) Include Endocrine history/problems--past pregnancies

1. _____ 4. _____ 7. _____

2. _____ 5. _____ 8. _____

3. _____ 6. _____ 9. _____

USE OF TOBACCO
☐ No ☐ Yes Type- Daily Amt.

USE OF ALCOHOL
☐ No ☐ Yes Type- Daily Amt.

HAVE YOU HAD ANY UNUSUAL PROBLEMS WITH ANESTHESIA?

FAMILY HISTORY

☐ Heart Disease ☐ Stroke ☐ Hypertension ☐ Asthma ☐ TB ☐ Diabetes ☐ Cancer ☐ Kidney Disease ☐ Allergy

☐ Epilepsy ☐ Blood Disorder ☐ Mental Disorder ☐ Other- ☐ Problems with Anesthesia

SOCIAL HISTORY

Religion: _____   Marital Status: ☐ Single ☐ Married

☐ Lives with family ☐ Lives alone ☐ No family LIVES IN: ☐ House ☐ Apartment ☐ Other-

Occupation ☐ Full time ☐ Part time ☐ Retired ☐ Other-

ECONOMIC/FINANCIAL STATUS

☐ Medicare ☐ Supplemental Insurance ☐ Economic Problem Referred to Social Service/Financial Counselor ☐ Yes ☐ No

FUNCTIONAL HISTORY

☐ ADL ☐ Independent Needs assist with: ☐ Ambulation ☐ Eating ☐ Bathing ☐ Dressing ☐ Toileting

☐ Other-

Physical Handicaps: ☐ None ☐ Walker ☐ Cane ☐ Prosthesis Type: ☐ Other-

*NOTIFY IN EMERGENCY: Home Phone# _____

_____ Relation _____ Work. Phone# _____

Info Obtained from
☐ Patient ☐ Family ☐ Other *Nearest Relative- _____ Hm. Ph.# _____ WK _____

Home Phone# _____   Work Phone# _____

ADMITTING NURSE/P.A.T. NURSE _____ LPN/RN

PART III - SYSTEM ASSESSMENT: Place on (X) in area of abnormality/(X) requires explanation/if unable to assess, indicate reason.   * ICCU   Only

ASSESS EYES, EARS, NOSE, THROAT FOR ABNORMALITY   ____ No Problem

____ Impaired vision ____ Blind ____ Pain ____ Reddened ____ Drainage ____ Gums ____ Aphasic

____ Hard of hearing ____ Deaf ____ Burning ____ Edema ____ Lesion ____ Teeth ☐ Capped Teeth ☐ Loose Teeth ☐ Dentures

Explain: _____

Language Barrier ☐ No ☐ Yes, Explain: _____

ASSESS CHEST CONFIGURATION, RESP. RATE, RHYTHM, DEPTH, PATTERN, BREATH SOUNDS, COMFORT   ____ No Problem

____ Asymmetric ____ Tachypnea ____ Apnea ____ Rales ____ Cough ____ Absent ____ Barrel Chest ____ Bradypnea ____ Shallow

____ Rhonchi ____ Sputum ____ Diminished ____ Dyspnea ____ Orthopnea ____ Labored ____ Wheezing ____ Pain ____ Cyanotic

Explain: _____

FIGURE 2-5.   Sample structured nursing assessment form.

(Courtesy of Hackettstown Community Hospital, Hackettstown, NJ.)

ASSESS HEART SOUNDS, RATE RHYTHM, PULSE, BLOOD PRESSURE, CIRC., FLUID RETENTION, COMFORT ___ No Problem

___ Arrhythmia ___ Tachycardia ___ Rub* ___ Numbness ___ Diminished Pulses ___ Edema ___ Irregular ___ Bradycardia

___ Murmur* ___ Tingling ___ Absent Pulses ___ JVD* ___ Pain ___ S_3 or S_4* ___ Fatigue

Explain: _____

ASSESS WT., ABDOMEN, BOWEL SOUNDS, COMFORT ___ No Problem

Home diet/Food habits/Caffeine amt.- _____ Stool Color _____

___ Wt. loss ___ N or V ___ Anorexia ___ Diarrhea ___ Distention ___ Hypoactive BS ___ Mass ___ Colostomy ___ Obese

___ Thirst ___ Dysphagia ___ Constipation ___ Rigidity ___ Hyperactive BS ___ Pain ___ Date Last BM _____

Usual Bowel Pattern _____ Explain: _____

ASSESS URINE FREQ., CONTROL, COLOR, CONSISTENCY, ODOR, COMFORT/GYN-BLEEDING, DISCHARGE, PREGNANCY ___ No Problem

Birth Control Method -

___ Pain ___ Hesitancy ___ Oliguria ___ Dysuria ___ Urine Color ___ Vaginal Bleeding ___ Frequency ___ Incontinent

___ Nocturia ___ Hematuria ___ Discharge ___ Pregnancy ___ Catheter ___ Type ___ Texas ___ Indwelling

___ Suprapubic ___ Ileoconduit
Explain: _____

ASSESS MOTOR FUNCTION, SENSATION, LOC, STRENGTH, GRIP, GAIT, COORDINATION, ORIENTATION, SPEECH, VISION ___ No Problem

___ Weakness ___ Numbness ___ Headache ___ Paralysis ___ Stuporous ___ Pupils ___ Forgetful ___ Unsteady ___ Tingling

___ Seizures ___ Lethargic ___ Comatose ___ Speech ___ Vertigo ___ Pains ___ Tremors ___ Confused ___ Grip

Oriented: ___ Time ___ Place ___ Person ___ Self Understands Directions: ☐ Yes ☐ No

Explain: _____

EMOTIONAL STATUS:

___ Calm ___ Anxious ___ Angry ___ Withdrawn ___ Fearful ___ Irritable ___ Restive ___ Euphoric Other: _____
(SPECIFY)

CONCERNS/EXPECTED OUTCOMES ACCORDING TO PATIENT: _____

NURSE'S PERCEPTION OF CONCERNS/EXPECTED OUTCOMES: _____

ASSESS SKIN INTEGRITY: _____ Intact _____ Lesion/Decubitus Describe _____

GOSNELL SCALE: DATE

Mental Status	Continence	Mobility	Activity	Nutrition	TOTAL SCORE
1. Alert	1. Fully Controlled	1. Full	1. Ambulatory	1. Good	
2. Apathetic	2. Usually Controlled	2. Slightly Limited	2. Walks with Assistance	2. Fair	
3. Confused	3. Minimally Controlled	3. Very Limited	3. Chairfast	3. Poor	
4. Stuporous	4. Absence of Control	4. Immobile	4. Bedfast		
5. Unconscious					

Description Lesion: _____

Prevention Protocol _____ Initiated ☐ Yes ☐ No

HIGH-RISK FALL ASSESSMENT		Risk Points
Confusion/Disorientation	Age < 70	+ 8
	Age ≥ 70	+ 1
Depression		+ 10
Elimination (incontinence, nocturia, frequency)		+ 4
Fall History	Age < 70	+ 12
	Age ≥ 70	+ 1
Mobility, (decreased in lower extremities)		+ 5
Surgery, (24 hrs post-op)		+ 3
Temperature elevation (0 >100° R > 101°)		- 3
Weakness, (generalized)		+ 4
	FINAL RISK SCORE =	SCORE

	Final Risk Score	Intervention Class	
K	Less than 4	Normal/Low Risk	K
E	4 - 7	Level 1	E
Y	More than 7	Level 2	Y

☐ Normal / Low Risk
☐ Level 1 Prevention Protocol Initiated
☐ Level 2 Prevention Protocol Initiated

TABLE 2-2   Guidelines for Interviewing

1. Select the environment carefully, ensuring privacy and comfort. Avoid noises, odors, interruptions, inadequate lighting, and temperature extremes.
2. Defer the interview when indicated because of the client's condition or environmental barriers.
3. Create an environment of trust, caring, and concern with a calm, unhurried approach.
4. Utilize the client as the primary source of data whenever possible; address by name, and avoid talking around the client to family or others.
5. Begin with introductions, a handshake, and an explanation of the purpose of the interview, including its relationship to nursing care.
6. Use terminology appropriate to the client's level of understanding. Speak clearly and distinctly.
7. Discuss the client's chief complaint early in the interview. Focus on this complaint and determine its effects on the client.
8. Encourage verbalization by using open-ended questions and supportive statements. Discuss general nonthreatening information before asking personal questions. Avoid interruptions, "why" questions, and biased questions.
9. Verify perceptions of the client's responses by using the reflective techniques of repetition and rephrasing.
10. Provide realistic reassurance if necessary. Avoid giving advice, opinions, or unrealistic reassurance.
11. Listen actively, maintain eye contact, and observe the nonverbal behavior of the client.
12. Conclude the interview with a brief summary of the client's problems, including anticipated nursing interventions.
13. Document as soon as possible away from the client's bedside, utilizing notations written briefly during the interview.

Each of the individual findings identified during observation requires further investigation, which may either substantiate or negate your initial impressions.

Physical Examination

The third major method of collecting data during the assessment process is physical examination. The focus of the physician's physical examination is the diagnosis of disease. The nurse's examination concentrates on

- further defining the client's response to the disease process, particularly those responses amenable to nursing interventions.

- establishing baseline data for comparison in evaluating the efficacy of nursing or medical interventions.

- substantiating subjective data obtained during interview or other nurse-client interactions.

TABLE 2-3   Observation: Use of Senses

SIGHT

Abrasions, absence of body part, absent or broken teeth, baldness, bandages, bitten nails, bleeding, blinking, blisters, boils, books, braces, bunions, burns, calluses, canes, casts, catheter, cleanliness of client or environment, clenched fists, clothing, convulsions, corns, crusting, crutches, crying, cyanosis, decubitus, dentures, diaphoresis, diarrhea, distention, drainage, drooling, ecchymosis, edema, eyeglasses, feces, fidgeting, fistula, flaking, flared nares, flies, flowers, frowning, gait, hangnail, hearing aids, hives, intravenous device, jaundice, jewelry, lighting, make-up, moles, monitor electrodes, mottling, newspaper, ostomy, paresis, petechiae, pimples, position—sitting, standing, or lying, posture, pregnancy, ptosis, purulent drainage, redness, room—type, size, and temperature, scabs, scars, scratches, scratching, shivering, significant other, skin color, slings, sneezing, squinting, stairs, sternal retraction, striae, support stockings, tatoo, telephone, television, tension, toilet articles, twitching, ulcerations, urine, vaccination, varicosities, vomiting, walker, warts, wheelchair, yawning

HEARING

Banging, barking, blood pressure, bruit, burping, clicking, coughing, crying, dripping, eructation, esophageal speech, expressions of pain, anger, sorrow, or depression, gargling, gasping, groaning, grunting, gurgling, harsh cough, heart rate and rhythm, hiccough, hissing, hoarseness, hyperactive or hypoactive bowel sounds, knocking, laughing, loudness, moaning, panting, radio, scratching, screaming, sighing, sirens, sneezing, squeaking, stammering, stuttering, sucking, telephone ringing, television, tone of voice, wheezing, whispering, whistling, yawning

TOUCH

Coarseness, coldness, dryness, edema, goose bumps, hardness, heat, lumps, masses, moisture, pain, pulsation, relaxation, roughness, skin texture, smoothness, softness, subcutaneous emphysema, swelling, tautness, temperature, tension, tremors, warmth, wetness

SMELL

Alcohol, axillary odor, bleeding, breath or body odor, disinfectants, feces, flowers, foot odor, garlic, gas, hair spray, marijuana, medicine, onion, perfume, perspiration, pubic odor, purulent drainage, tobacco, urine, vomitus

Techniques.   Four specific techniques are used during the examination: inspection, palpation, percussion, and auscultation.

Inspection refers to the visual examination of the client to determine normal, unusual, or abnormal conditions or responses. It is a type of observation that focuses on specific behaviors or physical features. Inspection is also more systematic and detailed than observation, because it defines characteristics such as size, shape, position, anatomical location, color, texture, appearance, movement, and symmetry.

INTRODUCTION
DATA COLLECTION
Priorities in Data Collection
Methods of Data Collection
Interview

Observation
Physical
Examination
Inspection
Palpation

Generally, inspection refers to the use of the unaided eye; however, the expanded role of the nurse in a variety of settings may incorporate the use of instruments. Those used most frequently are the otoscope and ophthalmoscope. These tools allow you to complete a more comprehensive and accurate examination of the eye or ear when indicated.

Palpation is the use of touch to determine the characteristics of body structure under the skin. This technique allows you to evaluate size, shape, texture, temperature, moisture, pulsation, vibration, consistency, and mobility. Your hands are the tools of palpation, and specific parts are used to assess particular characteristics. The back of your hand is most useful in assessing temperature because the skin in this area is thinner and allows discrimination of temperature differences. The fingertips are used to determine texture and size, since nerve endings are concentrated there. The palmar surfaces of the metacarpal joints are the most sensitive to vibration and therefore are particularly useful in detecting phenomena such as thrills over the heart or peristalsis.

Light palpation is the method used to examine most body parts. The use of your dominant hand is preferred. Hold your hand parallel to the body part being examined, with fingers extended. Exert gentle pressure downward while moving your hand in a circular motion. This technique is frequently used in breast examination to detect the presence and characteristics of abnormal masses. Deep palpation is particularly effective when examining the abdomen to locate organs or identify unusual masses. This technique requires both hands, one for pressure application and the other as a sensor. Place your dominant hand over the area to be palpated; it becomes the passive sensor. The other hand is positioned on top and is used to apply pressure. The client's facial expression and body movements during palpation provide you with additional information to assist in evaluating variables such as the degree of pain or discomfort.

INTRODUCTION
DATA
COLLECTION
Priorities in Data
Collection
Methods of Data
Collection
Interview
Observation
Physical
Examination
Inspection
Palpation
Percussion
Auscultation

Percussion involves striking of a body surface with your finger or fingers to produce sounds. This allows determination of size, density, organ boundaries, and location. Direct percussion occurs when you strike or tap the body surface directly with one or more fingers of one hand. This method is often used to define the cardiac border. Indirect percussion is used more frequently. Place your index or middle finger of one hand firmly on the skin and strike with the middle finger of the other hand.

The sounds resulting from percussion may be described as flat, dull, resonant, or tympanic. Flat sounds are low-pitched and abrupt and are produced when muscle or bone is percussed. Dull sounds are medium-pitched and thudding and may be heard over the liver and spleen. Resonance is a clear, hollow sound produced by percussion over a normal air-filled lung. Tympany is a loud, high-pitched sound heard over a gas-filled stomach or puffed out cheek.

Auscultation involves listening to the sounds produced by the organs of the body. You may use direct auscultation (with the unaided ear) to detect

---

BOX 2-2
Physical Assessment Techniques

Inspection	Visual examination of the client to determine normal, unusual, or abnormal conditions or responses
Palpation	The use of touch to determine characteristics of structures of the body
Percussion	Striking a body surface with your fingers to produce sounds
Auscultation	Listening to sounds produced by the body with the naked ear or a stethoscope

---

sounds such as wheezing. Generally, however, sounds are evaluated indirectly by using a stethoscope. This technique is used most frequently to determine the characteristics of lung, heart, and bowel sounds. It enables you to identify the frequency, intensity, quality, and duration of auscultated sounds.

Each of the four techniques—inspection, palpation, percussion, and auscultation—may be performed independently. However, the most effective method of physical examination is a comprehensive approach including a combination of techniques. Box 2-2 summarizes the techniques used in physical assessment.

Methods of Enhancing Data Collection

A number of variables affect your ability to collect data. These include environmental factors, data collection techniques, and verbal and nonverbal communication.

Environmental Factors

Data collection is dependent on effective nurse-client interaction. The environment in which data collection takes place frequently affects the ability of the client and the nurse to participate in this process. You may control the environment by manipulating several physical factors.

The physical area should be arranged to allow comfortable face-to-face interaction between the nurse and the client or family. The client should be positioned comfortably in bed or in a chair. Seat yourself opposite the client. Standing over the client should be avoided if possible, since this may convey superiority, disinterest, or haste.

Privacy should be ensured, since you will be asking many personal questions and physically observing and examining the client. This may be

---

BOX 2-3
Types of Questions Used to Collect Data

Open	Used to obtain a description from the client; requires more than a one- or two-word response
Closed	Used to obtain specific facts and to focus data collection; requires brief one- or two-word response
Biased	Slanted to obtain a specific response; includes loaded and leading questions
Leading	Imply that a particular response is preferred
Loaded	Designed to elicit the client's reaction to a certain situation or topic

---

accomplished by finding a quiet spot, or closing a door. Privacy also increases the potential for obtaining accurate, complete information and assists in creating a trusting relationship. To facilitate your ability to concentrate as well as that of your client, select a data collection area free from noise, odors, and interruptions. The temperature of the area should be comfortable, and lighting should allow both participants to observe each other clearly.

Data Collection Techniques

Data collection is most effective when you use both verbal and nonverbal techniques to obtain data. The combination of both approaches facilitates the acquisition of an accurate, complete data base.

Verbal Techniques.   The most commonly used verbal techniques include questioning, reflection, and supplementary statements. If you use these approaches during the interview you are more likely to be successful in obtaining the most significant information from the client.

1. *Questioning* allows the nurse to obtain information from the client, clarify perceptions of client responses, and validate other subjective or objective data. Questions may be open, closed, or biased. Box 2-3 summarizes the types of questions used to collect data.

   Open questions are those that by their nature elicit the client's perception of an event or description of concerns or feelings. Open questions stimulate the client to respond, tend to be less threatening, and encourage more honest replies. Generally, these questions require more than a one or two word response.

Examples

- ☐ "What happened today that made you come to the emergency department?"
- ☐ "How did you feel when the doctor told you about your blood pressure?"
- ☐ "Which medications do you take on a regular basis?"
- ☐ "What do you usually do when the pain occurs?"

Questions beginning with "what," "how," or "which" tend to result in the most detailed client response. "Why" questions tend to put the client in a defensive position.

Examples

- ☐ "Why did you do that?"
- ☐ "Why didn't you see a doctor sooner?"

Closed questions are those that require brief one or two word responses. They are used most frequently to obtain specific facts, and to focus data collection.

Examples

- ☐ "Did you take your blood pressure medicine today?"
- ☐ "How long did the pain last?"
- ☐ "When was your last menstrual period?"
- ☐ "How many times did you have diarrhea yesterday?"

Closed questions may also be used to clarify responses to open questions.

Example

Nurse: What do you usually do when the back pain occurs? (Open)

Client: Well, I usually lie down and take two pain pills.

Nurse: Did you do that today before you came to the hospital? (Closed)

Client: Yes.

Biased questions are those that tend to elicit a specific response or reaction from a client. They may be either open or closed. The most commonly used are **leading** or **loaded** questions. Leading questions imply that a particular response is preferred. Clients tend to answer these questions with responses they believe are desirable.

Examples

- ☐ "You don't take drugs, do you?"
- ☐ "There's no history of mental illness in your family, is there?"
- ☐ "You're feeling better today, aren't you?"

Loaded questions are used to elicit the client's reaction to a specific topic. You might use these when trying to evaluate the client's nonverbal response rather than the content of the actual reply to the question.

Examples

☐ "Do you think that your pain increases after your husband visits?"
☐ "Does your drinking interfere with your work?"

When asking questions of this nature, watch for squirming, lack of eye contact, or other signs of uneasiness. This nonverbal behavior may be more revealing than the client's verbal response. Biased questions tend to intimidate clients and frequently block the communication process. Clients often provide responses that they believe are expected; therefore, the information may be inaccurate. Biased questions should be used only when other techniques have been unsuccessful. Ideally, the use of a mixture of open and closed questioning will result in accurate, complete data, eliminating the need for biased questions.

Enhancing Data Collection
Environmental Factors
Data Collection Techniques
Verbal Questioning
Reflection

2. *Reflection* is the second verbal interviewing technique that can be used when collecting data. Your perception of the client's response is repeated or rephrased. Repetition encourages the client to continue discussion of a particular area of content. When you repeat key words from the client's statement, you assist the client to respond to the topic more completely.

Example

Nurse: How did you feel when the doctor told you about your high blood pressure?

Client: I was really afraid.

Nurse: You were really afraid? (Repetition of key words.)

Client: Yes, I thought I might have a stroke and die or be an invalid.

Since rephrasing provides the client with the nurse's interpretation of the information discussed, this allows both you and client to expand, clarify, or correct your perception of the data you have collected.

Example

Client: I found this lump in my breast last week when I was taking a shower. My mother had them too before she died from cancer.

Nurse: You're afraid that you might have cancer?

Client: Yes. I'm too young to die; my children need me.

In this case the client verified your perceptions, but there are times when reflection allows the client to correct your inaccurate perceptions.

Example

Client: I never had this dizziness or nausea until the doctor started me on that new blood pressure medicine.

Nurse: You think that the medicine is the cause of the problems you're having now?

Client: No, not really, but I think it may be part of the problem.

Here, the client clarified your interpretation of the initial statement.

After reflective statements, clients may seek advice or reassurance or ask you to validate their feelings. The client might respond with "What do you think?" "It's OK, isn't it?" or "What would you do?" Such responses may also be the client's attempt to obtain additional information. Avoid providing advice, unrealistic reassurance, or opinions since this tends to shift the accountability for decision-making from the client to you. The most effective method of dealing with this type of interaction is to use reflection to redirect the question.

Example

Client: The doctor told me that I can either have my hysterectomy the day after tomorrow or go home and come back in six weeks. What would you do, nurse?

Nurse: You're not sure whether you should have the surgery now or later? Let's look at the pros and cons of each.

This approach allows you to (1) rephrase the client's concerns, (2) clarify the decision that needed to be made by the client, and (3) create an environment that would encourage the client to look at her options objectively before making a decision.

3. *Supplementary statements* is the third technique that encourages the client to continue verbalization throughout the data collection process. Short phrases such as "Um-hm," "Yes," "Go on," "I see," and "What happened next?" send a clear message. These brief responses let the client know that you are interested and they frequently stimulate further communication. They are particularly effective when accompanied by nonverbal cues such as touch, eye contact, and nodding the head.

Enhancing Data Collection
Environmental Factors
Data Collection Techniques
Verbal Questioning
Reflection
Supplementary Statements

Examples

Client: "I had chest pain and I took a nitroglycerin tablet just like my doctor told me to."

Nurse: "What happened next?"

Client: "The pain didn't go away, so I called the doctor."

Nurse: "Go on."

Nonverbal Techniques. Nonverbal methods may also facilitate or enhance communication during the data collection. The nonverbal components of a nurse-client interaction frequently convey a message more effectively than the actual spoken words. In fact, if the verbal and nonverbal messages differ, the nonverbal message tends to be accepted more readily. The most common nonverbal components include facial expression, body position, touch, voice, silence, and active listening.

1. *Facial expressions* often reveal important information. Watch for appropriateness of expression, frowning, and lack of eye contact. **Appropriateness of expression** suggests that facial expression should be congruent with the words being spoken and to the context of the conversation. Be particularly alert to situations in which the expression on the client's face does not match the verbal message. For example, when a client describes himself as depressed, you would not expect to see a smile on his face. Similarly, when a woman talks about how happy she is in her marriage, her facial expression usually indicates sincerity. You might question this sincerity if her statement is accompanied by a smirk.

   You should also be concerned if the facial expression is not appropriate to the context of the message. For example, you might encounter a client who smiles when discussing a serious problem. The smile, which may be resulting from uneasiness, could mislead you into believing that the client is not concerned about the problem.

   Frowning may indicate disagreement, lack of understanding, pain, anger, or unhappiness. For example, when you are explaining to Mrs. Kuroishi that she should take her pulse each day before taking her digoxin, she frowns. You might interpret this as an indication of unwillingness to carry out this step. In reality, Mrs. Kuroishi does not know how to take her pulse.

   Lack of eye contact may mean that the client is uncomfortable, shy, nonassertive, bored, intimidated, or withdrawn. For example, in a venereal disease clinic, you may frequently question clients about sexual contacts. In response to this question, Terry Williams turns his face away. You might interpret this change in eye contact as embarrassment. In reality, Terry is trying to remember a number of names.

   You may want to clarify discrepancies between facial expressions and verbal messages or context. For example, you might say, "I notice that you are smiling when you discuss your illness, but you seem really concerned. I'm confused. Could you clarify this for me?"

   Similarly, your facial expression may also convey mixed messages. For example, an inappropriate smile when very personal or sensitive information is shared may upset the client. In fact, you may feel uncomfortable discussing the topic. Likewise, frowning after a client's comments may be seen as being judgmental, when in reality you may

2-4 TEST YOURSELF
Verbal Communication Techniques

Read the following statements and identify them as open (O), closed (C), biased (B), reflective (R), or supplementary (S).

_____ "When did you first notice the lump in your breast?"

_____ "And then?"

_____ "You don't really believe that old wives' tale, do you?"

_____ "You're confused about how many times a day you should be taking this pill?"

_____ "How do you know when your blood sugar is low?"

_____ "When did you stop beating your wife?"

_____ "Oh, when you went to India you got malaria?"

_____ "What do you think you can do to assist in your recovery?"

_____ "Do you have any questions about what will be happening to you tomorrow?"

_____ "Go on."

2-4 TEST YOURSELF
Verbal Communication Techniques: Answers

Key: (O) open, (C) closed, (B) biased, (R) reflective, (S) supplementary

(C) "When did you first notice the lump in your breast?"

(S) "And then?"

(B) "You don't really believe that old wives' tale, do you?"

(R) "You're confused about how many times a day you should be taking this pill?"

(O) "How do you know when your blood sugar is low?"

(B) "When did you stop beating your wife?"

(R) "Oh, when you went to India you got malaria?"

(O) "What do you think you can do to assist in your recovery?"

(C) "Do you have any questions about what will be happening to you tomorrow?"

(S) "Go on."

Data Collection
Techniques
Verbal
Nonverbal
Facial Expression
Body Position and Stance

have a headache. Lack of eye contact because of preoccupation with a confused client in the other bed may be interpreted as lack of interest.

2. *Body position and stance* are elements of interaction that convey a nonverbal message. Observe the nonverbal messages communicated by the client's posture or stance throughout your data collection. The timing of specific behaviors may be particularly significant. A relaxed posture may indicate readiness to share information, just as a tense or rigid stance suggests unwillingness to share, pain, or anxiety. The relaxed client who tenses or shifts position when discussing family relationships or alcohol consumption may be communicating discomfort in discussing particularly sensitive information.

Gestures may also provide the nurse with information about the client.

Gesture		Interpretation
Finger-pointing		Anger; control
Hand-wringing	may suggest	Anxiety
Nodding		Agreement
Shoulder-shrugging		Uncertainty

Be particularly observant for discrepancies between the client's spoken words and the nonverbal messages communicated by posture or stance.

Your body position and stance send nonverbal messages too. Frequently you can help to create an environment of warmth and trust by a exhibiting a calm, relaxed posture. This position communicates interest and caring and tends to help the client feel comfortable in disclosing personal information. A hurried approach, an inappropriately warm or cold attitude, or a rigid or overly casual posture communicate disinterest, boredom, or preoccupation. These nonverbal messages tend to confuse the client and inhibit data collection.

3. *Touch* may also significantly affect your data collection. The individual's use or response to touch may effectively communicate specific attitudes, feelings, or responses. Clients may vary in their degree of comfort with touching or being touched. Your use of touch should be determined by the client's readiness to accept it. This is frequently evidenced by response to an introductory handshake or to the touching that accompanies taking a pulse or blood pressure. The client's tolerance of touch may be dependent on age, cultural background, social maturity, and past experiences. Some clients consider even simple touch an intrusion, and withdrawal from touch may demonstrate fear, pain, or resentment. On the other hand, the client who grasps your arm, squeezes hands, or touches your face may be communicating warmth, appreciation, or the need for support or reassurance.

You may convey caring, concern, and support by a simple touch on the client's arm, squeezing of a hand, or an arm around the shoulder. Similarly, rough, rushed, or insincere touch communicates the opposite message.

4. *Voice* is usually considered to be a verbal technique; however, nonverbal messages may be conveyed in response to vocal characteristics. Tone of voice, rate of speech, and volume may be significant in determining the perceptions of both nurse and client. When you speak calmly, relatively slowly, and at a comfortable level, you communicate relaxation, patience, and concern with privacy. The client may be intimidated, embarrassed, or uncomfortable when interviewed by the overly excited nurse who is loud or speaks too rapidly.

The client who speaks slowly, in a monotone, or with a flat affect may be worried or depressed. Conversely, loud or rapid speech suggests anger, pain, impatience, or hearing deficits. These may be particularly significant if observed at specific times during data collection.

Marginal notes, beside item 3:
Data Collection Techniques
Verbal
Nonverbal
Facial Expression
Body Position and Stance
Touch

Marginal notes, beside item 4:
Data Collection Techniques
Verbal
Nonverbal
Facial Expression
Body Position and Stance
Touch
Voice

Example

Nurse: How do you feel about your surgery?

Client: I told you, it's nothing to worry about, it's only a cyst. (Spoken loudly, through clenched teeth.)

Clearly this client is communicating some type of distress. It may be anger or impatience in response to repeated questioning or anxiety about the possible outcome of surgery.

There are a number of other sounds that may convey meaning. They may indicate impatience, sarcasm, pain, anxiety, embarrassment, emphasis, agreement, or disagreement.

Data Collection Techniques
Verbal
Nonverbal
Facial Expression
Body Position and Stance
Touch
Voice
Silence
Active Listening

5. *Silence* frequently causes discomfort in both nurses and clients. However, it is an important tool that provides an opportunity to (1) review what has transpired up to that point in the interview, (2) collect thoughts, and (3) begin to organize data. Frequently, inexperienced interviewers attempt to fill the gaps in conversation with multiple questions to avoid the discomfort associated with silence. This may communicate anxiety to the client and is often confusing. The client may feel pressured, rushed, or unable to respond.

Silence evidenced by the client may be significant in conveying discomfort, thoughtfulness, or embarrassment. Avoid filling silent periods too quickly. This indicates an acceptance of the client's feelings and may strengthen the nurse-client relationship.

6. *Active listening* is a communication technique used to enhance communication with clients, particularly during data collection. As previously discussed, both verbal and nonverbal messages are exchanged when interacting with clients. Active listening involves three stages:

- Listening to the verbal component.
- Identifying the existence of nonverbal cues.
- Carefully determining the significance of both.

When you learn to listen not only to what is spoken but also to what is left unsaid you are able to interpret the client's feelings and responses effectively and to identify specific areas requiring further exploration. Consequently, active listening:

- Allows more accurate reflection of these perceptions to the client.
- Encourages clarification or validation by the client.
- Promotes the acquisition of a more accurate and complete data base.

ANA Measurement Criteria I-4 (Standard of Care). The data collection process is systematic and ongoing.

Characteristics of Data Collection

There are two significant characteristics of data collection utilized during nursing assessment: it is **systematic** and **ongoing**.

Systematic

Systematic data collection is vital to accurate and complete assessment. There are a variety of useful and practical approaches used by nurses to assess clients

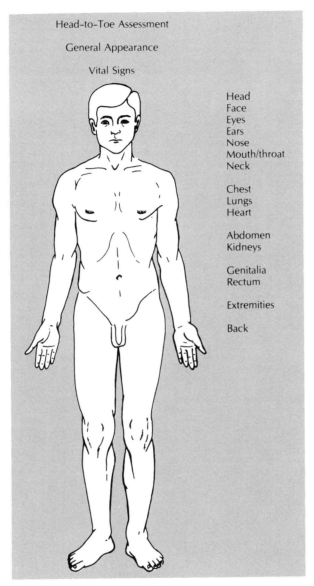

Head-to-Toe Assessment

General Appearance

Vital Signs

Head
Face
Eyes
Ears
Nose
Mouth/throat
Neck

Chest
Lungs
Heart

Abdomen
Kidneys

Genitalia
Rectum

Extremities

Back

FIGURE 2-6.   Head-to-toe assessment.

systematically. The head-to-toe, major body systems, functional health patterns, and human response patterns approaches are described below.

Head to Toe.   This approach begins with the client's head and systematically and symmetrically progresses down the body to the feet. The components of the physical examination are outlined in Figure 2-6.

Major Body Systems.   In this approach, the nurse examines the body by

INTRODUCTION
DATA
COLLECTION
Priorities in Data
Collection
Methods of Data
Collection

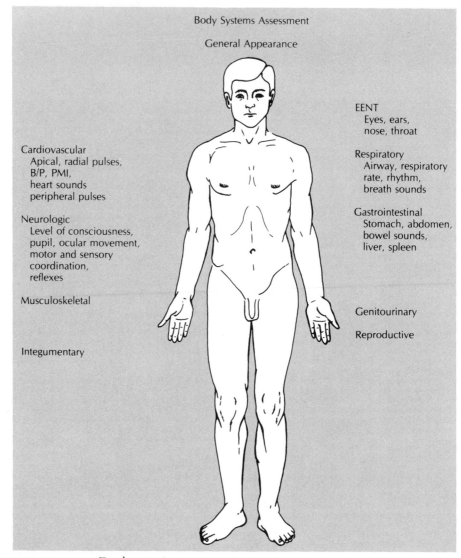

FIGURE 2-7. Body systems assessment.

systems rather than by individual body parts. Information from the interview and observation assists the nurse to determine which systems require particular emphasis. The components of this system are identified in Figure 2-7.

Functional Health Patterns. This approach allows the nurse to collect data systematically by evaluating the functional health patterns of the client. The nurse attempts to identify patterns and to focus the physical examination on particular functional areas. The list in Table 2-4 identifies the patterns evaluated.

TABLE 2-4   Functional Health Patterns Assessment Guide

NAMES OF PATTERNS	PHYSICAL EXAMINATION
Health perception/health management	General appearance
Nutritional/metabolic	Vital signs, height, weight
Elimination	Eyes
Activity/exercise	Mouth
Sleep/rest	Hearing
Cognitive/perceptual	Pulses
Self-perception	Respirations
Sexuality/sexual functioning	Skin
Coping/stress management	Functional ability
Value/belief systems	Mental status

Human Response Patterns.   This methodology allows the nurse to examine the client based on the nine human response patterns that reflect the client's interaction with the environment. Table 2-5 lists assessment categories under each of the nine patterns.

Comparison of these approaches reveals that the information obtained is identical. Therefore, you should select the method that is found to be most effective or more appropriate to your particular practice setting. Regardless of the approach selected, skilled assessment requires discipline and practice to perfect interview, observation, and physical examination techniques.

Ongoing

The initial assessment enables you to accumulate comprehensive data about the client. It also establishes your relationship with the client and facilitates the completion of the remaining phases of the nursing process. It also helps to identify health responses and the specific factors that contribute to the existence of these responses in the individual client. This encourages collaboration between the nurse and the client in the development of client outcomes and appropriate nursing interventions designed to achieve them. Ongoing reassessments validate the existence of previously identified concerns and document the client's progress toward the outcomes. These data also determine whether you should change, expand, or discontinue nursing interventions. Because assessment is an ongoing process, reassessment data also allow you to identify additional responses that may have developed as a result of hospitalization, the disease process, or treatment modalities. This is accomplished through a process that compares current information to previously acquired baseline data. Table 2-6 lists the Joint Commission on Accreditation of Healthcare Organizations (JCAHO) standards that relate to assessment.

TABLE 2-5   Human Response Patterns Assessment Guide

EXCHANGING

Cardiac
Peripheral
Oxygenation
Nutrition
Cerebral
Skin integrity
Physical regulation
Elimination

COMMUNICATING

Read/write/understand English,
  other languages, impaired speech,
  other forms of communication

RELATING

Relationships
Socialization

VALUING

Religious preference, important
  religious practices, spiritual
  concerns, cultural orientation,
  cultural practices

CHOOSING

Coping
Judgment
Participation in health regimen

MOVING

Activity
Recreation
Health maintenance
Rest
Environmental maintenance
Self-care
Sensory-perception

PERCEIVING

Self-concept
Sensory-perception
Meaningfulness

KNOWING

Current health problems
Current medications
Readiness to learn
Memory
Health history
Risk factors
Mental status

FEELING

Pain/discomfort associated/
  aggravating/alleviating factors
Emotional integrity/status

INTRODUCTION
DATA
COLLECTION
CRITICAL
THINKING AND
ASSESSMENT

CRITICAL THINKING AND ASSESSMENT

The nurse's ability to think critically is key to systematic and ongoing assessment. Clearly, you must be able to determine what type of data should be collected, by which method it can best be obtained, in what priority it should be collected, what the best sources of information might be, and which communication strategies are most effective in each individual situation for a particular client.

Example. Maria Rosselli, the 30-year-old mother of a 2-year-old child, is admitted to the hospital for scheduled lung surgery.

TABLE 2-6   JCAHO Standards That Affect Assessment

PE.1	Each patient's physical, psychological, and social status is assessed.
PE 1.1	There is an initial assessment/screening of each patient's physical, psychological, and social status to determine the need for and type of care or treatment and/or the need for further assessment.
PE 1.2	The scope and intensity of any further assessment is determined by:
	PE 1.2.1 The patient's diagnosis
	PE 1.2.2 The treatment setting
	PE 1.2.3 The patient's desire for treatment
	PE 1.2.4 The patient's response to any previous treatment
PE 1.3	The need for assessment of the nutritional status of the patient is determined.
PE 1.4	The need for assessment of the functional status of the patient is determined.
PE 1.5	The need for education of the patient and the patient's family in care or treatment of the patient is assessed.
PE 1.7	The need for a discharge planning assessment of the patient is determined.

Applying the critical-thinking process to Maria, you would ask the following questions:

1. *What is the issue?*
   In the assessment phase of the nursing process, you are interested in collecting a comprehensive data base about the client in order to best plan her care.

2. *What information do I need?*
   In order to acquire a comprehensive data base, some questions you might ask include:
   a. What information do I need to begin to develop a plan of care?
   b. How much does the client understand about her condition and the reason for the anticipated surgery?
   c. What is her reaction to this hospitalization and the need for surgery?
   d. Are there significant factors in her health history that might hasten or interfere with her recovery?

3. *What is the best source of the information?*
   Some questions you would ask include:
   a. Is Maria able to provide the data? If not why and who can provide it?
   b. Are there any reasons why the data should not be collected at this time?
   c. From what sources can I obtain additional information?

4. *What is the most important data to collect?*
   Frequently, you will initiate your admission assessment with very little background information about the client. Therefore you may use the principles of Maslow's hierarchy to determine priorities in assessment. You might ask:

a. What data do I need to acquire about Maria's physical condition?

b. Does she have safety or comfort needs?

c. Who are her significant others and social supports?

d. How does she feel about herself and her abilities to deal with her hospitalization and surgery?

e. What impact will her surgery have on her ability to reach her potential?

5. *Is there other information I need?*

Throughout your assessment of Maria, you should be asking yourself whether your information is complete. For example, when you ask the client to tell you about her family, she mentions her husband and her daughter. You may ask about her parents and siblings and whether they have lung problems as well. Maria indicates that she has been in the hospital five times in the past. Ask her to tell you about those experiences to determine if they were related to her lung problem and if her previous experiences in the hospital were positive.

6. *Is this the best way to deal with the issue?*

During your assessment of Maria, you explain the purpose of your data collection and create an environment that is conducive to acquiring the necessary information. You use verbal and nonverbal strategies to communicate your interest and concern about her while accumulating the data necessary to plan her care. You observe her carefully during your interactions and complete a systematic and comprehensive physical assessment. You involve her actively in the process and respond honestly to her questions. When appropriate you are both creative and flexible in your approach by adapting your usual data collection procedures to her special needs or concerns. **Yes, this is the best way to collect data!**

In summary, the first step of the assessment phase, data collection, involves the accumulation of subjective, objective, current, and historical information from primary and secondary sources. The nurse sets priorities for the collection of data and utilizes methods such as interviewing, observation, and physical examination to collect data. Critical-thinking principles promote the acquisition of an organized, accurate, and systematic data base about the individual client.

INTRODUCTION
DATA
COLLECTION
CRITICAL
THINKING AND
ASSESSMENT
DOCUMENTATION
Purposes

DOCUMENTATION

The second component of the assessment phase is documentation of the data base. Although the following discussion of documentation is primarily directed toward the recording of data accumulated during the assessment, documentation is integral to all phases of the nursing process.

2-5 TEST YOURSELF
Critical Thinking and Assessment

Refer to the case study of Ted Alexander. This exercise will focus on Ted's love and belonging needs. You note that Ted is tense and concerned about his separation from his children, the unfamiliar doctor, and job demands. You know that Ted is alone in an unfamiliar city and is facing a life-threatening illness: gastric bleeding.

Use the critical-thinking format presented below to identify additional assessment data that will be needed to address his love and belonging needs. The first question is answered for you.

1. *What is the issue?*
   In order to help Ted become less anxious, I need to obtain more information from him about his concerns.

2. *What information do I need?*
   a.
   b.
   c.
   d.
   e.

3. *What is the best source of information?*

4. *What is the most important data to collect?*

5. *Is there other information that I need?*

6. *Is this the best way to deal with the issue?*

> ✔ **2-5 TEST YOURSELF**
> # Critical Thinking and Assessment: Answers

1. *What is the issue?*
   In order to help Ted become less anxious, I need to obtain more information from him about his concerns.

2. *What information do I need?*
   a. How old are Ted's teenage children? Are they 12 or 13, or a more independent age—18 or 19?
   b. What is the involvement of the children's mother in their care?
   c. What arrangements have been made for supervision while Ted is away on his business trip?
   d. Can these arrangements be extended?
   e. What is Ted's normal support system at home?
   f. Is there a significant other who can be contacted?

3. *What is the best source of information?*
   At this point, Ted is the best source, but he may be able to provide you with some contacts that may help to answer some of these questions.

4. *What is the most important data to collect?*
   The first concern he mentioned in addition to his physical condition was associated with his children. He needs to know that they are taken care of in order to refocus on his physiological needs.

5. *Is there other information that I need?*
   a. Who needs to be contacted at his place of work?
   b. What is the name and telephone number of his physician in Las Vegas? It may help Ted to feel more secure if the attending physician in Atlantic City can talk to Ted's doctor.

6. *Is this the best way to deal with the issue?*
   Yes, it is important that Ted have his concerns addressed. In order to do that, you need more information. He is your only source of information, therefore, until you make additional contacts, questions must be directed to Ted.

ANA Measurement Criteria I-5 (Standard of Care). Relevant data are documented in a retrievable form.

Purposes of Documentation

The recording of data in the client's medical record is an important part of the nursing process for a variety of reasons, which are summarized in Box 2-4.

BOX 2-4
Purposes of Documentation

- Encourages communication
- Facilitates delivery of quality client care
- Provides mechanism for evaluation of care
- Forms permanent legal record
- Source of data for research

---

1. It establishes a mechanism for communication among the members of the health care team. This provides a variety of disciplines with pertinent, accurate, and current data about the client as an individual. A common frustration of clients in health care systems is repeated questioning and examination by a variety of personnel: physicians, nurses, therapists, dietitians. Complete documentation assists in eliminating this repetition and prevents gaps in data. It also helps to create positive relationships between the client and health care providers.

2. Documentation of assessment data facilitates the delivery of quality client care. The information collected allows the nurse to develop preliminary nursing diagnoses, outcomes, and nursing interventions. Accurately documented baseline findings form the standard for comparison of subsequent data collection, allowing the nurse to validate, clarify, or update preliminary diagnoses and to facilitate the provision of consistent individualized care.

3. Documentation ensures a mechanism for the evaluation of individual client care. Medical records are reviewed by a variety of internal systems and external regulatory agencies. These may include quality assurance and risk management committees, State Departments of Health (DOH), Professional Review Organizations (PRO), and the Joint Commission on Accreditation of Healthcare Organizations (JCAHO). These committees and organizations have developed standards for the delivery of nursing care. Careful documentation, beginning with the assessment data base, assists in demonstrating compliance with these accepted standards.

4. Documentation creates a permanent legal record of the care provided to the client. Although the medical record is confidential, it is available as a legal document in a number of situations. Obviously, the chart may be used to evaluate liability in a malpractice litigation. However, it may also be used to document client competence, determine the extent of injury in accident or compensation claims, or substantiate the provision of specific treatment modalities for reimbursement purposes. Therefore, detailed

accurate documentation, beginning with assessment findings, may protect the client, the care providers (particularly nurses), and the institution or agency. Additional information on legal and ethical considerations can be found in Chapter 10.

5. Documentation provides the foundation for nursing research. The information found in the medical record may be utilized as a source for identification of research topics specific to nursing practice. Validation of nursing diagnoses, comparison of client responses to nursing interventions, and development of nurse-client relationships are potential areas of exploration. The accumulation of a body of research associated with nursing practice helps to define nursing as a science and to refine the nursing process.

The documentation of the nursing assessment should clearly identify those findings that necessitate nursing interventions. These include a variety of factors affecting the client's health status or ability to function. The client's responses, perceptions, feelings, and coping mechanisms are particularly significant in the formulation of nursing diagnoses and the identification of specific nursing interventions.

INTRODUCTION
DATA COLLECTION
DOCUMENTATION
CRITICAL THINKING AND ASSESSMENT
Purposes
Guidelines

Guidelines for Documentation

The format for recording the nursing assessment varies among practice settings. Regardless of the type and structure of the documentation tool, there are some general guidelines that should be considered. These are summarized in Box 2-5.

1. **Write entries objectively without bias, value judgments, or personal opinion.** Refrain from using judgmental words such as "obnoxious," "drunk," "turkey," and so on. Provide objective descriptions of the behaviors the client is exhibiting.

Example.   In the case of the client in whom alcohol intoxication is suspected: "Client exhibits staggering gait and slurred speech, and has odor of alcohol on breath."

2. **Include important information shared with you by the client or family.** Use quotation marks to clearly identify these types of statements.

Example.   Client's description of illness: "My diabetes is out of control, and I'm here to have tests and get it regulated."

3. **Document sufficient information to support your interpretations of the client's appearance and behavior.**

Example.   Emotional status: Depressed, sits in darkened room with curtain

---

BOX 2-5
Guidelines for Documentation

- Write entries objectively without bias, value judgments, or personal opinion.
- Include important information shared with you by the client or family.
- Document sufficient information to support your interpretations of the client's appearance and behavior.
- Avoid generalizations, including "basket" terms such as "good," "fair," "usual," "normal."
- Describe findings as thoroughly as possible, including defining characteristics such as size and shape.
- Document data clearly and concisely, avoiding superfluous information and long, rambling sentences.
- Write or print entries legibly in nonerasable ink.
- Do not tamper with the medical record.
- Entries should be correct in grammar and spelling.
- Do not leave spaces that allow others to insert content into your entry.
- Identify late entries correctly.
- Be precise in documenting information you have reported to a physician.
- Provide complete descriptions when the client is uncooperative or chooses not to follow the recommended treatment regimen.

---

pulled around bed, rarely initiates conversation, responds in monotone with short answers when questioned, limited eye contact, cries softly.

These findings support the nurse's interpretation of depression.

4. **Avoid generalizations,** including "basket" terms such as "good," "fair," "usual," "normal." These descriptions are open to broad interpretation based on the reader's point of reference.

Example. "Abdomen moderately distended" may be interpreted differently by each nurse reading the entry. More specific documentation might include the exact measurement of abdominal girth.

"Fair mobility" may suggest that the client was able to perform activities of daily living effectively. In reality, the nurse may mean that the client was able to turn independently in bed but required assistance with bathing, feeding, and ambulating.

"Normal bowel patterns" is more clearly defined by "moves bowels every other day without the use of laxatives."

5. **Describe findings as thoroughly as possible, including defining characteristics such as size and shape.**

For example, the description of a client's decubitus ulcer should include measurements, depth, color, odor, and drainage. This is particularly important when documenting the initial assessment, since this information is the baseline for evaluating the effectiveness of nursing interventions.

6. **Document data clearly and concisely,** avoiding superfluous information and long, rambling sentences.

Example. "The client indicates that she didn't feel good for five days, so she went to the doctor and told him about her symptoms. He gave her three medications, including antihistamine, antibiotic, and cough medicine. These didn't help so she went to the emergency department, and the doctor there admitted her."

This could be reworded as: "History of fever, cough, and nasal congestion × 5 days, unrelieved by antihistamine, antibiotic, antitussives prescribed by family physician."

7. **Write or print entries legibly in nonerasable ink.** Errors in documentation should be corrected in a manner that does not obscure the original entry. The most commonly used method involves drawing a single line through the incorrect item, writing "mistaken entry," and initialing the entry. The use of correction fluid, erasure, or crossing out to obliterate the entry is not acceptable.

8. **Do not tamper with the medical record.** This includes destroying pages, falsifying information, omitting significant data, or rewriting your entries at someone else's direction. Tampering with the record is a serious act that can destroy the credibility of the record and mislead others involved in the care of the client.

9. **Entries should be correct in grammar and spelling.** The nurse should incorporate only those abbreviations approved for use in the particular practice setting. Slang, clichés, and labels should be avoided except in the context of a direct quotation.

10. **Do not leave spaces that allow others to insert content into your entry.** Draw a line through unused space. Do not leave a space for others to chart their entry. Other health care professionals can add their entries after yours, even if the information is out of sequence.

11. **Identify late entries correctly.** If you have to include additional

information because the chart was not available at the time you needed it or you realize that you forgot to include important information, follow this procedure:

- Add the entry to the next available line in the progress notes or to the appropriate section of a form.
- Label the entry "late entry" to indicate that it was added out of sequence.
- Record the time and date of the entry.

12. Be precise in documenting information you have reported to a physician.

Example. "Dr. Wilson notified of low blood sugar of 40, unresponsiveness. Order for IV glucose received."

13. Provide complete descriptions when the client is uncooperative or chooses not to follow the recommended treatment regimen. When the client does not follow instructions relating to activity or intake or tampers with medical equipment, describe the behavior. Also, be sure to document that you have warned the client of the consequences of these actions.

Example. In the case of a teenage client who adjusted his IV flow rate: "IV found running wide open. Client indicates that he opened it "so he could get it over with." Rate adjusted as ordered and client instructed regarding the dangers of excessive IV fluid over a short period of time."

Figure 2-8 demonstrates how the information obtained from Ted Alexander, the man described in Test Yourself 2-2, would be documented.

COMPUTERS

Computer applications that automate all phases of the nursing process have been designed and implemented. These applications include both components of the assessment phase: data collection and documentation.

Data Collection

Many automated systems provide for computerized history-taking. This may be accomplished directly or indirectly. In direct systems, the client uses a computer terminal to respond to a series of questions. These histories have been demonstrated to be valid when compared with those taken indirectly and are frequently more complete and accurate (Andreoli and Musser, 1985). In indirect systems, the nurse obtains the information from the client and enters it into a bedside terminal.

MERCER MEDICAL CENTER
NURSING HISTORY AND PHYSICAL

Date __6/11/95__   Time __10__   (A.M.)/P.M.

BP __104/60__   TPR __98.2 - 120 - 26__

Admitting Diagnosis __Bleeding gastric ulcer__

PAST MEDICAL HISTORY (medical, surgical, trauma)   Height __6'2"__   Weight __196__

__Cirrhosis - 2 years ago__   ALLERGIES AND REACTIONS
__Denies surgery__   __denies__

MEDICATIONS
Name & Dosage	Usual Time Taken	Time of Last Dose
denies		

REASONS FOR HOSPITALIZATION (onset, character, methods used to resolve problem)

__3 Days prior to admission, developed pain in upper abdomen, took Alka-Seltzer with little relief. Pain worsened today, associated with vomiting bloody fluid.__

Signature __J Henderson Rn__

COMMUNICATION

SUBJECTIVE
- ☐ Hearing Loss   Comments: __left glasses__
- ☑ Visual Changes   __& contact lenses__
- ☐ Denied   __in hotel__

OBJECTIVE
- ☑ Glasses
- ☑ Contact Lens
- ☐ Language Barrier
- ☐ Hearing Aide
- ☐ Speech Difficulties

Pupil Size _____ R   L
Reaction _____

OXYGENATION

- ☐ Dyspnea   Comments: _____
- ☑ Smoking History __2 packs/day__
- ☐ Cough
- ☐ Sputum
- ☐ Denied

Resp ☑ Regular   ☐ Irregular
Describe: _____
R _____
L _____

CIRCULATION

- ☐ Chest Pain   Comments: _____
- ☐ Leg Pain
- ☐ Numbness of Extremities
- ☑ Denied

Heart Rhythm ☑ Regular   ☐ Irregular
Ankle Edema _____

Pulse	Car.	Rad.	DP	Fem.*
R	+	+	+	
L	+	+	+	

Comments: _____
*If applicable

NUTRITION

Diet: __low fat__
- ☐ N   ☐ V   Comments: __Has eaten little__
- Character   __in last two days__
- ☑ Recent change in weight, appetite
- ☐ Swallowing difficulty
- ☐ Denied

☑ Dentures   ☐ None

	Full	Partial	With Patient
Upper	☐	☐	☐
Lower	☐	☑	☐

__4 caps on upper teeth__

13122 11-84

FIGURE 2-8.   Documentation of client Ted Alexander.

(Courtesy of Mercer Medical Center, Trenton, NJ.)

ELIMINATION

SUBJECTIVE

Usual bowel pattern _daily_
- ☐ Constipation
  Remedy _occasional laxatives_
  Date of last BM _6-9_
- ☐ Diarrhea
  Character _____
- ☐ Urinary Frequency
- ☑ Urgency
- ☐ Dysuria
- ☐ Hematuria
- ☐ Incontinence
- ☐ Polyuria
- ☐ Foley in place
- ☐ Denied

OBJECTIVE

Comments: _several episodes nocturia & urgency in last few months_

Bowel Sounds _absent_
Abdominal distention present:
- ☐ Yes   ☑ No

Urine* (color, consistency, odor)
_____
_____
_____
*If foley in place

MGT. OF HEALTH AND ILLNESS

- ☐ Alcohol   ☑ Denied
  (Amount, frequency) _Has history of heavy drinking for 15 yrs. Quit 2 years ago_
- ☐ BSE   Last Pap Smear _____
  LMP: _____

Briefly describe patient's ability to follow treatments (diet, meds, etc.) for chronic health problems (if present). _Compliant_

SKIN INTEGRITY

- ☐ Dry   Comments: _____
- ☐ Itching
- ☐ Other
- ☑ Denied
*Use Skin/body Stamp on Progress Notes

- ☐ Dry   ☑ Cold   ☐ Pale
- ☐ Flushed   ☐ Warm
- ☑ Moist   ☐ Cyanotic
*Rashes, ulcers, decubitus (describe size, location, drainage)

ACTIVITY/SAFETY

- ☐ Convulsions   Comments: _____
- ☐ Dizziness
- ☐ Limited motion
  of joints
Limitations in
  ability to:
- ☐ Ambulate
- ☐ Bathe self
- ☐ Other
- ☑ Denied

- ☑ LOC and Orientation _alert & oriented_

Gait: ☐ Walker   ☐ Cane   ☐ Other
- ☑ Steady   ☐ Unsteady _____
- ☐ Sensory and motor losses in face or extremities _____

- ☐ ROM limitations _____

COMFORT SLEEP/WAKE

- ☑ Pain   Comments: _____
  (Location,   _Abdominal_
  frequency,   _tenderness_
  remedies)   _unrelieved by_
               Alka Seltzer
- ☐ Nocturia
- ☐ Sleep Difficulties
- ☐ Denied

- ☐ Facial Grimaces
- ☐ Guarding
- ☑ Other signs of pain _Rigid abdominal wall_

- ☐ Siderail release form signed (60 + years)

COPING

Occupation _____
Members of household _Divorced - lives with two teenage children (Jim & Lauri)_

Most supportive person _Children_

Observed non-verbal behavior _anxious_
_____

Person and phone number that can be reached at any time
Jim or Lauri
_702-788-7117_

R.N. Signature _J. Henderson Rn_

```
┌─────────────────────────────────────────────────────────────────────────┐
│                          Enter Assessment                                 │
├─────────────────────────────────────────────────────────────────────────┤
│  Bed:    030902        Patient: 000030000326        Cromwell, Maureen     │
├─────────────────────────────────────────────────────────────────────────┤
│  Screen:  General Admission Assessment Data                               │
├─────────────────────────────────────────────────────────────────────────┤
│    Mode of Arrival  :  Ambulatory      Admitted From  :  Admitting Office │
│    Accompanied by :                     Arrival D/T     :                  │
│    Informant       :                    Oriented to     :                  │
│                                                                           │
│  # *Temperature    :  102.2            *Pulse          :   80             │
│    *Respirations   :   20              *Blood Pressure :  120/80          │
│    *Height         :  5'6"             *Weight         :  125             │
│                                                                           │
│    Prosthesis      :                    ADL Needs       :                  │
│    Valuables?      :                                                       │
│                                                                           │
│   *Pt. Complaint   :                    Recur Illness?  :                  │
│   *Medication?     :                    Allergies       :  Penicillin     │
├─────────────────────────────────────────────────────────────────────────┤
│  F7 - Abnormal(#)   F10 Pt. Information   F12 View Past VS   F13 View Past I/O │
├─────────────────────────────────────────────────────────────────────────┤
│  Enter mnemonic or use FIND to select pt's mode of arrival.               │
└─────────────────────────────────────────────────────────────────────────┘
```

FIGURE 2-9.   Computerized assessment screen.

(Courtesy of Shared Medical Systems Corporation, Malvern, PA.)

Computerized systems are particularly valuable in automating physical examination. Computer terminals located at the bedside prompt the nurse to complete examinations using the body systems, head-to-toe, functional health, or human response patterns. Figure 2-9 demonstrates a sample screen used in a body systems approach.

Computers frequently provide objective data when located in technologically advanced areas, such as critical care units. Automated readings of vital signs and abnormal heart rhythms are frequently used by critical care nurses to provide both initial and subsequent data. "Computerized monitoring systems can detect arrhythmias, generate alarms for vital signs ranging out of safe

```
                    CliniCom Medical Center - QA          06/12/90 10:39

              PATIENT ADMISSION ASSESSMENT REPORT (pat_adasm)
                     From 06/12/90 00:00  To 06/12/90 10:38
              ------------------------------------------------
```

Admission Assessment

Neurological (normal parameters)
 06/12 10:30 Alert & oriented to person, place and time. Verbalization clear and understandable
             (exclude speech impediments). Able to follow and understand directions. Pupils
             equal & reactive to light. Equal strength and voluntary movement in all
             extremities.. (AMJ)
Respiratory (normal parameters)
 06/12 10:30 Respirations quiet and regular, rate within patient's norm. (AMJ)
       10:30 Respirations appear effortless. Nasal passages appear clear. (AMJ)
Respiratory (OUTSIDE normal parameters)
 06/12 10:30 Breath sounds (by auscultation): scattered fine crackles bilateral base(s). (AMJ)
       10:30 Cough description: intermittent and harsh. Cough can be precipitated by:
             exertion. (AMJ)
       10:30 Description of Sputum: small amount, cloudy and thick. (AMJ)
Cardiovascular (normal parameters)
 06/12 10:30 Regular apical pulse within patient's normal rate. Absence of edema. Neck veins
             flat at 45 degrees. Absence of pain/discomfort in chest, neck, jaw, left arm. Cap
             refill < 3 sec. Peripheral pulses palpable and equal. No calf tenderness. (AMJ)
Gastrointestinal (normal parameters)
 06/12 10:30 Abdomen soft and non-distended. Bowel sounds high-pitched, gurgling and
             active.(5-34/min.) No abdominal pain reported with or without palpation. Tolerates
             prescribed diet without nausea or vomiting. Having BMs within own normal pattern
             and consistency. Stools are normal coloration. Well-nourished appearance. (AMJ)
Renal/Urinary (normal parameters)
 06/12 10:30 Empties bladder without dysuria. Bladder not distended after voiding. Urine clear,
             yellow to amber in color, normal urine odor. Able to void in last 8 hours. Volume
             voided is normal for patient. Frequency of voiding is normal for patient. (AMJ)
Renal/Urinary (OUTSIDE normal parameters)
 06/12 10:30 Patient's control - stress incontinence (cough/sneeze/activity). (AMJ)
Skin/Lymphatic (normal parameters)
 06/12 10:30 Skin color within patient's norm. Skin is warm, dry, smooth, soft, and flexible.
             Good tissue turgor present, no edema noted. Mucous membranes moist. Skin integrity
             is intact. (AMJ)
Musculoskeletal (normal parameters)
 06/12 10:30 Absence of joint swelling, erythema and tenderness. Active and passive ROM of all
             joints is normal. Absence of muscle weakness or atrophy. Normal muscle tone. All
             movement is pain free. Able to participate in normal activity without fatigue.
             (AMJ)
Reproductive/Male (normal parameters)
 06/12 10:30 Genitals are not swollen. Absence of pain with or without palpation. Absence of
             purulent urethral discharge. Absence of erythema or rash. (AMJ)

Psychological/Social (normal parameters)
 06/12 10:30 Mood and affect are expressed appropriately for situation. Thoughts are clear,
             reality-based, and progress logically. Interpretation of reality is appropriate.
             Support system present and adequate to meet patient's needs. Has not recently
             attempted suicide or verbalized a plan for suicide. Absence of recent problems
             with or treatment for drug/alcohol use. (AMJ)
Care Providers:
JONES, ANNE (AMJ) NRN

    0500-A   Name: SMITH, CHARLEY B. MD: SILVER,JOHN
    Sex: M Age: 41Y Adm: 05/21/90 21:18 Patient Id: 456456456 Med Rec No: 654654654
```

```
     SMITH, CHARLEY B.  PATIENT ADMISSION ASSESSMENT REPORT (pat_adasm) -
```

FIGURE 2-10. Documentation of computerized assessment.

(Courtesy of Clinicom Inc., Boulder, CO.)
```

bound, store records of unusual events, provide graphic representation of vital sign trends, and correlate vital signs to reveal unsuspected relationships.

Documentation

Nurses may also use computers to document the data obtained in the interview or examination. The nurse enters the data either at the bedside or in a central location. When a significant health problem is identified, the computer assists the nurse to document it accurately and completely. For example, if the nurse enters data indicating a reddened area on the client's skin, the computer will prompt for information such as location, size, and drainage. Figure 2-10 demonstrates a sample of a computerized documentation of a nursing assessment.

The principal advantages of computerized data collection are thoroughness and ease of recording data. The step-by-step design of the assessment process ensures that no significant areas are overlooked. Use of the computer reduces the amount of clinical time required to enter information using the traditional pen-and-paper format, thus improving efficiency.

The primary disadvantages of computerized client records include the expense, the time required to develop or adapt program components, and the training required prior to use. Additionally, some object to the restrictions imposed by standardized screens, formats, and limited vocabulary.

SUMMARY

The assessment phase of the nursing process consists of the accumulation and documentation of information about a client. Data collection involves interviewing, observation, and physical examination and concludes with documentation of the information obtained in the client's medical record. Assessment involves interaction between the nurse and the client and requires a broad knowledge base as well as specific interpersonal, technical, and critical-thinking skills. Assessment is a continuous activity that begins at the time of admission and continues during each client contact. It forms the foundation for subsequent phases of the nursing process: diagnosis, planning, implementation, and evaluation.

REFERENCES

American Nurses' Association: Nursing: A Social Policy Statement. Kansas City, MO: American Nurses' Association, 1980.

American Nurses' Association: Standards of Clinical Nursing Practice, Washington, DC: American Nurses' Association, 1991.

Andreoli K and Musser L: Computers in nursing care: The state of the art. Nurs Outlook 1985; 33(1):16–25.

Kalish R: The Psychology of Human Behavior, 5th ed. Monterey, CA: Brooks/Cole, 1983.

Maslow A: A theory of human motivation. Psychol Rev 1943; *50*:370.

BIBLIOGRAPHY

Barry C and Gibbons L: Information systems technology: Barriers and challenges to implementation. J Nurs Admin 1990; *20*(2):40–42.

Bates B: A Guide to Physical Examination, 4th ed. Philadelphia: JB Lippincott, 1987.

Benner P: From Novice to Expert: Excellence and Power in Clinical Nursing Practice. Menlo Park, CA: 1984.

Brown M: How do you spell assessment? A simple mnemonic device to organize your work. Am J Nurs 1991; *91*(9):55–56.

Carnevali D: Nursing Care Planning, 3rd ed. Philadelphia: JB Lippincott, 1983.

Carpenito LJ: Nursing Diagnosis—Application to Clinical Practice, 3rd ed. Philadelphia: JB Lippincott, 1989.

Eggland ET: Documentation do's and dont's. Nursing 1993; *23*(8):30.

Fiesta J: The Law and Liability—A Guide for Nurses, 2nd ed. New York: John Wiley & Sons, 1988.

Gehring PE: Physical assessment begins with a history. RN 1991; *54*(11):26–32.

Gordon M: Nursing Diagnosis: Process and Application, 2nd ed. New York: McGraw-Hill, 1987.

Guzzetta CE, Bunton S, Prinkey L, et al: Unitary person assessment tool: Easing problems with nursing diagnoses. Foc Crit Care 1988; *15*(2):12–24.

Hartman D and Knudson J: Documentation: A nursing data base for initial patient assessment. Oncol Nurs Forum 1991; *18*(1):125–130.

Hildeman TB and Ferguson GH: Registered nurses' attitudes toward the nursing process and written/printed nursing care plans. Nurs Admin 1992; *22*(5):5.

Holmes SB et al: Development of an automated documentation system. Orthop Nurs 1992; *11*(1):55–70.

Iyer P and Camp N: Nursing Documentation: A Nursing Process Approach, 2nd ed. St Louis: Mosby Year Book, 1995.

Rundio A and Cericola D: The role of the assessment nurse: One hospital's vision for meeting Joint Commission Standards: Health Care Superv 1992; *10*(4):12–19.

Stearns L: Nursing diagnosis: An assessment form. Nurs Manage 1988; *19*(4):101–102.

Yura H and Walsh MB: The Nursing Process, 5th ed. New York: Appleton Century Crofts, 1988.

THREE

THE DIAGNOSTIC PROCESS

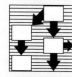

OBJECTIVES

After reading this chapter, you will be able to:

1. Define nursing diagnosis and discuss its historical evolution.
2. Name four steps in the diagnostic process.
3. Identify three errors that may be made in the diagnostic process.
4. Describe the role of critical thinking in the diagnostic process.
5. Describe the role of computers in the diagnostic process.

INTRODUCTION

The diagnostic process, the second phase of the nursing process, is a complex intellectual function. There are four steps in this phase: data processing, formulation of the nursing diagnostic statement, validation, and documentation. The outcome of the diagnostic process, the nursing diagnosis, forms the foundation for the remaining phases of the nursing process: planning, implementation, and evaluation. This chapter will explore the concept and evolution of nursing diagnosis as well as the data processing component of the diagnostic process. Chapter 4 will describe how to write, validate, and document a nursing diagnosis.

NURSING DIAGNOSIS

Before attempting to describe the diagnostic process, it may be helpful to describe its evolution and to define the concept of nursing diagnosis.

Historical Evolution of the Diagnostic Process

Chapter 1 described the historical evolution of the nursing process; the diagnostic process had a similar evolution. The term *nursing diagnosis* was first used in the 1950s. In 1960, Faye Abdellah introduced a classification system for identifying 21 client clinical problems. This system was used in the curriculum of nursing schools in the 1960s to assist students to diagnose client responses to health and illness requiring nursing intervention.

In the 1970s, several nursing leaders recognized the need to develop terminology to describe the health problems diagnosed and treated by nurses. In 1973, the First National Conference on the Classification of Nursing Diagnoses was held at the St. Louis University School of Nursing. The group began to formulate nursing diagnoses and published a tentative list. Since then, the group has continued to work to develop and refine nursing diagnoses.

The American Nurses' Association (ANA) endorsed and legitimated the use of the term *nursing diagnosis* and the diagnostic process in 1973 in the published *Standards of Nursing Practice* (ANA, 1973). Standard II stated "Nursing diagnoses are derived from the data of the health status of the client." Subsequently, several states began incorporating the concept into their nurse practice acts. This provided nurses with a legal right and professional obligation to use the diagnostic process to determine appropriate nursing diagnoses. At this time, a nursing diagnosis was viewed as an outcome or label that resulted from the diagnostic process. The development of the nursing diagnosis through the initiation of the diagnostic process became the second step of the five-phase nursing process.

Throughout the 1970s and into the 1980s, nursing research and literature explained the concept of nursing diagnosis and supported the diagnostic process as a phase of the nursing process. The 1980s also saw the addition of new diagnoses (including the first that were wellness oriented), refinement of existing diagnoses, and continued efforts to validate diagnoses through nursing research. The North American Nursing Diagnosis Association (NANDA) agreed on a method of organizing the diagnoses and the ANA adopted the NANDA diagnoses as the official system of nursing diagnosis. The National League for Nursing (NLN), in its approval criteria for schools of nursing, also required that the concept of nursing diagnosis be incorporated into the curriculum as a component of the nursing process. The ability of graduate nurses to use the diagnostic process was also evaluated in the NCLEX examination for licensure of registered nurses.

The expectations for nursing diagnosis in the 1990s include refinement of existing diagnoses, development of additional diagnoses (including expansion of those related to well clients), and continued research and validation. Nursing diagnoses may also be one of the essential components of financial systems designed for direct reimbursement for nursing services.

Definitions of Nursing Diagnosis

A *diagnosis* is essentially a statement that identifies the existence of an undesirable state. This definition applies whether the diagnostician is a health care worker, lawyer, electrician, or mechanic. The subject matter of the diagnosis is derived from those areas in which the diagnostician possesses a level of expertise. Lawyers write diagnoses pertaining to elements of law, physicians diagnose disease states, and electricians identify electrical system malfunctions.

Nurses, by virtue of their nurse practice acts, are responsible for diagnosing and treating human responses to actual and potential health problems (ANA, 1980). Nursing expertise that is developed as a result of education and experience identifies those nursing functions which can be ordered independently without collaboration with physicians or other health care professionals. These functions may include (1) *preventive* approaches, such as education, changes in position, and detection of potential complications, or (2) *corrective* approaches, such as forcing fluids, skin care, and counseling. This focus on independent nursing actions not only avoids duplication and overlap with other disciplines but also continues to define and validate the elements of nursing practice.

NANDA has identified three types of nursing diagnoses: actual, high-risk, and wellness. They are defined as follows:

Nurses are responsible for diagnosing and treating human responses to actual and potential health problems.

Actual

An actual nursing diagnosis is a clinical judgment about an individual, family, or community response to actual or potential health problems or life processes.

An actual nursing diagnosis is a clinical judgment about an individual, family or community response to actual or potential health problems/life processes.

Examples

- ☐ Hopelessness
- ☐ Parental role conflict
- ☐ Fatigue

High Risk

A high-risk nursing diagnosis is a clinical judgment that an individual, family, or community is more vulnerable to develop a problem than others in the same or a similar situation. High-risk diagnoses include risk factors (behaviors, conditions, or circumstances) that guide nursing interventions to reduce or prevent the occurrence of the problem.

A high-risk nursing diagnosis is a clinical judgment that an individual, family, or community is more vulnerable to develop a problem than others in the same or a similar situation.

Examples

- ☐ High risk for infection
- ☐ High risk for peripheral neurovascular dysfunction
- ☐ High risk for caregiver role strain

A wellness nursing diagnosis is a clinical judgment about an individual, family, or community in transition from a specific level of wellness to a higher level of wellness.

Wellness

A wellness nursing diagnosis is a clinical judgment about an individual, family, or community in transition from a specific level of wellness to a higher level of wellness.

Examples

☐ Health-seeking behaviors

☐ Effective breast-feeding

☐ Altered family coping: potential for growth

The remaining information in this chapter will describe the diagnostic process by which the nurse determines correct nursing diagnoses for individual clients.

ANA Standard II. Diagnosis (Standard of Care). The nurse analyzes assessment data in determining diagnoses.

STEPS IN THE DIAGNOSTIC PROCESS

As mentioned earlier, there are four steps involved in the diagnostic phase: data processing, formulation of the nursing diagnosis, validation, and documentation. The remaining information in this chapter will describe the diagnostic process by which you determine the correct human response demonstrated by your client. Chapter 4 describes guidelines for writing nursing diagnoses as well as validation and documentation.

Data Processing

The information collected by the nurse about a client is vital to the development of the appropriate nursing diagnosis and subsequent nursing care planning, implementation, and evaluation. Before planning can occur, collected data must be processed: classified, interpreted, and validated. Although data processing will be examined as the first step of the diagnostic phase, it is not so specifically isolated. These types of activities occur continuously throughout the nursing process.

Classification

While assessing a client, the nurse accumulates a large volume of data. The nurse may find it extremely difficult to manage this volume in total. The classification process begins following the nursing assessment and allows the nurse to develop more manageable categories of information. It also stimulates discrimination between data, which helps the nurse to focus on data that are pertinent to the client's needs.

Classification involves sorting information into specific categories. Examples include body systems, functional health patterns, historical data, and significant symptoms. The classification process that begins during data collection is facilitated by forms that are organized into specific categories.

DATA	CLASSIFICATION
Appendectomy three years ago	Past medical history
Sleeps during day	Sleep/rest pattern
Full range of motion	Motor ability
Colostomy	Gastrointestinal system
Mother died of cancer	Family history
Chest pain	Significant symptom
Laxatives every other day	Bowel elimination pattern
Church elder	Spiritual history
Vomiting for three days	History of present illness
Sacral redness	Integumentary system

Placing data into categories also helps the nurse to complete the diagnostic process by identifying missing components that may require further data collection.

Example.   Joan Bennett is a 35-year-old woman who visits the Women's Health Care Center. During the interview she indicates that her mother died of cancer of the breast (family history) and that she had a breast biopsy two years ago (past medical history).

Classification of this information reveals a missing component: current status of breast disease. Therefore, the nurse might (1) question the client regarding the outcome of the biopsy and frequency of breast self-examination, (2) pay particular attention to palpation for breast masses during subsequent physical examination, and (3) assess the client's emotional response to this particular health problem.

Interpretation

The second step in data processing is interpretation, which involves identification of significant data, comparison with standards or norms, and recognition of patterns or trends. Cues and inferences developed from the scientific nursing knowledge base assist the nurse to interpret the data. A *cue* is a piece of information about an individual client obtained during the assessment process. It is the nurse's perception of what exists based on subjective and objective data obtained from the client and other secondary sources. Cues may include *signs*, which are objective data such as blood pressure and weight; or *symptoms*, which are subjective data such as pain and sadness.

Examples of Cues

☐ Temperature 102° F

☐ Grimacing

INTRODUCTION
NURSING
DIAGNOSIS
STEPS IN THE
DIAGNOSTIC
PROCESS
Data Processing
Classification
Interpretation

A cue is a piece of information about an individual client.

3-1   TEST YOURSELF

Classification of Data Human Response Patterns

Review the following case study on Ted Alexander. Take the *italicized* data and classify it according to the Human Response Pattern Framework presented in Chapter 2. Note that some data may fall into more than one category and some categories may not have data.

Mr. Ted Alexander, a *50-year-old white divorced salesman* from Las Vegas, was on a business trip to Atlantic City when he developed *pain in the left upper abdominal quadrant*. He took Alka-Seltzer with little relief, and the pain persisted for the next two days. He was busy with appointments during the day and evening and was able to ignore the pain. He ate very little and took *two sleeping pills* at night. On the afternoon of the third day, the pain became much more intense, and when it continued for several hours and he began to *vomit body fluid*, he went to the emergency department.

Physical examination and laboratory data at this time revealed an *alert, well-groomed* male with *generalized abdominal tenderness*, rigidity of the abdominal wall, *absent bowel sounds*, and a *hemoglobin level (Hgb) of 11.6* (normal = 16 ± −2) with a *hematocrit (Hct) of 38* (normal = 47 ± −5). The diagnosis of *bleeding gastric ulcer* was made. He was admitted to the hospital for initial medical management, with surgery anticipated at a later date.

Your examination of the patient reveals the following: *B/P 104/60, P 120, R 26, T 98.2*. The patient indicates that he is *6, 2 tall* and *weighs 196 lb*. He is *alert* and *oriented* and states, *"I've never had this bleeding before—it's serious isn't it?"* His skin is *cool to the touch and slightly diaphoretic*. The patient states that he has been a *heavy drinker for the past 15 years* and was admitted to the hospital with *cirrhosis two years ago* by his family doctor, Dr. Martland, but has never had surgery. He *denies drinking for the past two years* but *smokes two packs of cigarettes daily*.

Mr. Alexander is *tense* throughout your conversation but shares a number of concerns with you, including his *separation from his two teenage children* who *live with him*. He is also *anxious about being cared for by an unfamiliar physician*. The ED nurse indicates that he *wears contact lenses* and is concerned because he has left his case and supplies as well as his *glasses* in his hotel. He gives you $750.00 in cash and traveler's checks to deposit in the hospital safe. He has a *partial lower plate* of dentures and *caps* on his four front teeth. Further inquiry reveals that the patient prefers a *low-fat diet*, *occasionally uses laxatives*, and has had several occurrences of *urinary urgency and nocturia* in the last six months.

Continued.

3-1 TEST YOURSELF
Classification of Data Human Response Patterns—cont'd.

The physician states that his treatment plan includes gastric suction, antiulcer medications, and replacement therapy with IV fluid, blood, electrolytes, and vitamins until the patient is stabilized enough for exploratory surgery. Mr. Alexander *agrees to this plan* but is *concerned about his job demands* and wonders how he will deal with "getting back home after this is all over."

HUMAN RESPONSE PATTERN	DATA
EXCHANGING:	
COMMUNICATING:	
RELATING:	
VALUING:	
CHOOSING:	
MOVING:	
PERCEIVING:	
KNOWING:	
FEELING:	

☐ 6 ft, 375 lb

☐ White blood count 24,000 (normal 5000 to 9000)

Inferencing is the assignment of meaning to a cue. An *inference* is a judgment made by the nurse on the basis of education and experience. In the

An inference is a judgment made by the nurse about the meaning of a cue on the basis of education and experience.

3-1   **TEST YOURSELF**

Classification of Data Human Response Patterns: Answers

EXCHANGING:	Vomit body fluid, absent bowel sounds, alert, cool and diaphoretic Hgb 11.6, Hct 38, 6 ft 2 in., 196 lb, B/P 104/60, P 120, R 26, T 98.2, low-fat diet, urinary urgency and nocturia partial lower plate, caps
COMMUNICATING:	
RELATING:	50-year-old divorced salesman, separation from two children who live with him, concerned about job demands
VALUING:	
CHOOSING:	Denies drinking for past two years
MOVING:	Takes sleeping pills
PERCEIVING:	Contact lenses/glasses, well-groomed
KNOWING:	Bleeding gastric ulcer, "I've never had this bleeding before— it's serious isn't it?", smokes two packs cigarettes, heavy drinker for 15 years, no drinking for two years, diagnosis of cirrhosis two years ago, occasional laxatives, alert and oriented, agrees to plan of care
FEELING:	Pain left upper quadrant/abdominal tenderness, tense, anxious regarding unfamiliar physician

examples identified above, the nurse might make the following inferences based on the cues identified during the assessment of a client.

CUES	INFERENCE
Temperature 102° F	Elevated temperature
Grimacing	Possible pain, anxiety
6 ft, 375 lb	Obesity
White blood count 24,000	Probable infection

Clusters are groups of cues. The potential for making accurate judgments is increased when the nurse bases an inference on a cluster of cues rather than on a single cue. *Defining characteristics* are clusters of cues that are manifestations of particular nursing diagnoses. In the case of the client with a temperature elevation, note that two different inferences could be made based on the other cues identified during the assessment of a client.

Clusters are groups of cues.

Defining characteristics are clusters of cues that are manifestations of particular nursing diagnoses.

CLUSTER 1	INFERENCE
Temperature 102° F White blood count 24,000 Reddened incision Purulent drainage	Incision is infected

CLUSTER 2	INFERENCE
Temperature 102° F Decreased skin turgor Dry tongue Urine output 200 ml in 8 hours	Client is dehydrated

Theory, knowledge, experience, and data collected about the client are necessary to make correct inferences. Some inferences are very clearly based on clinical knowledge. For example, the presence of frequent loose stools, abdominal pain and cramping, and anal irritation suggest a bowel disorder, specifically diarrhea.

Other data may provide fewer concrete cues and clusters and require more interpretation. For example, the client with clenched fists and rigid body posture who is crying may be angry, frightened, or experiencing pain. Here, you may (1) make a preliminary interpretation and validate it with the client, or (2) continue to gather additional cues that may help to clarify the inferences based on the identified cues.

The interpretation of data based on cues and clusters is a complex process. Initially, the beginning practitioner may experience difficulty in identifying cues or correctly clustering related cues. However, as your nursing knowledge, skill, and expertise increase, accurate clinical judgments are made more consistently.

Example.   Joan Granberry works on a 24-bed critical care unit. She knows that anxiety is a common phenomenon in the client who has been admitted for a myocardial infarction (heart attack). Bob Agocs, a 48-year-old client, denies that he is experiencing anxiety. However, Joan observes that he is restless and diaphoretic, and that his pulse rate and blood pressure are elevated. Based on this cluster of cues, she concludes that Bob may be anxious and continues to gather additional data to support this judgment.

As you become more experienced in using the diagnostic process, the ability to anticipate, identify, and interpret specific client responses increases. For example, the experienced postpartum nurse recognizes that most first-time nursing mothers have questions about their ability to breast feed. On the basis of this knowledge, the nurse assesses for further cues that this response might be present.

Validation

The final step in data processing is validation. In this phase, the nurse attempts to verify the accuracy of the data interpretation. This is most often accomplished through direct interaction with the client or significant other(s), consultation with other health care professionals, or comparison of data with an authoritative reference.

Validation with the Client or Significant Others. Ideally, the nurse should validate findings with the client. This is generally accomplished through the use of reflective statements.

Example. Barbara Sabotka is a 30-year-old client admitted for a planned cesarean section. During the assessment interview, you notice that Barbara is easily distracted, paces intermittently while wringing her hands, and speaks very rapidly. These cues could lead you to infer that this client is nervous about the scheduled surgery.

Nurse: You seem anxious, Mrs. Sabotka.

Client: Yes, I am upset.

Nurse: Upset?

Client: I'm really worried about my 4-year-old. He had a high fever and bad cough so my husband took him to the doctor. He hasn't called me yet to tell me what the doctor found. I'm so afraid he has pneumonia.

In this situation, you validated the presence of fear in the client. The use of a reflective statement made you realize that your initial interpretation of the source of the client's fear was inaccurate. You were then able to identify that Mrs. Sabotka's concern was focused on her child.

There are times when you may find that it is not possible to validate interpretations with the client directly.

Example. The nurse admitting a comatose client, Danz Blasser, notices a small healed scar approximately 2½ in. long just below his left clavicle. There is also a small bulge under the patient's skin. Based on knowledge and past experience, the nurse interprets these findings to indicate the presence of a permanent cardiac pacemaker.

3-2 **TEST YOURSELF**
Identification of Inferences

Column 1 contains clues/clusters extracted from the Ted Alexander case study. Identify possible inferences in column 2.

CLUES/CLUSTERS	INFERENCES
1. Vomiting bloody fluid	1.
2. Hgb 11.6, Hct 3 (normal Hgb 16 ± 2, Hct 47 ± 5)	2.
3. B/P 104/60, P 120, R 26	3.
4. Cool, diaphoretic skin	4.
5. Tense tone: "it's serious, isn't it?"	5.
6. Concerned about unfamiliar physician, separated from children	6.
7. Generalized abdominal tenderness. Reports pain in abdomen	7.
8. Smokes two packs cigarettes daily	8.
9. Urinary urgency and nocturia	9.
10. Takes sleeping pills	10.
11. Contact lenses and glasses in hotel room	11.
12. Uses laxatives	12.
13. 196 lb; 6 ft, 2 in	13.
14. Heavy drinker for 15 years, no drinking for two years	14.
15. Well-groomed	15.

3-2 TEST YOURSELF

Identification of Inferences: Answers

COLUMN 1	COLUMN 2
1. Vomiting bloody fluid	1. Bleeding from some site
2. Hgb 11.6, Hct 3 (normal Hgb 16 ± 2, Hct 47 ± 5)	2. Low hemoglobin level and hematocrit
3. B/P 104/60, P 120, R 26	3. Low blood pressure, elevated pulse and respiration rates
4. Cool, diaphoretic skin	4. Abnormal skin temperature and moisture
5. Tense tone: "it's serious, isn't it?"	5. Fear
6. Concerned about unfamiliar physician, separated from children	6. Separated from support system
7. Generalized abdominal tenderness. Reports pain in abdomen	7. Acute pain
8. Smokes two packs cigarettes daily	8. Addicted to cigarettes
9. Urinary urgency and nocturia	9. Abnormal urinary patterns
10. Takes sleeping pills	10. Difficulty with sleep rest patterns
11. Contact lenses and glasses in hotel room	11. Abnormal vision without corrective lenses
12. Uses laxatives	12. Irregular bowel patterns
13. 196 lb; 6 ft, 2 in	13. Normal weight for height
14. Heavy drinker for 15 years, no drinking for two years	14. Unhealthful coping mechanism in the past
15. Well-groomed	15. Normal self-esteem

In this situation, the client is unable to confirm the nurse's judgment. Therefore, Mr. Blasser's daughter might be interviewed for confirmation.

Nurse: I noticed that your father has a small scar on his chest.

Daughter: Yes, he had a pacemaker put in six months ago after his heart attack. He has been checked every month, and it's been working fine.

Mr. Blasser's daughter has validated the presence of the pacemaker and in that process has provided additional important information about the client's past medical history as well as his compliance with suggested pacemaker follow-up.

Validation with Other Professionals. Another method of validation is collaboration with other health care professionals. In the case of Danz Blasser described previously, the presence of a cardiac pacemaker was validated through discussion with the client's daughter. In her absence, however, the nurse might have contacted the attending physician, inquired about old charts in the medical records department, or consulted with nurses in the coronary care unit.

Example. Nancy Abdels is a 48-year-old client with a diagnosis of cancer of the colon. She is four days postoperative after bowel surgery. Based on your observations of the client, you identify cues indicating that the client is denying her diagnosis. Subsequent discussion with the stomal therapist and the physician validates your interpretation.

Validation with Reference Sources. The nurse may also use reference sources to substantiate interpretations.

Example. Kathy Prihoda, a nurse in the clinic, is examining Jenny, an 8-month-old. She notices that the child does not turn over independently, sit unaided, or hold her bottle.

In this situation, the nurse might use a pediatric reference source to verify initial perceptions that Jenny is not at an appropriate developmental level for her age. Reference sources might include texts, journals, or developmental charts.

Validation is an important component of the diagnostic process. The approaches previously described facilitate verification of the accuracy and completeness of your interpretations. Validation assists you to recognize errors, isolate discrepancies, and identify the need for additional data. This phase in the processing of data forms the link between assessment and formulation of nursing diagnoses.

ERRORS IN THE DIAGNOSTIC PROCESS

Up to this point, the text has presented information on data collection, classification, interpretation, and validation. These are the components necessary for the diagnostic process to be completed accurately. The nurse gathers data, identifies cues, makes inferences about the health status of the client, and validates these judgments with the client. The outcome of this process is a nursing diagnosis. If any of these steps are carried out incorrectly or incompletely, the label may be inaccurate.

There are three major sources of errors in the diagnostic process. They are

(1) inaccurate or incomplete data collection, (2) inaccurate interpretation of data, and (3) lack of clinical knowledge.

Inaccurate or Incomplete Data

The ability to formulate a nursing diagnosis is dependent on an accurate and complete data base. Several factors may interfere with the collection of data. These may include communication problems, withholding information, and distractions or interruptions.

Communication Problems

There are a variety of communication problems that may result in inaccurate or incomplete data collection.

Language Barrier. Either the client or the nurse may have a language barrier that interferes with the collection of data.

Example.   When Juan Rivera came to the emergency department, the nurse noted that he was obviously anxious, diaphoretic, grimacing, and holding his abdomen. When the nurse, Jeff Halter, began to question Juan, he determined that the client did not speak English.

Jeff recognized that additional information was necessary to accurately determine the client's problem. If available, family members who understand English or staff who speak the client's language might be utilized to collect additional pertinent data.

Slang or Jargon. Even when the nurse and client speak the same language, either may use language that confuses the other. The client's age, environment, or cultural background may involve the use of expressions that are foreign to the nurse.

Example

Nurse: Mr. Blass, have you had prostate problems in the past?

Client: No, I haven't, but my "night work" hasn't been too good lately.

Further questioning revealed that Mr. Blass was describing a recent history of sexual dysfunction.

The nurse may also use technical jargon or terminology that is foreign to the client.

Example

Nurse: Mrs. Connor, have you ever had an IVP?

Client: An IV what?

Biased Questions. This type of question, as described in Chapter 2, tends to intimidate clients and may result in inaccurate or incomplete data.

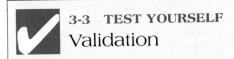

3-3   TEST YOURSELF

Validation

Identify methods that you might use to validate inferences related to Ted Alexander in column 1 (refer to previous exercise)

COLUMN 1	COLUMN 2
1. Low hemoglobin level and hematocrit	1.
2. Low blood pressure	2.
3. Abnormal vision/perceptual problem	3.
4. Irregular bowel habits	4.
5. Difficulty with sleep/wake patterns	5.
6. Normal weight	6.
7. Fear	7.

3-3 TEST YOURSELF
Validation: Answers

COLUMN 1	COLUMN 2
1. Low hemoglobin level and hematocrit	1. Standard lab normals for hemoglobin level and hematocrit
2. Low blood pressure	2. Ask Ted what is normal for him
3. Abnormal vision/perceptual problem	3. Ask Ted how badly his vision is impaired
4. Irregular bowel habits	4. Collaborate with social worker
5. Difficulty with sleep/wake patterns	5. Ask Ted about his normal sleep pattern
6. Normal weight	6. Consult a height/weight chart

Clients may give the response they believe is expected or choose not to respond at all.

Examples

☐ "You're not frightened, are you?"

☐ "Does being obese interfere with your work?"

Withholding Information.   Clients may not share information for a number of reasons. They may be anxious, embarrassed, suspicious, or unaware of the importance of the information.

Example.   Cathy Whitsell is admitted to an ambulatory surgery center for an elective breast biopsy. You ask the client if she has any allergies. Assuming that you mean allergies to medications, Cathy says, "No."

In reality, the client has a shellfish allergy that could predispose her to reactions if iodine-based skin preparations are used to cleanse her skin before surgery.

Distractions.   There are a number of distractions that may interfere with the concentration required to collect data. These may include interruptions, a noisy nonprivate environment, or thoughts that are preoccupying the nurse or client.

The nurse who is harried may not listen carefully to the information provided.

Example.   When Steven Samuel was admitted with emphysema, he said he had no family. The nurse, who was rushed, did not pursue this by asking if he had friends who would be visiting him. When Mr. Samuel became progressively more depressed as his hospitalization continued, the nurses assumed that his depression was related to his chronic illness. However, when encouraged to talk about his feelings, Steven revealed that he was upset because no one had visited him. The nurses then realized that his loneliness was the source of his withdrawal. The nurse who admitted the client might have anticipated this problem if inquiries had been made about his support systems.

Frequently, interruptions may also interfere with complete data collection.

Example.   Pat Murphy is interviewing Sam Madeira, a newly admitted client on a medical unit. During the course of the interview, the telephone rings four times with calls from Mr. Madeira's office. When Pat attempts to document her assessment, she realizes that she has not completed a portion of the interview. Perhaps this could have been avoided had she asked the operator to hold the client's calls.

At times, the client's preoccupation with other topics may lead to an incomplete data base.

Example

Client: Oh yes, I've had high blood pressure for years. I stopped watching my diet because it's too much trouble. I don't cook much since I live alone. I used to live with my sister, but she moved to Florida. She just loves it there.

Nurse: Where is she living in Florida?

Client: She lives in Orlando. The city is growing so fast because of the climate and the attractions. Now, that's a wonderful place. Have you ever been there?

Nurse: Yes.

Client: What I like best about it is the weather. I could spend months there. It's nicer than other places I've gone. Of course, I enjoy the Houston area too . . . .

In this situation, the nurse allowed the conversation to be directed away from the client's hypertension, which was the reason for her visit to the physician's office. Clearly, the client was preoccupied with other thoughts, but the nurse lost control of the interview process and did not investigate the client's nonadherence to the diet.

Inaccurate Interpretation of Data

Two different types of errors may lead to inaccurate interpretation of data: (1) using only one cue or observation to reach premature inferences, and (2) allowing personal prejudices or biases to influence the interpretation of data.

INTRODUCTION

NURSING DIAGNOSIS

STEPS IN THE DIAGNOSTIC PROCESS

ERRORS IN THE DIAGNOSTIC PROCESS

Inaccurate/Incomplete Data

Inaccurate Interpretation of Data

Premature Interpretation of Data

A common type of error is the development of a judgment before all the important information is collected or considered. Problems can occur when only one observation is used because clusters of information or patterns of behavior are more significant than single cues or episodes. This type of error occurs in the following situation:

Example.   Mrs. Rogers puts her call signal on at 3 AM and asks for something for cough. You notify the nurse in charge and indicate that you plan to call the physician to request an antitussive. The nurse suggests that you gather additional information about the client's lung sounds and heart rate. You find that the client has a rapid heart rate and her lungs are congested. To your dismay, you realize that the client's cough is related to fluid overload associated with heart failure.

Another type of error is jumping to inaccurate conclusions using the medical diagnosis as a cue. The nurse who expects a diabetic client to have specific responses because of the medical diagnosis may be unable to recognize the individuality of the client's needs.

Example.   Marge Chapman is a newly diagnosed insulin-dependent diabetic. You assume that because she was recently diagnosed as having diabetes, Mrs. Chapman requires instruction in insulin injection techniques. In reality, Mrs. Chapman is quite familiar with injection technique. Her mother and aunt require insulin injections, which Mrs. Chapman has administered for years.

In cases like Mrs. Chapman's, assumptions based on the client's medical diagnosis of diabetes might lead you to believe that she would require injection technique instruction. Therefore, diagnoses and interventions could be developed that have no bearing on the client's most pressing problem: adhering to the prescribed diet. To maintain a low rate of diagnostic error, you should take the time to validate interpretations of the client's responses.

Personal Prejudices

Personal prejudices and lack of awareness of cultural practices and beliefs can influence a nurse's interpretation of data. Sometimes the behavior of a client or family can become so annoying that the nurse is tempted to ignore important cues. Consider what could have happened in this situation:

Example.   Keith Fishbein was recovering well from gallbladder surgery. His family was very attentive but seemed overly concerned about his recovery. Although Mr. Fishbein himself never complained, his wife and two children had frequent requests that they expected to be accomplished immediately. One evening Mrs. Fishbein excitedly demanded that the nurse check her husband, who had pain in his left leg. The nurse thought, "What next?" as she went into the room fully expecting another false alarm. To her surprise, she was unable to find a pulse in Mr. Fishbein's leg. He was rushed to surgery for removal of a blood clot.

Lack of information regarding cultural diversity, customs, and norms of behavior may also influence your interpretation of data.

Example. You arrive on duty to find a group of 40 gypsies in the waiting room of your unit. Your inquiries of other staff reveals that one of the patients on the unit is the gypsy queen. Unaware of the custom that requires their presence, Susan requests that the group leave the unit. This is particularly distressing to the client.

In this case your lack of understanding of the client's cultural norms created undue stress for the client and her visitors. You must be aware of personal values and biases, recognize how these influence perceptions, and attempt to overcome prejudices. When presented with unfamiliar cultural practices or beliefs, you should seek out resources to assist in understanding the client's responses. This will enhance your ability to interpret cues correctly.

Lack of Clinical Knowledge or Experience

Lack of clinical knowledge or experience may affect the collection and interpretation of data. It can result in any of the following: (1) critical data not being collected, (2) incorrect clustering of cues, or (3) inaccurate interpretation of cues.

The inexperienced nurse may simply overlook important assessment data because of inadequate clinical knowledge. For example, an inexperienced nurse may fail to recognize that an elderly client with sacral edema is at risk for skin breakdown.

In other cases, the nurse may focus entirely on one aspect of care and ignore another set of cues.

Example. An 80-year-old woman who had been in the hospital for 10 days fell while getting out of bed at midnight to go to the bathroom. The woman had received flurazepam (Dalmane) about an hour before. Although the bedrails at her head were elevated, those by her legs were down. The manufacturer of Dalmane warns that dizziness, drowsiness, lightheadedness, staggering, ataxia, and falls have occurred with its use, particularly in elderly or debilitated persons (Cushing, 1985).

In this example, the nurse did not identify the client's potential for falling associated with the use of the drug. The nurse's lack of experience with the drug and subsequent failure to initiate adequate preventive measures contributed to the client's injury.

Example. As a new graduate, you are making rounds on your patients at the beginning of the night shift. When you approach Mr. Gray, the client tells you that a large man has been watching him from the hall for the last two hours. You look in the hall and detect only a housekeeping cart. Assuming that his condition was due to his age, the unfamiliar environment, or electrolyte imbalance, you review the client's chart and call the physician to report your findings. You did not observe the client's eyeglasses lying on the bedside cabinet. In reality, the client had very poor visual acuity without his glasses and thought that the cleaning cart, which had been left in the hall across from his room, was a human form.

The nurse who lacks adequate clinical knowledge or experience can compensate for these deficits by seeking information and guidance from more experienced nurses or other resources. Careful development of an organized approach for data classification and interpretation is also critical for accurate diagnosis.

CRITICAL THINKING AND THE DIAGNOSTIC PROCESS

The diagnostic process requires critical-thinking skills. You examine assessment data, classify and cluster significant cues, and interpret and validate them. The outcome of this process is the development of an accurately stated actual, high-risk, or wellness nursing diagnosis.

Example. In Chapter 2, Maria Roselli, a 30-year-old client, was admitted to your unit for scheduled lung surgery. During your assessment of the client, you identified the following data: Maria tells you that over the past three years her right lung has collapsed six times. She says that her doctor told her that these were the result of blebs (blisters) on the surface of her lung and that surgery is now necessary to avoid further incidence of collapse and permanent lung damage. She also indicates that she has been hospitalized for each of the six episodes, for the birth of her 2-year-old daughter, and for a concussion when she was 5 years old. She tells you that she smokes a pack of cigarettes a day because she tends to be nervous and smoking helps to deal with her stress. She also mentions that she has developed infections in three of her previous hospitalizations. She says she fears the surgery because of her low tolerance for pain, the possibility that they may find something other than blebs, and that she dreads having that big tube in her chest after the surgery. You observe that she is restless, avoids eye contact when talking about her smoking habits and her previous hospitalizations, and paces around the room periodically during your conversation. She says that she has not slept well for the past week worrying about the surgery and how her daughter will do while she is in the hospital.

Your physical examination reveals that Maria is 5 ft, 6 in. tall and weighs 110 lb. Her vital signs are T 98.4, B/P 142/70, P 108, R 32. You note that her respirations are shallow and that breath sounds are decreased over the right upper lobe. Her skin is cool to touch and moist over her hands and feet. You also observe that she coughs frequently throughout your examination, particularly when she takes a deep breath.

As you begin to classify the data, you ask yourself these questions:

1. Which data are relevant to Maria's care?
2. Which data go together?
3. What do Maria's behaviors mean?
4. Have I gathered enough data?

Classification of the data reveals the following:

CUE/CLUSTER	CATEGORY
Planned surgery.	Anticipated invasive procedure.
Six episodes of collapsed lung, child-birth, concussion, previous infections.	Past medical history.
Nervous. Not sleeping. Smokes one pack a day.	Client's statement of current health habits.
Verbalizations about postoperative pain, outcome of surgery and chest tube, daughter's well-being.	Client's statement of concerns.
Restlessness, pacing, avoids eye contact.	Client's behaviors.
Height 5 ft, 6 in. Weight 110 lb.	Body characteristics.
B/P 142/70, P 118.	Cardiovascular system.
Respirations shallow, breath sounds decreased, rate 32, cough.	Respiratory system.

As you begin to interpret the data, you ask yourself the following questions:

1. What data is related?
2. Do I need additional data?
3. What does the data mean?
4. What inferences are suggested by the data?

Further clustering of the data identifies the following inferences:

CLUSTER	INFERENCE
Respirations shallow, rate 32, decreased breath sounds, cough.	Abnormal breathing pattern for age.
History of previous infections, planned invasive procedure.	Client may be at risk for infection following surgery.
Restlessness, pacing, elevated blood pressure and pulse, verbalized concerns about pain, chest tube, and outcome.	Client is fearful and is able to identify sources of her fear.

Applying the critical-thinking model to this example, you ask yourself:

1. *What is the issue?*
   In this case, the issue is identification of inferences that form the basis for Maria's care.

2. *What information do I need and how can I obtain it?*
   You may need additional information regarding Maria's respiratory status, such as the results of her arterial blood gases drawn at the time of admission, and whether she is short of breath or uses accessory muscles to breathe. You may also want to determine whether the elevations of her blood pressure, pulse rate, and respirations are transient manifestations associated with hospitalization. These may also be indications of her fear or associated with other processes, such as infection or recurrent lung collapse. This information may be found in the medical record or through discussions with or observations of the client.

3. *Are the data valid?*
   The most effective method of validating your findings is to discuss them with the client. After you share your findings with Maria, she agrees that her breathing patterns are of concern and indicates that although they differ from her normal patterns, they are not the same as those she experienced in the past when her lung collapsed. She admits that the anticipation of pain, the insertion of a chest tube postoperatively, and the outcome of surgery are causing her to be fearful. She also agrees that based on her past history, postoperative infection is a potential complication. You may also wish to use a reference source to validate that the inferences you have made are consistent with cues you have identified.

4. *What do the data mean?*
   The data suggest that, while a number of responses may be present, the focus of Maria's care should be directed toward managing her fear, her altered breathing patterns, and her risk of infection.

3-4 TEST YOURSELF

Critical Thinking and the Diagnostic Process

Refer back to the case of Ted Alexander. You are attempting to interpret the data and have decided that the cues of vomiting, bloody fluid, and B/P 104/60, P 120, R 26 may be related. You make the initial inference that there is an abnormal loss of body fluid but decide you need further data.

Use the critical thinking format listed below in order to resolve this issue. The first question is answered for you.

1. What is the issue?

   In this case I need to collect more data related to his condition before making a definite inference of abnormal fluid volume.

2. What information do I need and how can I obtain it?

3. Are the data valid?

4. What do the data mean?

5. Based on the data, what should I do?

6. Is this the best way to deal with the issue?

5. *Based on the facts, what should I do?*
   In Maria's case you should gather the additional data suggested in question 2 above. Then, you should reclassify and reinterpret the data to determine that your findings remain valid with the new data. If so, your next step is the formulation of a nursing diagnosis that reflects Maria's situation and will guide the management of her care.

6. *Is this the best way to deal with the issue?*
   You have classified and interpreted the data gathered through the interview, observation, and physical examination during your assessment of Maria. You have also acquired additional data and validated your findings with the client. You have identified three inferences of concern in Maria's case. This is precisely the method identified in the diagnostic phase of the nursing process.

3-4 TEST YOURSELF
Critical Thinking and the Diagnostic Process: Answers

1. What is the issue?

In this case I must collect more data relating to his condition before making a definite inference of abnormal fluid volume.

2. What information do I need and how can I obtain it?

INFORMATION NEEDED	METHOD OF OBTAINING INFORMATION
A. How many times did he vomit?	**A.** Ask Ted
B. Can he approximate how much fluid he vomited?	**B.** Ask Ted
C. What do his BP and pulse normally run?	**C.** Ask Ted
D. How much urine output has he had? (When was the last time he urinated?)	**D.** Ask Ted
E. What does the urine look like? Is it concentrated?	**E.** May need to obtain a urine specimen
F. Are his lab values consistent with effects of fluid loss?	**F.** Look at chart/call lab for results
G. Are his mucous membranes dry?	**G.** Physical exam

3. Are the data valid?

Ted may be unable to tell you the volume of fluid he vomited. However, by finding out Ted's normal vital signs you will be able to judge if the low blood pressure and increased pulse and respiration rates are indications of loss of circulating fluid volume. The results of the lab work would also validate the presence of a fluid deficit.

4. What do the data mean?

Continued.

3-4   TEST YOURSELF

Critical Thinking and the Diagnostic Process: Answers—cont'd.

After examining the data I conclude that the data are consistent with an abnormal fluid volume loss.

5. Based on the data, what should I do?

The next step would be to formulate a nursing diagnostic statement.

6. Is this the best way to deal with the issue?

Yes. I have gathered the data, made an inference, and validated it.

COMPUTERS AND THE DIAGNOSTIC PROCESS

Computers are being used by nurses during the diagnostic process to organize and interpret data collected during assessment. Computer systems may be designed to assist in clinical diagnosis by processing assessment data. Most commonly, data are entered by the nurse at the nurses' station. However, in more sophisticated systems, data may be entered at the client's bedside using a terminal, mouse, keypad, or voice.

After the data are entered, the software compares the cues identified during the assessment process with the defining characteristics for each nursing diagnosis in its data base. A list of possible diagnoses is generated and the nurse is able to accept or reject each entry on the list or enter other appropriate diagnoses. Figure 3-1 demonstrates an example of a computer-assisted nursing diagnosis generated from a nursing assessment.

The chief advantages of computer-assisted nursing diagnosis center on the system's ability to identify patterns that might be overlooked by the nurse. These systems use consistent, organized processes to organize, analyze, and interpret data. The computer is not affected by distraction, fatigue, headaches, or any of the other human variables that impact on the processing of data.

However, the ability of any software to generate nursing diagnoses is only as good as the program on which it is based. Some nursing diagnoses lack large reliable data bases, which may make accurate diagnoses difficult. Additionally, clients can display an infinite variety of responses to health problems, making it difficult to anticipate all such responses. Nurses using programs that suggest certain diagnosis need to exercise professional judgment in evaluating the conclusions developed by the software.

```
DFALT-G981            NYUMC HOSP 4
05/28/85  11:55 AM              PAGE 001                  00000   000   00000
                                                         0    0  0   0  0    0
                                                         00000  0   0  00000
=== === === === === === === === ===                      0      0   0  0
DEMONSTRATION DAN-1        1336                          0        000  0
4342877 85464  04/02/40   44 M                           ===== ===== ===== =====
MARKS CLEMENT MD                                         DEMONSTRATION DAN-1
=== === === === === === === === === === === === === === === === === === ===


PRIMARY DIAGNOSIS:  GI BLEED...

NURSING DIAGNOSIS
 05/22   ACTUAL SKIN BREAKDOWN R/T....INCONTINENCE OF URINE/FECES      JBKA
EXPECTED OUTCOMES                                            R/P   R/D
 05/22   DECREASE IN SIZE OF DECUBITUS ULCER                  QD    5/30   JBKA
NURSING ORDERS
 05/22   TURN & POSITION Q2H                                               JBKA
 05/22   FOLLOW SCHEDULE--RT-BACK-LT                                       JBKA
 05/22   DO NOT ELEVATE HOB MORE THAN 30 DEG                              JBKA
 05/22   USE APPROPRIATE PRESSURE-RELIEVING DEVICE:
         WATER MATTRESS                                                   JBKA
 05/22   OOB IN STRETCHER CHAIR TID                                       JBKA
 05/22   PAD BEDPAN                                                       JBKA
 05/22   PASSIVE ROM TO ALL EXTREMITIES Q4H                               JBKA
 05/22   DIETARY CONSULT REGARDING ASSESSMENT OF
         NUTRITIONAL STATUS                                               JBKA
 05/22   CHECK FOR FECAL/URINARY INCONTINENCE
         Q1/2H. (NA TO CHECK Q1H ON THE 1/2H & RN TO
         CHECK Q1H ON THE HOUR)                                           JBKA
 05/22   CLEAN SKIN THOROUGHLY & PAT DRY POST VOID/BM                     JBKA
 05/22   METHOD OF TREATMENT: STAGE 3- STOMA ADHESIVE
         METHOD                                                           JBKA
 05/22   WEAR STERILE GLOVES WHEN IN CONTACT W/
         WOUND.
         CLEANSE AREA, USING A STERILE IRRIG TRAY W/
         1/2 STRENGTH PEROXIDE & NS.
         RINSE THOROUGHLY W/ NS & PAT DRY W/ STERILE
         GAUZE                                                            JBKA
 05/22   APPLY HEAT LAMP X15 MINS 12 INCHES FROM SKIN
         & AT THE SIDE OF BED SO THAT INADVERTENT PT
         MOVEMENT WILL NOT CAUSE LAMP TO CONTACT
         SKIN.
         PAT ANTACID OVER THE AFFECTED AREA USING
         STERILE GAUZE. ALLOW TO DRY THOROUGHLY                           JBKA
 05/22   APPLY MYCOSTATIN POWDER AS ORDERED BY MD.
         REMOVE EXCESS POWDER BY BRUSHING W/ STERILE
         GAUZE.
         APPLY A LIGHT COAT OF SKIN PREP. ALLOW AREA
         TO DRY THOROUGHLY                                                JBKA
 05/22   APPLY STOMA ADHESIVE TO COVER THE ENTIRE
         AREA EXTENDING 1 INCH BEYOND THE REDNESS ON
         ALL SIDES. ROUND THE CORNERS W/ A SCISSOR TO
         PREVENT WRINKLING.
         SECURE THE EDGES OF THE STOMA ADHESIVE W/ 1
         INCH PAPER TAPE                                                  JBKA
 05/22   LEAVE DSG IN PLACE 2-3 DAYS IF THE INTEGRITY
         OF THE DSG REMAINS INTACT                                        JBKA


=== === === === === === === === === === === === === === === === === === ===
DEMONSTRATION DAN-1                                         PATIENT CARE PLAN
```

FIGURE 3-1.   Computer Sample of Nursing Diagnosis.

(Courtesy of New York University Medical Center.)

SUMMARY

The diagnostic process is a critical phase of the nursing process. In this phase, which follows assessment, data are processed, classified, interpreted, and validated. The outcome of this diagnostic process is a nursing diagnosis. The steps of the diagnostic process can be affected by several types of errors, including inaccurate or incomplete data, inaccurate interpretation of data, or lack of knowledge or experience. Errors can result in nursing diagnoses that are not appropriate for the client.

Software is available for computer systems with the capability of classifying and interpreting assessment data. This chapter has explored the organization and interpretation of data accumulated during the assessment phase. Chapter 4 will address the formulation, validation, and documentation of the nursing diagnosis.

REFERENCES

Abdellah F, Martin A, Beland I, and Matheney R: Patient Centered Approaches to Nursing: New York: Macmillan, 1960.

American Nurses' Association: A Social Policy Statement. Kansas City, MO: American Nurses' Association, 1980.

American Nurses' Association: Standards of Nursing Practice. Kansas City, MO: American Nurses' Association, 1973.

Cushing M: First, anticipate the harm . . . . Am J Nurs 1985 Feb; 85(2):137–138.

BIBLIOGRAPHY

Allen CJ: Incorporating a wellness perspective for nursing diagnosis in practice. In Carroll-Johnson RM (ed): Classification of Nursing Diagnoses: Proceedings of the Eighth Conference. Philadelphia: JB Lippincott, 1989, pp 37–42.

Fredetta SL: Common diagnostic errors. Nurse Educ 1988; 13(3):31–35.

Harvey RM: Nursing diagnosis by computers: An application of neural networks. Nurs Diag 1993; 4(1):26–34.

Popkiss-Vawter S: Wellness nursing diagnoses: To be or not to be? Nurs Diag 1991; 2(1):19–25.

Snyder M: Critical thinking: A foundation for consumer-focused care. J Cont Educ Nurs 1993; 24(5):206–210.

Thomas NM and Newsome GG: Factors affecting the use of nursing diagnosis. Nurs Outlook 1992; 40(4):182–186.

Tribulski J: Nursing diagnosis: Waste of time or valued tool. RN 1988; 51(12):30–34.

Weber C: Making nursing diagnosis work for you and your client: A step-by-step approach. Nurs Health Care 1991; 12(8):424–430.

FOUR

Writing a Nursing Diagnosis

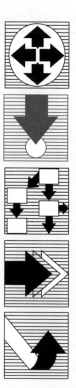

After completing this chapter, you will be able to:

1. Name two components of a nursing diagnosis.
2. Identify four variations of the nursing diagnosis.
3. List 10 guidelines for writing a nursing diagnosis.
4. Describe the importance of validation of the nursing diagnosis.
5. Document a nursing diagnosis accurately.

INTRODUCTION

The assessment phase of the nursing process provides the basis for the diagnostic process. As described in Chapter 3, collected data are organized, analyzed, interpreted, and validated by the nurse. The outcome of the diagnostic process is the nursing diagnosis, which becomes the framework for subsequent phases of planning, implementation, and evaluation. This chapter focuses on how to develop, validate, and document the nursing diagnosis.

THE NORTH AMERICAN NURSING DIAGNOSIS SYSTEM

There are several ways to state nursing diagnoses using a number of diagnostic systems. The most commonly used system was developed by the North

American Nursing Diagnosis Association (NANDA). The NANDA system of diagnosis was adopted by the American Nurses' Association (ANA) as the official system of diagnosis for the United States in 1988, and it is the system that will be utilized throughout this text. Before exploring how to write a diagnosis, it might be helpful to discuss the NANDA organization and the system as it has evolved.

The First National Conference on Classification of Nursing Diagnosis was held in 1973 and resulted in publication of the first list of approved diagnoses. NANDA evolved from the group formed at the First National Conference and has been in existence in its current form since 1982. Conferences have been held approximately every two years since that time. The members of the organization have continued to develop and refine the list of approved diagnoses.

A nursing diagnosis is a clinical judgment about an individual, family, or community response to actual or potential health problems/life processes.

The process by which new diagnoses are submitted and approved by NANDA is going through a process of being changed. Presently, the proposed diagnosis is submitted to NANDA and placed into the diagnosis review cycle. In order to enter the cycle, each proposed diagnosis may include some or all of the following elements, including label, definition, defining characteristics, and related/risk factors. The proposed diagnosis must be consistent with the NANDA definition of a nursing diagnosis. The **label** provides a name for the diagnosis. The **definition** provides a clear, precise description of the diagnosis, delineates its meaning, and differentiates it from other diagnoses. **Defining characteristics** are the critical behaviors or signs and symptoms that are manifestations of the diagnosis. **Related factors** are conditions or circumstances that can cause or contribute to the development of the diagnosis. **Risk factors** are environmental factors and physiological, genetic, or chemical elements that increase vulnerability to an unhealthful event. Ideally, the proposed diagnoses include references from the literature or research studies to support the rationale for the diagnostic label, defining characteristics, and related/risk factors. Table 4-1 is a sample of a NANDA diagnosis with its name, definition, defining characteristics, and related factors.

New proposed diagnoses are labeled as "Diagnoses in Progress." Figure 4-1 lists the first set of "Diagnoses in Progress" which were submitted at the 1994 NANDA biannual conference. Information about the new diagnoses is disseminated by NANDA. After the diagnoses are used for 2 years, they will be discussed at the next biannual meeting.

At present, the NANDA-approved diagnoses are usually found in an alphabetical table (Table 4-2) or are classified according to the Taxonomy, which was proposed by the Nurse Theorist Group convened by NANDA in 1978. These 14 nursing theorists, through a democratic process, agreed upon some basic conclusions and proposed that the nine human response patterns of the "Unitary Person" should form the framework for organizing the diagnoses. These nine patterns reflect how individuals interact with the environment that surrounds them. The nursing diagnoses categorized under each pattern describe how they respond to particular states of health or illness. The patterns include exchanging, valuing, perceiving, feeling, relating, communicating,

TABLE 4-1   Sample of a NANDA-Approved Nursing Diagnosis

DIAGNOSIS NAME: FATIGUE

DEFINITION:

The state in which an individual experiences an overwhelming sense of exhaustion and decreased capacity for physical and mental work

DEFINING CHARACTERISTICS:

Major:
   Verbalization of an unremitting and overwhelming lack of energy
   Inability to maintain usual routines
Minor:
   Perceived need for additional energy to accomplish routine tasks
   Increase in physical complaints
   Impaired ability to concentrate
   Decreased performance
   Lethargy or listlessness
   Disinterest in surroundings/introspection
   Decreased libido
   Accident prone

RELATED FACTORS:

   Decreased/increased metabolic energy production
   Increased energy requirements to perform activities of daily living
   Overwhelming psychological or emotional demands
   Excessive social and/or role demands
   States of discomfort
   Altered body chemistry
      Medications
      Drug withdrawal
      Chemotherapy

Modified with permission from Taptich BJ, Iyer P, Bernocchi-Losey D: Nursing Diagnosis and Care Planning, 2nd ed. Philadelphia, WB Saunders, 1994.

moving, knowing, and choosing. Table 4-3 identifies the patterns and their definitions, and gives an example of a nursing diagnosis that is included in the pattern. Each of the existing NANDA-approved diagnoses have been placed under these nine categories (Table 4-4). Subcategories are used when diagnoses require more specificity. For example, in the Exchanging pattern *Fluid Volume* includes two subcategories: *Fluid Volume Deficit* and *Fluid Volume Excess*. The list of diagnoses continues to expand as nurses identify and validate labels that describe the realm of nursing practice. Taxonomy IR can also be expected to change as nurses continue to clarify the concept of nursing diagnosis and to develop effective methods of organization.

Alcohol Drinking Patterns, Dysfunctional
Community Coping, Ineffective
Community Coping, Potential for Enhanced
Confusion, Acute
Disorganized Behavior, Infant
Disorganized Infant Behavior, High Risk For
Environmental Interpretation Syndrome, Impaired
Family Processes, Altered: Addictive Behavior (Individual and Family)
Idiopathic Fecal Incontinence
Impaired Skin Integrity, High Risk For: Pressure Ulcer
Labor Pain
Loneliness, High Risk For
Organized Infant Behavior, Potential for Enhanced
Parent/Infant Attachment, Altered
Preservation/Quality of Life, Alteration in
Self Care Deficit, Medication Administration
Spasticity
Spiritual Well Being, Opportunity for Enhanced
Therapeutic Regimen, Ineffective Management of (Families)
Terminal Illness Response
Urinary Filtration Syndrome, Impaired

FIGURE 4-1   North American Nursing Diagnosis Association
1994 Diagnoses in Progress

INTRODUCTION
NANDA SYSTEM
COMPONENTS OF
NURSING
DIAGNOSIS
Part I: Human
Response

COMPONENTS OF THE NURSING DIAGNOSIS

A nursing diagnosis consists of two parts joined by the phrase "related to." The diagnosis begins with a determination of the human response of concern to the client (Part I). It also includes the factors that contribute to the presence of the response in the individual (Part II). Actual nursing diagnoses have related factors as the second part of the statement, whereas high-risk diagnoses have risk factors.

ANA Measurement
Criteria Standard
II-1 (Standard of
Care). Diagnoses
are derived from
the assessment
data.

Part I: The Human Response

A *human response*, in the context of nursing diagnosis, identifies how the client responds to a state of health or illness. The first part of the diagnostic statement specifies a particular human response of concern identified by the nurse during the diagnostic phase, based on the assessment data. This clause

TABLE 4-2   Alphabetical Listing of NANDA-Approved
Nursing Diagnoses
_____

Activity intolerance
Activity intolerance, high risk for[+]
Adjustment, impaired
Airway clearance, ineffective
Anxiety
Aspiration, high risk for[+]
Body image disturbance
Body temperature, high risk for altered[+]
Breast-feeding, effective
Breast-feeding, ineffective
Breast-feeding, interrupted*
Breathing pattern, ineffective
Cardiac output, decreased
Care-giver role strain*
Care-giver role strain, high risk for*
Communication, impaired verbal
Conflict, decisional (specify)
Conflict, parental role
Constipation
Constipation, colonic
Constipation, perceived
Coping, defensive
Coping, family: ineffective, compromised
Coping, family: ineffective, disabling
Coping, family: potential for growth
Coping, individual: ineffective
Denial, ineffective
Diarrhea
Disuse syndrome, high risk for[+]
Diversional activity deficit
Dysreflexia
Family processes, altered
Fatigue
Fear
Fluid volume deficit
Fluid volume deficit, high risk for[+]
Fluid volume excess
Gas exchange, impaired
Grieving, anticipatory
Grieving, dysfunctional
Growth and development, altered
Health maintenance, altered
Health-seeking behaviors (specify)
Home maintenance management, impaired
Hopelessness
Hyperthermia
Hypothermia
Incontinence, bowel

Incontinence, functional
Incontinence, reflex
Incontinence, stress
Incontinence, total
Incontinence, urge
Infant feeding pattern,
    ineffective*
Infection, high risk for[+]
Injury, high risk for[+]
Knowledge deficit (specify)
Mobility, impaired physical
Neurovascular dysfunction, high
    risk for*
Noncompliance (specify)
Nutrition, altered: less than body
    requirements
Nutrition, altered: more than body
    requirements
Nutrition, altered: high risk for
    more than body requirements[+]
Oral mucous membrane, altered
Pain
Pain, chronic
Parenting, altered
Parenting, altered: high risk for[+]
Personal identity disturbance
Poisoning, high risk for[+]
Post-trauma response
Powerlessness
Protection, altered
Rape-trauma syndrome
Rape-trauma syndrome: compound
    reaction
Rape-trauma syndrome: silent
    reaction
Relocation stress syndrome*
Role performance, altered
Self-care deficit (bathing/hygiene,
    dressing/grooming, feeding,
    toileting)
Self-esteem, chronic low
Self-esteem disturbance
Self-esteem, situational low
Self-mutilation, high risk for*
Sensory/perceptual alterations
    (specify) (visual, auditory,
    kinesthetic, gustatory, tactile,
    olfactory)

*New diagnoses, 1992.
[+]Modified label terminology, 1992.

_____

Continued.

TABLE 4-2   Alphabetical Listing of NANDA-Approved
Nursing Diagnoses–cont'd

Sexual dysfunction	Tissue perfusion, altered (specify
Sexuality patterns, altered	type) (cardiopulmonary, cerebral,
Skin integrity, impaired	gastrointestinal, peripheral,
Skin integrity, high risk for impaired[+]	renal)
Sleep pattern disturbance	Trauma, high risk for[+]
Social interaction, impaired	Unilateral neglect
Social isolation	Urinary elimination, altered
Spiritual distress	patterns of
Suffocation, high risk for[+]	Urinary retention
Swallowing, impaired	Ventilation, inability to sustain
Therapeutic regimen (individual),	spontaneous[*]
ineffective management of[*]	Violence, high risk for: self-
Thermoregulation, ineffective	directed or directed at others[+]
Thought processes, altered	Weaning response, dysfunctional
Tissue integrity, impaired	ventilatory[*]

[*]New diagnoses, 1992.
[+]Modified label terminology, 1992.

indicates what needs to change in an individual client as a result of nursing intervention. For example, if you determine that the client is experiencing difficulties in deciding among a number of ways to treat a medical problem, the human response might be termed "decisional conflict." The first part of the statement also determines the client-centered outcomes that will measure the change.

When writing the first part of the diagnostic statement, consider the following:

1. What is the human response suggested by the assessment data?

2. To what degree is the human response problematic?

The human response can be selected from the list of accepted nursing diagnoses approved by NANDA.

Examples

☐ **Hypothermia**

☐ **Altered protection**

☐ **High risk for self-mutilation**

The degree to which the human response is present or the type of response identified may be clarified by the use of modifiers or qualifying statements (Table 4-5).

TABLE 4-3   NANDA Taxonomy I: Human Response Patterns

PATTERN	DEFINITION AND EXAMPLE
EXCHANGING	A human response pattern involving mutual giving and receiving
	Fluid volume excess may occur as a result of the *exchange* of fluid and electrolytes at the cellular level when the client consumes excessive fluid or sodium
COMMUNICATING	A human response pattern involving sending messages
	Impaired verbal *communication* may occur when the client does not speak the dominant language
RELATING	A human response pattern involving establishing bonds
	Altered parenting may result when a new mother is unable to *bond* with her premature infant
VALUING	A human response pattern involving the assigning of relative worth
	Spiritual distress may be found in individuals who are unable to attend *valued* religious services
CHOOSING	A human response pattern involving the selection of alternatives
	Decisional conflict may occur when clients are given numerous treatment options and are expected to *choose* one
MOVING	A human response pattern involving activity
	Impaired physical mobility may result when a child is unable to *move* normally because of traction
PERCEIVING	A human response pattern involving the reception of information
	Visual sensory *perceptual* alternatives may occur when the client doesn't wear or loses corrective lenses or glasses
KNOWING	A human response pattern involving the meaning associated with information
	Knowledge deficit exists when a client cannot identify the factors that precipitate angina
FEELING	A human response pattern involving the subjective awareness of information
	Anxiety may occur when a client *feels* uneasy when preparing for a first hospital experience

Examples

☐ **Decreased** cardiac output

☐ Fluid volume **excess**

☐ Feeding self-care **deficit**

TABLE 4-4   NANDA Taxonomy of Nursing Diagnoses

PATTERN 1:	EXCHANGING
1.1.2.1	Altered nutrition: more than body requirements
1.1.2.2	Altered nutrition: less than body requirements
1.1.2.3	Altered nutrition: high risk for more than body requirements[+]
1.2.1.1	High risk for infection[+]
1.2.2.1	High risk for altered body temperature[+]
1.2.2.2	Hypothermia
1.2.2.3	Hyperthermia
1.2.2.4	Ineffective thermoregulation
1.2.3.1	Dysreflexia
1.3.1.1	Constipation
1.3.1.1.1	Perceived constipation
1.3.1.1.2	Colonic constipation
1.3.1.2	Diarrhea
1.3.1.3	Bowel incontinence
1.3.2	Altered patterns of urinary elimination
1.3.2.1.1	Stress incontinence
1.3.2.1.2	Reflex incontinence
1.3.2.1.3	Urge incontinence
1.3.2.1.4	Functional incontinence
1.3.2.1.5	Total incontinence
1.3.2.2	Urinary retention
1.4.1.1	Altered (specify type) tissue perfusion (renal, cerebral, cardiopulmonary, gastrointestinal, peripheral)
1.4.1.2.1	Fluid volume excess
1.4.1.2.2.1	Fluid volume deficit
1.4.1.2.2.2	High risk for fluid volume deficit[+]
1.4.2.1	Decreased cardiac output
1.5.1.1	Impaired gas exchange
1.5.1.2	Ineffective airway clearance
1.5.1.3	Ineffective breathing pattern
1.5.1.3.1	Inability to sustain spontaneous ventilation*
1.5.1.3.2	Dysfunctional ventilatory weaning response*
1.6.1	High risk for injury[+]
1.6.1.1	High risk for suffocation[+]
1.6.1.2	High risk for poisoning[+]
1.6.1.3	High risk for trauma[+]
1.6.1.4	High risk for aspiration[+]
1.6.1.5	High risk for disuse syndrome[+]
1.6.2	Altered protection
1.6.2.1	Impaired tissue integrity
1.6.2.1.1	Altered oral mucous membrane
1.6.2.1.2.1	Impaired skin integrity
1.6.2.1.2.2	High risk for impaired skin integrity[+]
PATTERN 2:	COMMUNICATING
2.1.1.1	Impaired verbal communication

*New diagnostic categories, approved 1992.
[+]Categories with modified label terminology.

Continued.

TABLE 4-4   NANDA Taxonomy of Nursing Diagnoses–cont'd.

PATTERN 3:	**RELATING**
3.1.1	Impaired social interaction
3.1.2	Social isolation
3.2.1	Altered role performance
3.2.1.1.1	Altered parenting
3.2.1.1.2	High risk for altered parenting[+]
3.2.1.2.1	Sexual dysfunction
3.2.2	Altered family processes
3.2.2.1	Care-giver role strain*
3.2.2.2	High risk for care-giver role strain*
3.2.3.1	Parental role conflict
3.3	Altered sexuality patterns
PATTERN 4:	**VALUING**
4.1.1	Spiritual distress (distress of the human spirit)
PATTERN 5:	**CHOOSING**
5.1.1.1	Ineffective individual coping
5.1.1.1.1	Impaired adjustment
5.1.1.1.2	Defensive coping
5.1.1.1.3	Ineffective denial
5.1.2.1.1	Ineffective family coping: disabling
5.1.2.1.2	Ineffective family coping: compromised
5.1.2.2	Family coping: potential for growth
5.2.1	Ineffective management of therapeutic regimen (individual)*
5.2.1.1	Noncompliance (specify)
5.3.1.1	Decisional conflict (specify)
5.4	Health-seeking behaviors (specify)
PATTERN 6:	**MOVING**
6.1.1.1	Impaired physical mobility
6.1.1.1.1	High risk for peripheral neurovascular dysfunction*
6.1.1.2	Activity intolerance
6.1.1.2.1	Fatigue
6.1.1.3	High risk for activity intolerance[+]
6.2.1	Sleep pattern disturbance
6.3.1.1	Diversional activity deficit
6.4.1.1	Impaired home maintenance management
6.4.2	Altered health maintenance
6.5.1	Feeding self-care deficit
6.5.1.1	Impaired swallowing
6.5.1.2	Ineffective breast-feeding
6.5.1.2.1	Interrupted breast-feeding*
6.5.1.3	Effective breast-feeding
6.5.1.4	Ineffective infant feeding pattern*
6.5.2	Bathing/hygiene self-care deficit

*New diagnostic categories, approved 1992.
[+]Categories with modified label terminology.

Continued.

TABLE 4-4   NANDA Taxonomy of Nursing Diagnoses–cont'd.

PATTERN 6:	**MOVING**
6.5.3	Dressing/grooming self-care deficit
6.5.4	Toileting self-care deficit
6.6	Altered growth and development
6.7	Relocation stress syndrome*
PATTERN 7:	**PERCEIVING**
7.1.1	Body image disturbance
7.1.2	Self-esteem disturbance
7.1.2.1	Chronic low self-esteem
7.1.2.2	Situational low self-esteem
7.1.3	Personal identity disturbance
7.2	Sensory/perceptual alterations (specify) (visual, auditory, kinesthetic, gustatory, tactile, olfactory)
7.2.1.1	Unilateral neglect
7.3.1	Hopelessness
7.3.2	Powerlessness
PATTERN 8:	**KNOWING**
8.1.1	Knowledge deficit (specify)
8.3	Altered thought processes
PATTERN 9:	**FEELING**
9.1.1	Pain
9.1.1.1	Chronic pain
9.2.1.1	Dysfunctional grieving
9.2.1.2	Anticipatory grieving
9.2.2	High risk for violence: self-directed or directed at others[+]
9.2.2.1	High risk for self-mutilation*
9.2.3	Post-trauma response
9.2.3.1	Rape-trauma syndrome
9.2.3.1.1	Rape-trauma syndrome: compound reaction
9.2.3.1.2	Rape-trauma syndrome: silent reaction
9.3.1	Anxiety
9.3.2	Fear

*New diagnostic categories, approved 1992.
[+]Categories with modified label terminology.

Punctuation marks such as commas, colons, and parentheses are often used in the first part of the diagnostic statement to separate or clarify the diagnosis.

Example

☐ Altered nutrition: more than body requirements

☐ Altered (cerebral) tissue perfusion

☐ Rape trauma syndrome: compound reaction

TABLE 4-5   Nursing Diagnosis Modifiers

MODIFIER	DEFINITION	EXAMPLE
ALTERED	A change from the usual optimum for a particular client	Altered body temperature
HIGH RISK	The individual is at risk for a problem	High risk for infection
INEFFECTIVE	Not producing the desired effect; not capable of performing satisfactorily	Ineffective thermoregulation
DECREASED	Smaller; lessened; diminished; lesser in size, amount, or degree	Decreased cardiac output
IMPAIRED	Made worse, weakened; damaged, reduced; deteriorated	Impaired swallowing
DEFICIT	Amount or quantity that is less than is necessary, desirable, or usable	Diversional activity deficit
EXCESS	Amount or quantity that is more than is necessary, desirable, or usable	Fluid volume excess
DYSFUNCTIONAL	Abnormal; impaired or incompletely functioning	Sexual dysfunction
DISTURBANCE	The state of being agitated, interrupted, or interfered with	Sleep pattern disturbance
ACUTE	Severe, but of short duration	Acute urinary retention
CHRONIC	Lasting a long time; recurring; habitual; constant	Chronic pain
LESS THAN	A smaller amount	Altered nutrition: less than body requirements
MORE THAN	A larger amount	Altered nutrition: more than body requirements
ANTICIPATORY	Occurring in advance	Anticipatory grieving
COMPROMISED	To lay open to danger; to endanger the interests of	Ineffective family coping; compromised

Source: Webster's New World Dictionary, College Edition, Cleveland: The World Publishing Company, 1959. Modified with permission from North American Nursing Diagnosis Association Taxonomy Committee: Diagnosis Qualifiers. St. Louis, North American Nursing Diagnosis Association, 1986.

The information gathered during the assessment phase provides data to validate that the defining characteristics of diagnoses are present.

Example. Mrs. James is a 72-year-old client who had a total hip replacement this morning as a result of chronic arthritic changes in her hip. During your assessment, she complains of postoperative incisional pain and indicates that she would like a laxative because she will be in bed for a while. She states that she has become constipated in the past when she wasn't "up and around" but knows that a high-fiber diet will help.

This information suggests three nursing diagnoses that reflect the presence of human responses of concern in this client. The first parts would be written as:

HUMAN RESPONSE	INFERENCE
1. **Pain**	Indicates that the client is actually experiencing pain
2. **High risk for constipation**	Identifies the possibility that the client will become constipated
3. **Health-seeking behaviors (high-fiber diet)**	Demonstrates client's interest in positive health practices

Part II: Related/Risk Factors

The related/risk factors (etiology) are identified in the second part of the nursing diagnosis. In order to prevent, minimize, or alleviate a response in the client, the nurse must know why it is occurring. *Related factors* identify the physiological, psychological, sociocultural, environmental, or spiritual factors believed to be causing or contributing to the response seen in the client. Box 4-1 lists examples of related factors.

Risk factors are those that predispose an individual, family, or community to an unhealthful event. They are used with high-risk diagnoses to define the specific situations that place the client at risk for developing the unhealthful response. For example, decreased immune responses place the client at risk for infection and prolonged immobility predisposes the client to altered skin integrity.

In the preceding case of Mrs. James, three responses were identified. The second parts of the diagnostic statements could be written as follows:

HUMAN RESPONSE		RELATED FACTOR
1. Pain		**effects of surgery**
2. High risk for constipation	*related to*	**prolonged immobility**
3. Health-seeking behaviors		**fear of constipation**

BOX 4-1
Examples of Related Factors

Physiological	Immobility
	Effects of sensory deficit
	Side effects of medications
Psychological	Fear of death
	Feelings of loneliness
	Separation from family
Sociocultural	Decreased ability to procure food
	Language barrier
	Lack of support systems
Environmental	Excessive noise
	Noxious odors
	Sensitivity to light
Spiritual	Inability to practice religious beliefs
	Challenged beliefs about God
	Conflict between religious beliefs and prescribed health regimen

---

Remember that the related factors help to identify the variables that contribute to the presence of the human response. They also suggest specific nursing interventions that will prevent, correct, or alleviate the response. For example, the following nursing diagnoses identify the same human response but have quite different related factors.

HUMAN RESPONSE		RELATED FACTORS
1. Altered nutrition: less than body requirements		difficulty in swallowing
2. Altered nutrition: less than body requirements	*related to*	decreased appetite
3. Altered nutrition: less than body requirements		feelings of loneliness

Because the nursing interventions are dependent on the related/risk factors, those suggested by each of the diagnostic statements listed above are also quite different. The nursing interventions that might be initiated in the presence of swallowing difficulties might include the following:

1. Sit the client in an upright position, 60 to 90 degrees.
2. Encourage the client to:

■ take small amounts of semisolid food
■ place food at the back of the mouth
■ think about swallowing.

If the client is experiencing decreased appetite, the following interventions may help:

1. Determine food preferences.
2. Serve food in an appealing manner.
3. Provide small, frequent feedings.

For the client who does not eat because she is lonely following her husband's death, the nurse may include these interventions:

1. Encourage the client to verbalize feelings about the death of her husband.
2. Explain the hazards of continued decreased intake.
3. Arrange consultation with a psychiatric clinical specialist.
4. Provide information about support groups such as Widows and Widowers or I Can Cope.

Summary of Components of the Diagnostic Statement

The nursing diagnosis consists of two parts joined by the words "related to." Part I includes the human response identified by the nurse during the assessment phase of the nursing process. It determines the outcomes that will measure progress in preventing, minimizing, or alleviating the client's health problem. Part II consists of the related/risk factors that contribute to the response. This part suggests the interventions that may be appropriate in the management of the client's care. Figure 4-2 illustrates the relationship between the components of a nursing diagnosis. Sample nursing diagnoses are listed in Table 4-6.

INTRODUCTION
NANDA SYSTEM
COMPONENTS
OF NURSING
DIAGNOSIS
VARIATIONS
OF NURSING
DIAGNOSIS
Many Related/Risk
Factors

VARIATIONS OF THE NURSING DIAGNOSIS

There are four common variations of the nursing diagnosis, including many related/risk factors, unknown related/risk factors, one-part diagnoses, and three-part diagnoses.

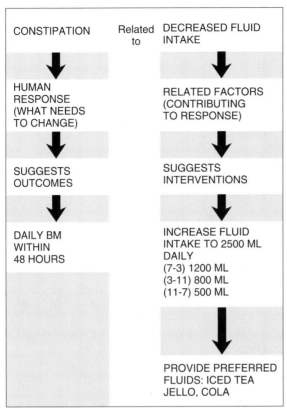

FIGURE 4-2   Flowchart of a sample nursing diagnosis illustrating the relationship of its components.

Many Related/Risk Factors

Clients' health care problems are rarely simple. The responses seen in clients frequently have a number of related factors that contribute to their existence. For example, care-giver role strain may be related to severity of illness of the care receiver, duration of care requirements, and immaturity of care-giver.

Example.   Although Jose Esposito is hypertensive, when admitted to the hospital he tells the nurse that he has discontinued his medication because it was interfering with his sex life. He is 5 ft, 4 in. and weighs 190 lb. In reviewing the client's typical eating habits, the nurse determines that his caloric intake is excessive. Jose also indicates that his favorite leisure activities are watching TV and drinking beer. He also smokes three packs of cigarettes daily.

In Jose's case, obesity, smoking, and discontinuance of the antihypertensive medication are all contributing to his hypertension. This illustrates the

TABLE 4-6   **Examples of Correctly Written Nursing Diagnoses**

- ☐ Impaired verbal communication related to language barrier
- ☐ High risk for injury related to impaired visual perception
- ☐ Sexual dysfunction related to fear of rejection
- ☐ Diversional activity deficit related to inability to participate in usual activities
- ☐ Impaired skin integrity related to irritating wound drainage
- ☐ High risk for aspiration related to decreased level of consciousness
- ☐ Altered growth and development related to effects of prolonged hospitalization
- ☐ Impaired adjustment related to effects of recent relocation
- ☐ High risk for peripheral neurovascular dysfunction related to prolonged immobilization (cast)
- ☐ Dysfunctional ventilatory weaning response related to pain, anxiety

complex nature of his illness. Imagine how redundant the client's plan of care would be if each of the related factors were identified in a separate nursing diagnosis.

"Ineffective management of therapeutic regimen related to lack of knowledge of effects of medication on hypertension"

"Ineffective management of therapeutic regimen related to lack of knowledge of effects of smoking on hypertension"

"Ineffective management of therapeutic regimen related to lack of knowledge of effects of obesity on hypertension"

Combination of all of the factors related to Jose's hypertension allows the nurse to develop one comprehensive diagnosis. This will encourage the implementation of a number of nursing interventions to effectively manage this client's response to his illness. Jose's diagnosis should be written as:

- ☐ "Ineffective management of therapeutic regimen related to lack of knowledge of effects of medication, smoking, and obesity on hypertension"

At times, the second part of the diagnostic statement, the related/risk factors, may be divided into two parts to provide additional information. When this is done, the words "secondary to" or the abbreviation "2°" are used.

Examples

- ☐ Fluid volume deficit related to decreased intake of oral fluids **secondary** to weakness

- ☐ Altered nutrition: less than body requirements related to decreased appetite **2°** to effects of medication

☐ High risk for infection related to decreased immune response **secondary** to chemotherapy

Unknown Related/Risk Factors

At times the factors related to the existence of a particular client response may be unclear or unknown. It is acceptable to include the words "related to unknown factors" while continuing to identify or define the causative factors.

Examples

☐ Pain related to unknown factors
☐ Chronic low self-esteem related to unknown factors

One-Part Diagnoses

Usually nursing diagnoses are two-part statements joined by the words "related to." A few nursing diagnoses may be written with only one part, the human response, without the words "related to" or identified related factors. This usually occurs when the related factors are obvious or implied.

Examples

☐ Rape trauma syndrome
☐ Post trauma response

In the case of a person who is experiencing the signs of a traumatic response to being raped, it is usually clearly evident that the difficulties expressed by the client are the result of the rape. In this situation, it may not be necessary to identify rape as the related factor. Similarly, in the case of "post-trauma response," even though there may be numerous events that could precipitate this response, if the factor is known to all nurses caring for the client, it may not be necessary to identify it in the diagnostic statement. When there is any question about identification of the related factor, it should be included.

Three-Part Diagnoses

Many students in nursing programs and some practicing nurses use three-part nursing diagnoses. The first part is the human response, the second, related/risk factors, and the third, the cues, signs, and symptoms or defining characteristics that are present. The words "as evidenced by" or the abbreviation "AEB" is placed before the third part of the statement.

Examples

☐ Ineffective management of therapeutic regimen related to family conflict AEB client's statement, "I can't follow my diet if my wife won't cook for me"

☐ Effective breast-feeding related to previous positive experience as evidenced by infant satiation and verbalized maternal satisfaction

GUIDELINES FOR WRITING A NURSING DIAGNOSIS

Formulating a nursing diagnosis may be considered a new skill. As with any other new skill, it takes practice. The nurse will, with practice, find that the process of writing nursing diagnostic statements becomes easier. The following guidelines have been included to assist you in developing correctly written diagnoses.

1. Write the Diagnosis in Terms of the Client's Response Rather than Nursing Need

The first part of the diagnostic statement identifies the client's response to health or illness. Therapeutic or functional needs, such as "needs frequent turning" or "needs coughing and deep breathing," describe nursing interventions rather than client responses and should not be included in the diagnostic statement.

Example.   Stella Blackwell is a 45-year-old client who has a nasogastric tube following surgery. She tells her nurse that she is thirsty and that her mouth and lips are dry. The nurse recognizes that the client "needs additional fluids" and communicates this response in the diagnostic statement "fluid volume deficit related to decreased oral intake."

Examples

INCORRECT	CORRECT
Needs suctioning because she has many secretions	High risk for aspiration related to excessive oral secretions
Needs relief from care-taking because of own health problems	Care-giver role strain related to own new diagnosis of angina
Needs frequent rest periods because of shortness of breath	Fatigue related to persistent shortness of breath

2. Use "Related to" Rather than "Due to" or "Caused by" to Connect the Two Parts of the Diagnosis

Part I and Part II of the nursing diagnosis should always be linked by the words "related to" (r/t). This phrase does not necessarily mean that there is a direct cause-and-effect relationship between the two parts of the statement. Rather, it identifies a relationship between the human response and the related factors, implying that if one part of the diagnosis changes, the other part may also change.

Examples

INCORRECT	CORRECT
High risk for injury caused by change in mental status	High risk for injury related to change in mental status
Ineffective infant feeding pattern due to effects of prematurity	Ineffective infant feeding pattern related to effects of prematurity

3. Write the Diagnosis in Legally Advisable Terms

A nursing diagnosis such as "impaired skin integrity related to infrequent turning" is not legally advisable. This statement implies negligence or blame that may not be accurate and can create potential legal problems for the personnel caring for the client. This statement could be better phrased as "impaired skin integrity related to prolonged immobility." The therapeutic nursing orders would be similar in both instances, but the second statement is factual and does not imply fault.

Examples

INCORRECT	CORRECT
High risk for injury related to inadequately maintained skin traction	High risk for injury related to hazards associated with skin traction
Ineffective airway clearance related to excessive sedation	Ineffective airway clearance related to effects of sedation
High risk for self-mutilation related to inadequate supervision	High risk for self-mutilation related to feelings of self-contempt and guilt

GUIDELINES FOR WRITING A NURSING DIAGNOSIS
Describe Client's Response
Use "Related to"

GUIDELINES FOR WRITING A NURSING DIAGNOSIS
Describe Client's Response
Use "Related to"
Use Legally Advisable Terms

GUIDELINES
FOR WRITING
A NURSING
DIAGNOSIS

Describe Client's
Response

Use "Related to"

Use Legally Advis-
able Terms

*Avoid Value
Judgments*

4. Write Diagnoses Without Value Judgments

Nursing diagnoses should be based on objective and subjective data collected and validated in conjunction with the client or significant other. The behavior of the client should not be judged by the nurse's personal values and standards. Use of words such as "inadequate," "poor," and "unhealthy" in nursing diagnoses frequently imply value judgments.

Examples

INCORRECT	CORRECT
Altered parenting related to poor bonding with child	Altered parenting related to prolonged separation from child
Social isolation related to nasty, obnoxious behaviors	Social isolation related to fear of rejection
Impaired home maintenance management related to sloppy housekeeping habits	Impaired home maintenance management related to lack of knowledge regarding home safety measures

GUIDELINES
FOR WRITING
A NURSING
DIAGNOSIS

Describe Client's
Response

Use "Related to"

Use Legally Advis-
able Terms

Avoid Value Judg-
ments

*Avoid Reversing
Parts*

5. Avoid Reversing the Parts of the Diagnosis

Remember that the first part of the diagnosis identifies the human response and suggests outcomes. The second part of the diagnosis defines the related/risk factors and suggests nursing interventions (see Figure 4-2). Reversing the clauses may result in unclear communication about the client's response and its contributing factors, which makes the writing of appropriate outcomes and nursing interventions difficult.

Examples

INCORRECT	CORRECT
Sensory overload related to sleep pattern disturbance	Sleep pattern disturbance related to sensory overload
Decreased caloric intake related to altered nutrition: less than body requirements	Altered nutrition: less than body requirements related to decreased caloric intake

6. Avoid Using Single Cues in the First Part of the Diagnosis

The first part of the diagnostic statement is derived from a cluster of signs and symptoms observed by the nurse during the assessment of the client. An isolated cue is not a nursing diagnosis, but it may provide information to help define the response. Inaccurate diagnoses may occur if you focus on an isolated sign or symptom rather than on the entire clinical picture.

Example. William Ward, an elderly client admitted to a nursing home, has a history of lung problems. You observe that he is restless. Writing the diagnosis as "restlessness related to change in environment" suggests that restlessness is the response. In fact, the presence of restlessness may be a cue to other responses, such as ineffective airway clearance, altered coping, or fear.

A number of the approved diagnoses may appear to be isolated cues because of their one-word titles (pain, fear, anxiety). Remember that these are diagnostic terms that refer to a phenomenon that has a number of defining characteristics. For example, some of the characteristics for the diagnosis of pain include increased blood pressure, pulse, and respiratory rate, reports of pain, clutching of painful area, and facial mask of pain.

GUIDELINES FOR WRITING A NURSING DIAGNOSIS
Describe Client's Response
Use "Related to"
Use Legally Advisable Terms
Avoid Value Judgments
Avoid Reversing Parts
Avoid Single Cues

7. The Two Parts of the Diagnosis Should Not Mean the Same Thing

In some instances, nursing diagnoses are written in which the two parts are almost identical. Examine this statement: "ineffective airway clearance related to inability to clear airway." Both parts of the diagnosis have the same meaning. This is confusing and may result in difficulties when attempting to determine appropriate nursing interventions for the related factor. The diagnosis should be written as "ineffective airway clearance related to retained secretions."

Examples

GUIDELINES FOR WRITING A NURSING DIAGNOSIS
Describe Client's Response
Use "Related to"
Use Legally Advisable Terms
Avoid Value Judgments
Avoid Reversing Parts
Avoid Single Cues
Two Parts Should Not Be the Same

INCORRECT	CORRECT
Inability to feed self related to feeding problems	Feeding self-care deficit related to pain in fingers
Dysfunctional ventilatory weaning response related to inability to adjust to lowered levels of mechanical ventilation	Dysfunctional ventilatory weaning response related to uncontrolled pain

8. Express the Related Factor in Terms that Can Be Changed

One of the most common errors nurses make when writing nursing diagnoses is the inclusion of related factors that cannot be changed by nursing intervention. For example, nurses cannot change the fact that a client has had surgery or is dying of cancer. However, nurses can help the client to manage the effects of medical diagnoses, treatments, and life processes.

Keep in mind that the diagnostic statement identifies actual or potential client responses. These responses and the factors that contribute to their existence should be changeable by interventions that are within the realm of nursing practice.

Example. Shelby Donovan is a 6-year-old who is two days postoperative after an appendectomy. She is crying and points to the incisional area and says, "My tummy hurts." The diagnosis "pain related to surgical incision" is not accurate because nursing intervention cannot change the presence of a surgical incision. This can be restated as "pain related to the effects of surgery." Nursing interventions may relieve the effects of surgery: inflammation, immobility, anxiety, nausea.

Examples

INCORRECT	CORRECT
Dysfunctional grieving related to death of spouse	Dysfunctional grieving related to perceived loss of security
Ineffective airway clearance related to chronic pulmonary disease	Ineffective airway clearance related to copious, viscous secretions

9. Do Not Include Medical Diagnoses in the Nursing Diagnosis

The nursing diagnosis differs from the medical diagnosis in that it reflects the essence of nursing rather than medical practice. The following outline demonstrates the primary differences between medical and nursing diagnoses:

MEDICAL DIAGNOSIS	NURSING DIAGNOSIS
Identifies a specific illness	Identifies an actual or potential response to the illness
Clinical manifestations suggest medical need	Responses suggest a nursing need
Implies associated medical interventions	Implies associated nursing interventions

The following examples compare medical and nursing diagnoses that might be found in the same client.

Related Factors Changeable
Avoid Medical Diagnoses

MEDICAL DIAGNOSIS	NURSING DIAGNOSIS
Hepatitis	Ineffective individual coping related to prolonged isolation
Diabetes mellitus	Knowledge deficit (foot care) related to inability to retain information
AIDS	Altered protection related to effects of compromised immune system
Cancer	Altered oral mucous membranes related to effects of chemotherapy
Myocardial infarction	Ineffective denial related to fear of disability

As identified previously, the medical diagnosis suggests medical interventions; therefore, its use is inappropriate in either of the two parts of the nursing diagnostic statement.

Examples

INCORRECT	CORRECT
Ineffective breathing pattern related to emphysema	Ineffective breathing pattern related to retained secretions
Congestive heart failure related to failure to take medications	Noncompliance (cardiac medications) related to lack of knowledge about action and correct dosage

10. State the Diagnosis Clearly and Concisely

Clear, concise nursing diagnostic statements facilitate communication and allow you to concentrate on the specific factors contributing to a response exhibited by a client.

Example.   Kathleen Inman, the mother of a premature infant, reveals that she feels that *she* caused her premature labor. "I wouldn't be in this mess if I hadn't lifted that heavy can of paint—that's why my labor started." The client states that she is concerned about her 2-year-old son, because she spends a great deal of time at the hospital. She also indicates that she sees very little of her husband, which has created tension in their marriage.

GUIDELINES FOR WRITING A NURSING DIAGNOSIS
Describe Client's Response
Use "Related to"
Use Legally Advisable Terms
Avoid Value Judgments
Avoid Reversing Parts

4-1 TEST YOURSELF

Identification of Correctly and Incorrectly Written Diagnoses

The following is a list of nursing diagnostic statements. Decide whether each statement is correctly or incorrectly written. If incorrectly stated, identify the rule(s) violated, by number, from the list below.

GUIDELINES FOR WRITING NURSING DIAGNOSES

1. Write the diagnosis in terms of the client's response rather than nursing need.
2. Use "related to" rather than "due to" or "caused by" to connect the two parts of the diagnosis.
3. Write the diagnosis in legally advisable terms.
4. Write diagnoses without value judgments.
5. Avoid reversing the parts of the diagnosis.
6. Avoid using single cues in the first part of the diagnosis.
7. The two parts of the diagnosis should not mean the same thing.
8. Express the related factor in terms that can be changed.
9. Do not include medical diagnoses in the nursing diagnosis.
10. State the diagnosis clearly and concisely.

	CORRECT	INCORRECT	RULE
1. Inability to sustain spontaneous ventilations related to inability to breathe			
2. Needs skin care			
3. Fluid volume deficit related to decreased oral intake			
4. Altered nutrition: more than body requirements related to poor eating habits			
5. High risk for violence related to spouse's continuous verbal threats, arguing, belittling remarks, and physical beatings			

Continued.

4-1   TEST YOURSELF

Identification of Correctly and Incorrectly Written Diagnoses–cont'd.

	CORRECT	INCORRECT	RULE
6. Spiritual distress related to separation from religious ties			
7. Chronic pain related to arthritis			
8. Fear related to perceived threat of death			
9. High risk for trauma due to cataract surgery and corneal transplant			
10. Dribbling and diminished force of urinary stream related to urinary retention			
11. Altered role performance related to effects of change in health status			
12. High risk for infection related to poor use of aseptic technique by staff			
13. Effective breast-feeding related to previous positive experiences			
14. Constipation related to effects of codeine			

The following are examples of diagnostic statements that could be written for this client:

INCORRECT	CORRECT
Altered interactions between husband and wife and mother and two year old son related to mother's hospital visiting patterns	Altered family processes related to mother's hospital visiting patterns
Ineffective individual coping related to belief that she caused the onset of premature labor by lifting heavy paint can on day of delivery	Ineffective individual coping related to feelings of guilt

Avoid Single Cues
Two Parts Should Not Be the Same
Related Factors Changeable
Avoid Medical Diagnoses
State Clearly and Concisely

4-1 TEST YOURSELF

Identification of Correctly and Incorrectly Written Diagnoses: Answers

	CORRECT	INCORRECT	RULE
1. Inability to sustain spontaneous ventilations related to inability to breathe		✔	7
2. Needs skin care		✔	1
3. Fluid volume deficit related to decreased oral intake	✔		
4. Altered nutrition: more than body requirements related to poor eating habits		✔	4
5. High risk for violence related to spouse's continuous verbal threats, arguing, belittling remarks, and physical beatings		✔	10
6. Spiritual distress related to separation from religious ties	✔		
7. Chronic pain related to arthritis		✔	9
8. Fear related to perceived threat of death	✔		
9. High risk for trauma due to cataract surgery and corneal transplant		✔	2, 8
10. Dribbling and diminished force of urinary stream related to urinary retention		✔	5, 6
11. Altered role performance related to effects of change in health status	✔		
12. High risk for infection related to poor use of aseptic technique by staff		✔	3
13. Effective breastfeeding related to previous positive experiences	✔		
14. Constipation related to effects of codeine	✔		

4-2 TEST YOURSELF

Revision of Incorrectly Written Diagnoses

The nursing diagnoses that were incorrectly written in the previous exercise are listed below. Revise each statement to make it correct.

STATEMENT	REVISION
1. Inability to sustain spontaneous ventilation related to inability to breathe	
2. Needs skin care	
3. Altered nutrition: more than body requirements related to poor eating habits	
4. High risk for violence related to spouse's continuous verbal threats, arguing, belittling remarks, and physical beatings	
5. Chronic pain related to arthritis	
6. High risk for trauma due to cataract surgery and corneal transplant	
7. Dribbling and diminished force of urinary stream related to urinary retention	
8. High risk for infection related to poor use of aseptic technique by staff	

4-2 TEST YOURSELF
Revision of Incorrectly Written Diagnoses: Answers

There are a number of ways to revise the nursing diagnoses listed in this exercise. One example of a corrected revision for each diagnostic statement is provided below.

STATEMENT	REVISION
1. Inability to sustain spontaneous ventilation related to inability to breathe	Inability to sustain spontaneous ventilation related to respiratory muscle fatigue
2. Needs skin care	Impaired skin integrity related to immobility
3. Altered nutrition: more than body requirements related to poor eating habits	Altered nutrition: more than body requirements related to excessive caloric intake
4. High risk for violence related to spouse's continuous verbal threats, arguing, belittling remarks, and physical beatings	High risk for violence related to recurrent physical and emotional abuse
5. Chronic pain related to arthritis	Chronic pain related to effects of inflammatory process
6. High risk for trauma due to cataract surgery and corneal transplant	High risk for trauma related to impaired perception
7. Dribbling and diminished force of urinary stream related to urinary retention	Urinary retention related to effects of anesthesia
8. High risk for infection related to poor use of aseptic technique by staff	High risk for infection related to hazards associated with invasive monitoring

Neither of the incorrect examples shown is clear or concise. Although the client's comments are cues that suggest disrupted family interactions and feelings of guilt, it is not necessary to include her entire statements in the nursing diagnoses.

Clear and concise diagnostic statements facilitate communication and allow you to concentrate on the client's response and the related/risk factors. This approach promotes quality, individualized nursing care.

VALIDATION OF THE DIAGNOSIS

The third step in the diagnostic process is *validation*. Before committing the diagnosis to paper, it is helpful to verify its accuracy. This can be accomplished by asking the following questions:

- Do you have a comprehensive data base that reflects both history and physical assessment?
- Can you identify a pattern?
- Does the definition of the human response you have selected seem consistent with the pattern you have identified?
- Does the assessment data match the defining characteristics of the nursing diagnosis you have selected?
- Does (do) the related/risk factor(s) you have identified correspond to those associated with the human response?
- Does the nursing diagnostic statement identify a response and related factors that can be managed by nursing intervention?

After asking these questions, the nurse should validate the diagnosis with the client by describing what the nurse perceives the responses to be. The client should be asked if these are things of concern. If the concerns of the nurse and the client are not in agreement, the dialogue should continue until some consensus is reached.

DOCUMENTATION

After developing and verifying the nursing diagnostic statement, it is documented in the client's medical record by the nurse. The location may vary according to the agency, and institutional policies or guidelines should be followed. Most commonly, the nursing diagnosis is documented on the plan of care, nurses' notes, progress notes, discharge summaries, and interagency referral forms. Diagnostic statements should be reviewed at intervals and revised or eliminated as necessary.

SUMMARY

To summarize, nursing diagnostic statements are the outcome of the diagnostic process and usually consist of two parts joined by the words "related to." The

4-3   TEST YOURSELF

Writing Nursing Diagnoses from Case Studies

Develop correctly written nursing diagnoses for each of the case studies presented below by identifying significant cues/clusters and comparing them with the defining characteristics if possible. Use the guidelines listed previously to correctly phrase the diagnosis. Refer to the Appendix for definitions, defining characteristics, and related/risk factors for the NANDA diagnoses.

Case 1. Cassie Tilton is an 88-year-old woman transferred to your unit from a skilled nursing facility. Her history reveals that she had a "flu-like" syndrome for the past five days with persistent vomiting and diarrhea. Her vital signs are: B/P 108/56, P 112, R 28, and T 101.4. Her mucous membranes are dry and her skin turgor is decreased. She indicates that she feels weak, tired, and thirsty.

CUES

NURSING DIAGNOSIS

Case 2. Chip Ireland is a 35-year-old businessman admitted to the outpatient surgicenter for a tonsillectomy. He indicates that he has had recurrent tonsillitis for the last three years. Postoperatively, he complains of being thirsty and requests a cold drink. You observe that he has difficulty swallowing and coughs up the water. He states "my throat is too sore; it feels like it is swollen." Upon examination, you note the presence of redness and edema in the operative area.

CUES

NURSING DIAGNOSIS

Continued.

4-3 TEST YOURSELF
Writing Nursing Diagnoses from Case Studies—cont'd.

Case 3. Emily Fantin is an 86-year-old woman who calls the office nurse and requests free samples of laxatives. She complains, "I've spent so much money on laxatives at the drug store. I take them twice a day so that my bowels will move three times a day. My mother always told me to take laxatives to keep myself regular. By the way, do you have any sample enemas?" Upon further questioning you find out that Emily lives alone and does her own cooking. She eats mostly frozen dinners or prepared foods with few fruits and vegetables. In addition, she shops at a local convenience store with a limited supply of fresh produce. She relies on Metamucil daily, and Ex Lax and Milk of Magnesia approximately four times a week. She states that she gets very little exercise.

CUES

_____

_____

NURSING DIAGNOSIS

_____

_____

first part identifies the human responses to health or illness that may be prevented, altered, or alleviated by nursing intervention. This part forms the basis for client-centered outcomes by which progress can be measured.

The second part of the diagnostic statement includes the related/risk factors that contribute to the existence of the client's response. This part suggests nursing interventions that may be utilized to manage the client's care. Writing diagnostic statements is a skill that requires practice and may be facilitated by the use of consistent guidelines. A variety of resources are available to assist the nurse in acquiring these skills.

The *Nursing Diagnosis Journal*, published by Nursecom, Inc., assists NANDA in sharing information about nursing diagnoses. The journal encourages nurses to ask questions, exchange views, submit articles, and share experiences on the impact of diagnoses in practice, research, and education. Nurses may subscribe to the journal by contacting the North American Nursing Diagnosis Association, 1211 Locust Street, Philadelphia, PA 19107.

A number of handbooks have been developed—Taptich et al. (1994), Gordon (1993), and Kim et al. (1993)—that are helpful in formulating nursing diagnoses according to the NANDA system. Each of these sources include the

VARIATIONS OF NURSING DIAGNOSIS

GUIDELINES FOR WRITING A NURSING DIAGNOSIS

VALIDATION OF THE DIAGNOSIS

DOCUMENTATION

Case 1. Cassie Tilton

CUES

Weakness
Tired
Thirst
Dry mucous membranes
Decreased skin turgor
T 101.4
B/P 108/56
P 112
R 28
History of vomiting/diarrhea for five days

NURSING DIAGNOSIS

Fluid volume deficit related to vomiting and diarrhea

Case 2. Chip Ireland

CUES

Observed difficulty in swallowing
Cough
Complaints of sore throat
States "feels swollen"

NURSING DIAGNOSIS

Impaired swallowing related to edema, effects of surgery

Case 3. Emily Fantin

CUES

Expectation of bowel movement three times daily
Takes over-the-counter laxatives
Requesting enemas

NURSING DIAGNOSIS

Perceived constipation related to long-standing family health beliefs

4-4 TEST YOURSELF
Developing Nursing Diagnoses for Ted Alexander

In Chapter 3 you identified cues and made inferences based on the data presented on Ted Alexander. From this information develop nursing diagnoses. Compare the listed cues/clusters with the definitions and defining characteristics of the nursing diagnoses found in the Appendix. Refer back to the case study to assist you in identifying related factors.

CUE	INFERENCE	NURSING DIAGNOSIS
1. Concerned about unfamiliar physician Worried about separation from children	1. Separated from support systems	1.
2. Generalized abdominal tenderness Reports pain in upper quadrant	2. Pain	2.
3. Tense tone: "It's serious, isn't it?"	3. Fear	3.
4. Vomiting bloody fluid	4. Bleeding from some site	4.
5. Contact lenses and glasses in hotel room	5. Abnormal vision without corrective lenses	5.

4-4   TEST YOURSELF

Developing Nursing Diagnoses for Ted Alexander: Answers

CUE	INFERENCE	NURSING DIAGNOSIS
1. Concerned about unfamiliar physician Worried about separation from children	1. Separated from support systems	1. Ineffective individual coping r/t separation from support systems
2. Generalized abdominal tenderness Reports pain in upper quadrant	2. Pain	2. Pain r/t inflammatory process
3. Tense tone: "It's serious, isn't it?"	3. Fear	3. Fear r/t perceived threat of death
4. Vomiting bloody fluid	4. Bleeding from some site	4. Fluid volume deficit r/t active bleeding, diaphoresis
5. Contact lenses and glasses in hotel room	5. Abnormal vision without corrective lenses	5. Risk of sensory/perceptual alteration (visual) r/t absence of glasses/contact lenses

approved diagnoses, definitions, defining characteristics, and related/risk factors.

In review, here are the guidelines for writing a nursing diagnosis.

1. Write the diagnosis in terms of the client's response rather than nursing need.
2. Use "related to" rather than "due to" or "caused by" to connect the two parts of the diagnosis.
3. Write the diagnosis in legally advisable terms.
4. Write diagnoses without value judgments.
5. Avoid reversing the parts of the diagnosis.

6. Avoid using single cues in the first part of the diagnosis.

7. The two parts of the diagnosis should not mean the same thing.

8. Express the related factor in terms that can be changed.

9. Do not include medical diagnoses in the nursing diagnosis.

10. State the diagnosis clearly and concisely.

Completed diagnostic statements should be validated with the client whenever possible and documented in the medical record. Test Yourself exercises 4-1 through 4-4 will help you to apply the concepts covered in this chapter. If you have difficulty, reread the content and try again.

REFERENCES

Carroll-Johnson RM (ed): Classification of Nursing Diagnoses: Proceedings of the Eighth Conference. Philadelphia: JB Lippincott, 1989.

Gordon M: Manual of Nursing Diagnosis. New York: McGraw-Hill, 1993.

Kim MJ, McFarland GK, and McLane AM: Pocket Guide to Nursing Diagnosis, 3rd ed. St. Louis: CV Mosby, 1993.

Taptich BJ, Iyer P, and Bernocchi-Losey D: Nursing Diagnosis and Care Planning, 2nd ed. Philadelphia: WB Saunders, 1994.

BIBLIOGRAPHY

Briody ME et al: Toward further understanding of nursing diagnosis: An interpretation. Nurs Diagn 1992; 3(3):124-128.

Bulechek GM and McClosky TC: Nursing Diagnosis, Interventions and Outcomes: Nursing Interventions Essential Nursing Treatments. Philadelphia: WB Saunders, 1992.

Creason N: How do we define our diagnoses? Am J Nurs 1987; 87(2):230–231.

Henning M: Comparison of nursing diagnostic statements using a functional health pattern and health history/body systems format. In: Carroll-Johnson RM (ed): Classification of Nursing Diagnoses: Proceedings of the Ninth Conference. Philadelphia: JB Lippincott, 1991.

Larrabee JH et al: Developing and implementing computer-generated nursing care plans. J Nurs Care Qual 1992; 6(2):56-62.

Mitchell GJ: Diagnosis: clarifying or obscuring the nature of nursing. Nurs Sci Q 1991; 4(2):52.

Neel C: Making nursing diagnosis work for you . . . every day. Nursing 1986; 86(5):56–57.

Rantz MJ and Miller TV: Quality Documentation for Long-Term Care: A Nursing Diagnosis Approach. Gaithersburg, MD: Aspen Publishers, 1993.

FIVE

PLANNING: PRIORITY-SETTING AND DEVELOPING OUTCOMES

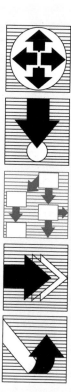

OBJECTIVES

After reading this chapter, you will be able to:

1. List four steps of the planning phase of the nursing process.
2. Set priorities for care using the human needs hierarchy.
3. Define client outcome and describe its purpose for the nurse and the client.
4. Name seven guidelines for writing outcomes.
5. Identify five types of human responses for which outcomes may be written.

INTRODUCTION

Planning involves the development of strategies designed to reinforce healthy client responses or to prevent, minimize, or correct unhealthy client responses identified in the nursing diagnosis. This phase begins after the formulation of the diagnostic statement and concludes with the actual documentation of the plan of care.

During the planning phase, outcomes and nursing interventions are developed. The outcomes indicate what the client will be able to do as a result of the nursing actions. The nursing interventions describe how the nurse can help the client to achieve the outcomes.

The planning component of the nursing process consists of four stages:

1. Setting priorities
2. Developing outcomes
3. Developing nursing interventions
4. Documenting the plan

This chapter will address the first two stages: priority-setting and developing outcomes. Chapter 6 will discuss nursing interventions and documentation.

STAGE 1: SETTING PRIORITIES

A thorough nursing assessment may identify many actual or potential responses that require nursing intervention, as shown in Chapter 4. The development of a plan incorporating all of these may be unrealistic or unmanageable. Therefore, a system must be established to determine which diagnosis or diagnoses will be addressed first. The most common mechanism is the human needs hierarchy, developed by Maslow (1943) and refined by Kalish (1983) as previously described in Chapter 2 (Figs. 5-1 and 5-2).

Survival Needs

Survival needs have been identified as those associated with food, air, water, manageable temperature, elimination, rest, and pain avoidance. These are the most basic needs and clients tend to utilize all available resources to satisfy them. Only then is it possible to focus on higher level needs.

Examples of survival needs in nursing diagnoses include the following:

NEED	NURSING DIAGNOSIS
Food	Altered nutrition: less than body requirements related to decreased appetite
Air	Impaired gas exchange related to retained secretions
Water	Fluid volume deficit related to persistent vomiting
Temperature	Hyperthermia related to effects of prolonged exposure to heat
Elimination	Diarrhea related to excessive intake of spicy food
Rest	Sleep pattern disturbance related to excessive noise
Pain	Pain related to muscle spasms

Stimulation Needs

Stimulation needs include those associated with sex, activity, exploration, manipulation, and novelty. When survival needs are met, the client will attempt to satisfy stimulation needs before moving up the hierarchy. This response is

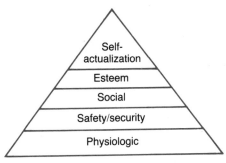

FIGURE 5-1. Maslow's model.

(Reprinted with permission from Maslow A: A theory of human motivation. Psychol Rev 1943; *50*:370.)

often seen in hospitalized clients who participate more actively in their care or request television, radio, magazines or other diversional activities when they are feeling better.

    Examples of stimulation needs in nursing diagnoses include the following:

NEED	NURSING DIAGNOSES
Sex	Sexual dysfunction related to discomfort secondary to decreased vaginal secretions
Activity	Diversional activity deficit related to effects of hospitalization
Exploration	Impaired physical mobility related to effects of right-sided weakness
Manipulation	Self-care deficit related to early morning pain secondary to inflammatory process
Novelty	Altered sensory perception related to stimulus deprivation secondary to isolation

Safety

The next levels in the hierarchy are the needs for safety, security, and protection. Clients focus on these needs after survival and stimulation needs have been satisfied. Remember that safety needs are of particular concern in the elderly or very young and may be exaggerated when they are exposed to an unfamiliar environment.

    Some examples of nursing diagnoses incorporating safety needs include the following:

NEED	NURSING DIAGNOSIS
Security	Impaired home maintenance management related to insufficient finances
Safety	High risk for trauma related to lack of awareness of environmental hazards
Protection	High risk for violence: self-directed related to feelings of hopelessness

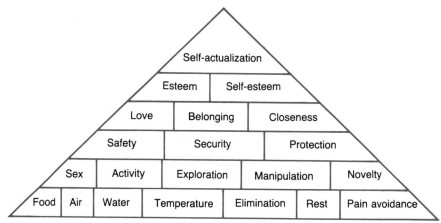

FIGURE 5-2.   Kalish's refinement of Maslow's model.

(Reprinted by permission of Brooks/Cole, Monterey, CA, from Kalish R: The Psychology of Human Behavior, 5th ed. by Wadsworth, Inc, 1983, 1977, 1973, 1970, 1966.)

Love and Belonging

Love, belonging, and closeness needs reflect an individual's ability to affiliate or interact with others in the environment and are met through involvement with family, friends, and coworkers. You will often encounter these needs in clients requiring prolonged hospitalization, those isolated for protection or because of infection, and those placed in areas where visiting privileges may be restricted.

Examples of nursing diagnoses reflecting love and belonging needs include the following:

NEED	NURSING DIAGNOSES
Love	Altered parenting related to impaired maternal infant bonding
Belonging	Altered family processes related to effects of terminal illness
Closeness	Social isolation related to prolonged hospitalization

Esteem

This level of the hierarchy relates to the need for the respect of oneself and others. The individual strives for recognition, usefulness, independence, dignity, and freedom. The health care system frequently magnifies deficits in these areas. Clients often perceive that it is necessary to surrender responsibility for elements of daily care to health care providers because they are hospitalized. The existing health care system perpetuates this perception as clients are expected to wear hospital attire and conform to the unit routine. As a result, individuals who are capable of self-care often expect nurses to pour their water, comb their hair, or shave them.

Examples of nursing diagnoses reflecting esteem needs include the following:

NEED	NURSING DIAGNOSES
Esteem	Powerlessness related to perceived lack of support systems
	Dysfunctional grieving related to change in body image secondary to mastectomy
	Personal identity disturbance related to persistent peer pressure

Self-Actualization

The highest level need in the hierarchy is self-actualization. Individuals strive to make the most of their physical, mental, emotional, and social abilities in order to feel that they are being what they wish to be. Most clients chose a lifestyle that utilizes their individual knowledge, talents, and skills. Clients in a hospital setting are frequently not concerned with self-actualization needs, because they are preoccupied with fulfilling lower level needs. However, clients may demonstrate concerns about their ability to achieve self-actualization as a result of changes that may have occurred during hospitalization. For example, clients who have experienced traumatic injuries may not be able to participate in work, recreational, and social activities that have provided self-fulfillment in the past.

Examples of nursing diagnoses that relate to self-actualization include the following:

NEED	NURSING DIAGNOSES
Self-Actualization	Altered thought processes related to effects of alcohol consumption
	High risk for violence directed at others related to inability to control behavior
	Family coping: potential for growth related to successful development of coping skills

In Chapter 2, you reviewed the example of Maria Roselli, who was admitted to the hospital for scheduled lung surgery. Your assessment data led you to identify three responses of concern: fear, altered breathing patterns, and high risk for infection. Using Maslow and Kalish's model, you would prioritize her diagnoses as follows:

NEED	CLIENT RESPONSES
Survival	Altered breathing patterns related to decreased lung expansion, fear
Safety	High risk for infection related to hazards of invasive procedure, history of previous infections
Security	Fear related to outcome of surgery, anticipated pain, need for chest tube postoperatively

Remember, however, that it is not necessary to completely resolve needs at one level before you move to another. In Maria's case, you would focus on her breathing patterns but would also try to help her to resolve some of her fears.

Maslow's hierarchy provides a constructive resource for the nurse to utilize in setting priorities for nursing diagnoses. Kalish's expansion of Maslow's model assists the nurse in differentiating more clearly between levels of needs. Ordinarily, clients progress up the hierarchy of needs, therefore you can prioritize nursing diagnoses according to their placement in the hierarchy.

ANA Measurement Criteria Standard III. Outcome Identification (Standard of Care): The nurse identifies expected outcomes individualized to the client.

STAGE 2: WRITING OUTCOMES

Outcomes are an important component of the planning phase of the nursing process. Outcomes are also referred to as *goals* or *behavioral objectives*. Regardless of what they are called, their purpose is the same: they define how the nurse and the client know that the human response identified in the diagnostic statement has been prevented, modified, or corrected. Therefore, outcomes also serve as a blueprint for the evaluation component of the process because well-written outcomes make it possible to determine the effectiveness of nursing interventions.

The following guidelines will help to develop well-written outcomes.

ANA Measurement Criteria Standard III.1 (Standard of Care): Outcomes are derived from the diagnosis.

1. Outcomes Are Derived from the Nursing Diagnosis

Nursing diagnostic statements identify actual or potential responses that are considered to be problematic for the client. This implies that alternative

5-1 TEST YOURSELF

Identification of Needs

Utilizing Maslow's Hierarchy, identify the type of need being addressed in each of the following nursing diagnostic statements.

NURSING DIAGNOSIS	NEED
1. High risk for violence directed at others related to effects of hallucinations	
2. Role performance disturbance related to effects of chronic pain	
3. Ineffective family coping: disabling related to recurrent marital discord	
4. Sleep pattern disturbance related to sensory overload	
5. Diversional activity deficit related to long-term confinement to home	
6. Spiritual distress related to inability to practice spiritual rituals	

5-1 TEST YOURSELF

Identification of Needs: Answers

NURSING DIAGNOSIS	NEED
1. High risk for violence directed at others related to effects of hallucinations	Safety/security
2. Role performance disturbance related to effects of chronic pain	Esteem
3. Ineffective family coping: disabling related to recurrent marital discord	Love and belonging
4. Sleep pattern disturbance related to sensory overload	Physiological (survival)
5. Diversional activity deficit related to long-term confinement to home	Physiological (stimulation)
6. Spiritual distress related to inability to practice spiritual rituals	Self-actualization

INTRODUCTION
SETTING
PRIORITIES
*WRITING OUT-
COMES*
*Derived from the
Diagnoses*

responses are required or preferred. For example, the nursing diagnosis "altered nutrition: less than body requirements related to chewing difficulties" suggests that the nutritional status of the client is less than optimal. This diagnosis indicates that improved nutrition is required. Similarly, the nursing diagnosis "high risk for infection related to prolonged weakness and immobility" suggests that the client is at risk for infection and requires nursing intervention or assistance to prevent its occurrence.

Outcomes should reflect the first half of the diagnostic statement by identifying alternative healthful responses that are desirable for the client. Outcomes also help to define specific behaviors that demonstrate that the problem has been prevented, minimized, or corrected. Answering the question "How will I know that the response has been changed?" will help to determine appropriate outcomes.

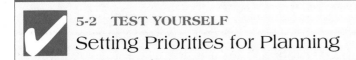
Ted Alexander was in the ICU for five days. His physical condition appeared to be stabilizing when he suddenly developed acute pain and bleeding through his nasogastric tube. A diagnostic gastroscopy discovered a tear in Ted's stomach. He underwent emergency surgery. This is Ted's first surgical experience. His social worker has informed you that one of Ted's children has become ill in Las Vegas, which has delayed their trip to Atlantic City by one week. Ted's employer has been making inquiries as to his progress and has expressed concern that the deal Ted was working on may fall through because of his illness. Ted has now returned to your unit after surgery and you are developing his care plan.

You have developed the nursing diagnoses listed in column 1. Identify the need addressed in column 2. For the purpose of this exercise, use Kalish's hierarchy to set priorities in dealing with these needs:

1. Survival
2. Stimulation
3. Safety
4. Love and belonging
5. Esteem
6. Self actualization

NURSING DIAGNOSIS	LEVEL OF NEED ACCORDING TO THE HIERARCHY
1. Situational low self-esteem r/t to fear of prolonged disability	1.
2. Ineffective breathing pattern r/t effects of anesthesia and history of smoking	2.
3. Parental role conflict r/t separation from children secondary to acute illness	3.
4. High risk for ineffective individual coping r/t effects of acute illness, lack of support system	4.
5. High risk for infection r/t hazards of invasive lines	5.
6. Self care deficit (bathing) r/t pain, activity intolerance	6.

5-2 TEST YOURSELF
Setting Priorities for Planning: Answers

NURSING DIAGNOSIS	LEVEL OF NEED ACCORDING TO THE HIERARCHY
1. Situational low self-esteem r/t to fear of prolonged disability	1. Esteem
2. Ineffective breathing pattern r/t effects of anesthesia and history of smoking	2. Survival
3. Parental role conflict r/t separation from children secondary to acute illness	3. Love and belonging
4. High risk for ineffective individual coping r/t effects of acute illness, lack of support system	4. Self-actualization
5. High risk for infection r/t hazards of invasive lines	5. Safety
6. Self-care deficit (bathing) r/t pain, activity intolerance	6. Stimulation

Example

Nursing Diagnosis Altered nutrition: less than body requirements related to chewing difficulties (broken dentures)

OUTCOME:

INCORRECT	CORRECT
No evidence of skin breakdown throughout hospitalization	Consumes 1800 calories of pureed and liquid foods each 24-hour period

In this example, the incorrectly stated outcome refers to skin integrity rather than to nutritional status. Certainly, there is a relationship between decreased nutritional status and the potential for skin breakdown. However, the correctly written outcome more appropriately answers the question "How will I know that the client's nutritional status is improved?" This outcome not only identifies the desirable limits of caloric intake for the client but also specifies that this intake be accomplished within each 24-hour period.

Example

OUTCOME:		Nursing Diagnosis
INCORRECT	CORRECT	High risk for infection related to prolonged weakness and immobility
Verbalizes decreased weakness within 24 hours	No evidence of infection throughout hospitalization	

In this example, the outcome is related to the second part of the diagnostic statement, referring to "weakness" rather than to the risk for infection. The correctly written outcome also demonstrates a broader, more long-term outcome than in the 24-hour period seen in the previous example.

Generally, outcomes are written to focus on the behavior of the client. The outcome should address what the client will do and when and to what extent it will be accomplished.

Example.   Consider the case of an 82-year-old woman who falls and fractures her hip. Because she will be on bedrest and unable to ambulate and move in her usual patterns, she is at risk for skin breakdown.

OUTCOME:		Nursing Diagnosis
INCORRECT	CORRECT	High risk for impaired skin integrity related to decreased mobility
Prevent skin breakdown	No evidence of skin breakdown over bony prominences throughout hospitalization	

The incorrectly written outcome is nurse-focused rather than client-centered. The correctly written outcome clearly identifies the criterion that will be used to determine whether or not the client's skin integrity has been maintained.

WRITING OUT-
COMES
Derived from
the Diagnoses
Measurable

ANA Measurement
Criteria Standard
III.2 (Standard of
Care): Outcomes
are documented as
measurable goals.

2. Outcomes Are Documented as Measurable Goals

Outcomes should address what the client will do, when it will be accomplished, and to what extent. Observable and measurable outcomes define the "what" and "to what extent."

Example

Nursing Diagnosis
Noncompliance
(1800 calorie ADA
diet) related to lack
of knowledge

OUTCOME:	
INCORRECT	CORRECT
Appreciates importance of adhering to 1800-calorie ADA diet	Prior to discharge, states intent to adhere to 1800-calorie ADA diet

It is difficult to evaluate an individual's appreciation of an activity. The client's recognition and acceptance of the behavior can be measured by statements or other similar responses.

When outcomes are measurable, observations can be made to determine whether they have been achieved. Compare the following and note that the second example is both measurable and observable:

Nursing Diagnosis
Fluid volume
deficit related to
excessive dia-
phoresis

OUTCOME:	
INCORRECT	CORRECT
Drinks adequate amounts of fluids	Drinks 2000 ml in 24 hours

Sometimes nurses write outcomes that are too broad or vague, or that may need to be broken down into more specific components.

Nursing Diagnosis
Knowledge def-
icit (disease
process—angina)

OUTCOME:	
INCORRECT	CORRECT
After the third teaching session:	After the third teaching session:
Knows about condition (angina)	Lists the cause of angina
	Identifies steps to alleviate pain
	Describes three activities that reduce anginal episodes

3. Outcomes Are Mutually Formulated with the Client and the Health Care Providers, When Possible

During the initial assessment, the nurse begins involving the client in the planning of care. In the interview, the nurse learns about what the client perceives as the primary health problem. This leads to the formulation of nursing diagnoses. The client and nurse should validate the diagnoses and outcomes. In the context of discussion, they can exchange expectations and modify any unrealistic or unacceptable outcomes. The inclusion of the client as an active participant in the plan of care will help to facilitate the achievement of the outcomes.

Example. Carol McAloon is caring for Mark Soffer, a diabetic with recurrent foot problems. During the interview the client expresses concern about his ability to care for his feet properly. Carol says, "Before you leave the hospital, we will review the proper way to wash and dry your feet, the signs of an infection, and what to do if you find an infection. How does this sound?" Mr. Soffer says, "Great, that's what I want to know!"

During this conversation, the nurse has set outcomes and validated them with the client. By the time of discharge, the client will:

- Demonstrate proper foot care
- Describe signs of infection
- State the course of action to follow if infection occurs

One of the consequences of failure to validate outcomes with a client may be the client's refusal to participate in the plan of care. This may occur if the client feels the outcomes are impossible to achieve or are in conflict with personal values.

Example. Reverend Johnson had a hernia repair four hours ago. You are caring for him in the ambulatory surgery unit and note that he is diaphoretic, pale, and lying in a rigid position. You repeatedly offer an injectable pain medication, which the client refuses.

Your outcome for the client: Asks for pain medication when needed	*The client's goal for himself:* Get through this without having to take a shot

In this case, your outcome and the client's outcome are in conflict. In this situation strategies must be used to resolve the disagreement and to formulate an outcome that is acceptable to both. By exploring the client's reasons for refusal of the injection and offering acceptable pain management techniques, you involve the client in choices about his care. Options might include oral analgesics, relaxation, or distraction techniques.

WRITING OUTCOMES

Derived from the Diagnoses

Measurable

Formulated with Client/Health Care Providers

ANA Measurement Criteria Standard III.3 (Standard of Care): Outcomes are mutually formulated with the client and health care providers, when possible.

Nursing Diagnosis Pain related to effects of surgery

Other health care providers should also be involved in formulating outcomes. Examples might include physicians, clinical nurse specialists, physical therapists, dietitians, speech therapists.

Example. Mike Esmond is recuperating after a knee replacement and goes to physical therapy twice daily for ambulation. You have developed a diagnosis related to his impaired physical mobility and wish to set a reasonable outcome. You meet with Mike and the physical therapist and determine that Mike needs to walk 50 feet four times daily using crutches within two days.

Here, you involved both the client and the therapist in formulating an outcome for the client's mobility needs. This type of dialogue promotes successful achievement of outcomes because the client is involved and the expertise of both the nurse and the physical therapist are utilized.

WRITING OUT-COMES

Derived from the Diagnoses

Measurable

Formulated with Client/Health Care Providers

Realistic

4. Outcomes Are Realistic in Relation to the Client's Present and Potential Capabilities

When writing outcomes, it is important that they be realistic in terms of the client's abilities. Factors to consider include the client's intelligence, level of education, and physical/emotional condition.

You should be aware of the client's level of intelligence and education when developing outcomes. For example, when caring for Peggy O'Malley, a 45-year-old severely retarded client, it is not realistic to write an outcome such as "Takes medications as ordered without assistance." A more reasonable outcome might be "Takes medications when assisted by home health aide." Education is an important component of nursing management, however, frequently materials prepared for clients may be difficult or impossible for them to understand. This is particularly evident in clients who have little or no formal education. Writing an outcome "Reads 'Tuberculosis and You' booklet by 11/30" is not realistic for a migrant worker who cannot read. A more appropriate outcome may be "After individual teaching on 11/30, describes tuberculosis."

When writing outcomes, you should also consider the client's physical condition. Often physical skills are required for clients to implement prescribed interventions and frequently their primary or secondary health problems may affect their ability to achieve outcomes.

ANA Measurement Criteria Standard III.4 (Standard of Care). Outcomes are realistic in relation to the client's present and potential capabilities.

Example. Bob Holder is a 78-year-old client who was recently diagnosed with coronary artery disease. Your knowledge of lifestyle changes required for management of this disease suggests that an exercise program is an important component of the client's postdischarge care. You develop an outcome of "Walks briskly for 30 minutes three times weekly." Further discussion with Mr. Holder reveals that he also has arthritis, which severely limits his walking capabilities. After discussion with the client, you develop an appropriate outcome of "Swims at least 20 laps in heated pool three times weekly."

The client's emotional status should also be a factor when developing outcomes. Clients who are emotionally unstable as a result of short- or long-term problems are often unable to accomplish tasks or acquire skills until their emotional issues are controlled or resolved.

Example. Joan Wilson is a 24-year-old married woman who has been diagnosed with cancer of the uterus and is admitted to your unit the morning of a scheduled hysterectomy. She is upset about her diagnosis, says she is afraid that she will die even though her cancer was diagnosed early, and is depressed about not being able to have children. An outcome of "Accepts diagnosis prior to discharge" is probably not realistic given the client's emotional state. A more realistic oucome might be "Verbalizes feelings about diagnosis to person of choice prior to discharge." Joan will probably require a substantial period of time to deal with the multiple issues surrounding her diagnosis and treatment.

Occasionally, outcomes are written for others when the client is unble to participate. In the case of 5-year-old David, a newly diagnosed insulin-dependent diabetic, his mother was identified as the person who will administer David's insulin until he is old enough to be taught to self-inject.

OUTCOME: Prior to discharge, David's mother will demonstrate correct insulin injection technique.

Nursing Diagnosis Knowledge deficit (insulin injection technique)

5. Outcomes Are Attainable in Relation to Resources Available to the Client

The outcomes you develop should be achievable considering the resources of the client. The client's ability to achieve outcomes may be affected by many factors, including finances, the capabilities of the care-giver and the setting in which care is provided.

Example. A diabetic hindered by a low income may be unable to purchase a home glucose monitoring system. Therefore, it may be unrealistic to write an outcome and develop a teaching plan encouraging the use of this system.

The strengths and weaknesses of the nursing staff should also be considered when formulating outcomes. Factors to evaluate may include the nurses' level of knowledge, autonomy, and availability.

Example. A woman who is pregnant with triplets is admitted to an obstetrical unit. None of the nurses working in the department has cared for a similar client. The perinatal clinical specialist has knowledge of the special care required in this situation. The specialist provides the information and helps the staff to formulate realistic client outcomes.

Finally, the resources of the setting must be considered when formulating attainable outcomes. Factors to take into account include the availability of equipment, facilities, and personnel.

WRITING OUTCOMES Derived from the Diagnoses Measurable Formulated with Client/Health Care Providers Realistic *Attainable*

ANA Measurement Criteria Standard III.5 (Standard of Care): Outcomes are attainable in relation to resources available to the client.

Examples

THE IDEAL	THE REAL
Spends four hours a day in a wheelchair	There are two wheelchairs and five clients who need them
Showers every day by 9:00 AM	There are 10 clients in a group home who need to use one shower by 9:00 AM each day

Clearly, the outcomes must be attainable given the resources that are available to the client. The abilities of the health care provider and the resources of the setting in which they are written are also important when developing outcomes. Additionally, the nurse must be able to identify and modify unrealistic or unachievable outcomes.

WRITING OUT-COMES
Derived from the Diagnoses
Measurable
Formulated with Client/Health Care Providers
Realistic
Attainable
Include Time Estimate

ANA Measurement Criteria Standard III.6 (Standard of Care): Outcomes include a time estimate for attainment.

6. Outcomes Include a Time Estimate for Attainment

The time allotted for achievement of the outcome should be stated. Time frames may be very limited, such as "within four hours," "on the first postop day," or "by the end of the first teaching session." These suggest a more specific time for evaluating the achievement of the outcome. Outcomes may also be stated to include broader perspectives, such as "by the time of discharge" or "throughout hospitalization." However, it must be pointed out that when these broader time periods are used, the nurse periodically evaluates the client's progress rather than waiting until the time of discharge or until the end of a hospitalization.

Examples

OUTCOME:	
INCORRECT	CORRECT
Ambulates with assistance in room	Ambulates with assistance in room within 48 hours

OUTCOME:	
INCORRECT	CORRECT
Moves bowels	Bowel movement within two days

7. Outcomes Provide Direction for Continuity of Care

A clearly written outcome enhances communication among care-givers and promotes continuity of care. Ambiguous or abstract wording should be avoided because it will tend to confuse rather than help the staff caring for a client. Simple terms and standard terminology will also help.

Examples

OUTCOME:

INCORRECT	CORRECT
CDBPDI q2	Coughs, deep breathes, and performs postural drainage independently q2h

Nursing Diagnosis
Ineffective airway clearance related to retained secretions

Outcomes should have as few words as possible yet still be clear. Long, involved outcomes can frequently be stated in fewer words. Compare the following outcomes. Which meets the criteria for being clear and concise, yet ensures that the correct information is communicated to other providers to ensure continuity of care?

OUTCOME:

INCORRECT	CORRECT
The client will discuss expectations of this hospitalization and previous hospital admissions and will discuss impending surgery with a basic knowledge of pre- and postop care	Prior to surgery, discusses expectations of hospitalization and surgery

Nursing Diagnosis
Knowledge deficit (hospitalization and surgical experience)

When writing outcomes, it is possible to eliminate the words "the client will . . ." at the beginning. It should be obvious from the way the outcome is stated that it is referring to the behaviors that the client will exhibit. At times, the outcome may include family members or others instead of or in addition to the client in order to ensure that care will be continuous:

OUTCOME: Prior to discharge, Manuel's mother discusses her feelings of inadequacy.

INDIVIDUAL RESPONSES AND OUTCOMES

Outcomes can be written to manage a variety of individual responses, including appearance and body function, specific symptoms, knowledge, skills, and emotions.

Appearance and Body Function

This category includes a number of observable manifestations. The following outcome written for a woman undergoing chemotherapy fits into this category: "Throughout chemotherapy, no evidence of ulcerations in oral cavity." This is a readily observable outcome that relates to the condition of her oral mucous membranes.

Examples

NURSING DIAGNOSES	OUTCOMES
Constipation related to decreased peristalsis and change in diet	Within 48 hours, bowel sounds present, expels flatus/BM
High risk for impaired gas exchange related to incisional pain	Lung sounds present and clear bilaterally each shift
Impaired corneal tissue integrity related to hazards associated with contact lenses	No evidence of corneal abrasion within the next three months

The outcomes illustrated above refer to the appearance and functioning of the client's body. It is important to note that a nursing diagnosis can be accompanied by more than one outcome. At times, several outcomes may be needed to define the prevention, modification, or resolution of a client response. In other situations, outcomes may change as the client progresses.

Specific Symptoms

Outcomes may be written to address the reduction or alleviation of symptoms that are interfering with the client's health status. Examples of symptoms include nausea, vomiting, diarrhea, constipation, burning sensation while urinating, frequent urination, pain, stiffness, weakness, and many others. The nurse identifies the symptoms during the assessment phase, develops appropriate nursing diagnoses during the diagnostic phase, writes outcomes to

Identification of Correctly and Incorrectly Written Outcomes

The following is a list of nursing diagnoses and outcomes. Decide whether each outcome is correctly or incorrectly written. If incorrectly stated, identify the guideline violated from the list that appears at the end of the chapter.

NURSING DIAGNOSIS	OUTCOME	CORRECT/INCORRECT RULE
1. Situational low self-esteem related to feelings of inadequacy 2° loss of job	Verbalizes positive feelings about self daily	
2. Altered health maintenance related to lack of knowledge about insulin injections	Injects self with insulin	
3. High risk for caregiver role strain related to age, inexperience in caring for sick (care giver indigent)	Takes vacation to Disneyland before mother comes home	
4. Fear related to unknown outcome of surgery	Before surgery, verbalizes fears regarding outcome of surgery	
5. Relocation stress syndrome related to age, frequent, traumatic moves in the past	Understands stress associated with frequent moves	
6. Altered nutrition: more than body requirements related to imbalance between caloric intake and activity	Loses 2 lb per week until weight of 110 lb is achieved	
7. Sleep pattern disturbance related to auditory/visual hallucinations	Decrease in number of auditory/visual hallucinations	

5-3 TEST YOURSELF

Identification of Correctly and Incorrectly Written Outcomes: Answers

NURSING DIAGNOSIS	OUTCOME	CORRECT/INCORRECT RULE
1. Situational low self-esteem related to feelings of inadequacy 2° loss of job	Verbalizes positive feelings about self daily	✔
2. Altered health maintenance related to lack of knowledge about insulin injections	Injects self with insulin	✔ 2,6
3. High risk for care-giver role strain related to age, inexperience in caring for sick (care-giver indigent)	Takes vacation in Disneyland before mother comes home	✔ 5
4. Fear related to unknown outcome of surgery	Before surgery, verbalizes fears regarding outcome of surgery	✔
5. Relocation stress syndrome related to age, frequent, traumatic moves in the past	Understands stress associated with frequent moves	✔ 4,6
6. Altered nutrition: more than body requirements related to imbalance between caloric intake and activity	Loses 2 lb per week until weight of 110 lb is achieved	✔
7. Sleep pattern disturbance related to auditory/visual hallucinations	Decrease in number of auditory/visual hallucinations	✔ 1,6

5-4 TEST YOURSELF
Revision of Incorrectly Written Outcomes

The outcomes that were incorrectly written in the previous exercise are listed below. Revise each outcome so that it is correctly stated.

NURSING DIAGNOSIS	OUTCOME	REVISED
1. Altered health maintenance related to lack of knowledge about insulin injections	Injects self with insulin	
2. High risk for care-giver role strain related to age, inexperience in caring for sick (care-giver indigent)	Takes vacation to Disneyland before mother comes home	
3. Relocation stress syndrome related to age, frequent, traumatic moves in the past	Understands stress associated with frequent moves	
4. Sleep pattern disturbance related to auditory/visual hallucinations	Decrease in number of auditory/visual hallucinations	

5-4 TEST YOURSELF
Revision of Incorrectly Written Outcomes: Answers

NURSING DIAGNOSIS	OUTCOME	REVISED
1. Altered health maintenance related to lack of knowledge about insulin injections	Injects self with insulin	Within 48 hours verbalizes need to learn health maintenance skills
2. High risk for care-giver role strain related to age, inexperience in caring for sick (care-giver indigent)	Takes vacation to Disneyland before mother comes home	Verbalizes confidence in ability to manage mother's care after attending care-giver's course
3. Relocation stress syndrome related to age frequent, traumatic moves in the past	Understands stress associated with frequent moves	Verbalizes decreased stress within two weeks after move
4. Sleep pattern disturbance related to auditory/visual hallucinations	Decrease in number of auditory/visual hallucinations	Within 24 hours, sleeps at least four hours uninterrupted q 24 hours

address them, and determines interventions to alleviate them during the planning phase.

Examples

NURSING DIAGNOSES	OUTCOME
Chronic pain related to inflammatory process	Takes pain medication when needed
Fear related to outcome of diagnostic studies	Verbalizes decreased fear within 48 hours

Knowledge

Outcomes may be formulated that involve the recall of information taught to the client. In order to determine whether the material has been mastered, outcomes should be developed that demonstrate comprehension and retention of certain information. Clients may be asked to list, describe, state, define, identify, or otherwise demonstrate knowledge acquisition and integration.

Example

OUTCOME: By the end of the first teaching session:

- ☐ defines diabetes
- ☐ explains relationship between diet and exercise

Psychomotor Skills

Psychomotor skills are often the subject of outcomes. Examples include the following:

- Injection of medications
- Transfer from bed to wheelchair
- Catheterization of self or others
- Counting pulse rate
- Performing CPR on mannequin
- Inserting intravenous catheters
- Testing urine or blood for glucose

The outcomes that are written for psychomotor skills identify what the client should be able to do as a result of the teaching plan.

Examples

NURSING DIAGNOSES	OUTCOMES
Altered health maintenance related to lack of knowledge about foot care	By the end of the second teaching session, demonstrates proper technique for foot care
Altered parenting related to lack of knowledge of newborn care	By the time of discharge, feeds, bathes, and diapers newborn

5-5   TEST YOURSELF

Developing Correctly Written Outcomes from Case Studies

Develop a correctly written outcome for each of the case studies presented below. Use the guidelines listed earlier in the chapter to correctly phrase the outcome.

Case 1. Cassie Tilton is an 88-year-old woman transferred to your unit from a skilled nursing facility. Her history reveals that she had a "flu-like" syndrome for the past five days with persistent vomiting and diarrhea. Her vital signs are B/P 108/56, P 112, R 28, and T 101.4. Her mucous membranes are dry and her skin turgor is decreased. She indicates that she feels weak, tired, and thirsty.

NURSING DIAGNOSIS:

Fluid volume deficit related to vomiting and diarrhea

OUTCOME:

Case 2. Chip Ireland is a 35-year-old businessman admitted to the outpatient surgicenter for a tonsillectomy. He indicates that he has had recurrent tonsillitis for the last three years. Postoperatively, he complains of being thirsty and requests a cold drink. You observe that he has difficulty swallowing and coughs up the water. He states "my throat is too sore; it feels like it is swollen." Upon examination, you note the presence of redness and edema in the operative area.

NURSING DIAGNOSIS:

Impaired swallowing related to edema and effects of surgery

OUTCOME:

Case 3. Emily Fantin is an 86-year-old woman who calls the office nurse and requests free samples of laxatives. She complains, "I've spent so much money on laxatives at the drug store, I take them twice a day so that my bowels will move three times a day. My mother always told me to take laxatives to keep myself regular. By the way, do you have any sample enemas?" Upon further questioning you find out that Emily lives alone and

Continued.

5-5 TEST YOURSELF
Developing Correctly Written Outcomes from Case Studies–cont'd.

does her own cooking. She eats mostly frozen dinners or prepared foods with few fruits and vegetables. In addition, she shops at a local convenience store with a limited supply of fresh produce. She relies on Metamucil daily, and Ex Lax and Milk of Magnesia approximately four times a week. She states that she gets very little exercise.

NURSING DIAGNOSIS:

Perceived constipation related to long-standing family health beliefs.

OUTCOME:

Emotional Status

Outcomes may be written about the emotional status of the client. These outcomes frequently address how the client or family is responding to a crisis or stressful event. This may be an illness, family disruption, or a maturational crisis. After assessing the emotional response, the nurse develops an outcome that identifies the desired behavior that should result from nursing interventions.

Examples

NURSING DIAGNOSES	OUTCOMES
Ineffective individual coping related to lack of support systems	Verbalizes planned coping strategies prior to discharge
Hopelessness related to perceived lack of alternatives	After third counseling session, verbalizes hope for the future

SUMMARY

Outcomes should be derived from the nursing diagnosis. They should also be measurable, formulated with the client and health care providers, realistic, and attainable, include time estimates, and provide direction for

5-5 TEST YOURSELF

Developing Correctly Written Outcomes from Case Studies: Answers

Case 1. Cassie Tilton

NURSING DIAGNOSIS:

Fluid volume deficit related to vomiting and diarrhea

OUTCOME:

Within 48 hours, moist mucous membranes, vital signs within normal limits for client

Case 2. Chip Ireland

NURSING DIAGNOSIS:

Impaired swallowing related to edema and effects of surgery

OUTCOME:

Before discharge from surgicenter, swallows at least 240 ml of fluid at a time

Case 3. Emily Fantin

NURSING DIAGNOSIS:

Perceived constipation related to long-standing family health beliefs

OUTCOME:

Within two months, verbalizes satisfaction with one bowel movement q one to two days

continuity of care. Outcomes may refer to individual responses, including appearance and functioning of the body, specific symptoms, knowledge, psychomotor skills, and emotional status. Consideration of these factors will enable the nurse to formulate outcomes that are individualized, and continue the nursing process by developing interventions to achieve them and evaluating their efficacy. In review, here are the guidelines for writing outcomes:

1. Outcomes are derived from the nursing diagnoses.

2. Outcomes are documented as measurable goals.

3. Outcomes are mutually formulated with the client and the health care providers, when possible.

4. Outcomes are realistic in relation to the client's present and potential capabilities.

5. Outcomes are attainable in relation to resources available to the client.

6. Outcomes include a time estimate for attainment.

7. Outcomes provide direction for continuity of care.

Exercises 5-3 through 5-5 provide you with the opportunity to practice the information you have learned in this chapter. If you have difficulty, reread the chapter and try again.

REFERENCES

Kalish R: The Psychology of Human Behavior, 5th ed. Monterey, CA: Brooks/Cole, 1983.

Maslow A: A theory of human motivation. Psychol Rev 50:370, 1943.

BIBLIOGRAPHY

Ferrell BR et al: Clinical decision making and pain. Cancer Nurs 1991; 14(6):289–297.

Fitzmaurice JB et al: High-volume high-risk nursing diagnoses as a basis for priority setting in a tertiary hospital. In Carroll-Johnson RM (ed): Classification of Nursing Diagnoses: Proceedings of the Ninth Conference. Philadelphia: JB Lippincott, 1991.

Inzer F and Aspinal MJ: Evaluating patient outcomes. Nurs Outlook 1981; 29:178–181.

Kerr ME et al: Human response patterns to outcomes in the critically ill patient. J Nurs Qual Assur 1991; 5(2):32–40.

Kingsley A: First step towards a desired outcome: preventing infection by risk recognition. Prof Nurse 1992; 7(11):725–729.

Kuhn RC: Development of outcome standards in critical care. AACN Clin Issues Crit Care Nurs 1991; 2(1):22–30.

Lang NM and Marek KD: The classification of patient outcomes. J Profess Nurs 1990; 6(3): 158–163.

Larson E and Jacox A: Methods of measuring patient outcomes. J Nurs Qual Assur 1991; 5(2):78–84.

Matz LB and Gary G: Patient outcomes measure home health care accomplishments. Nurs Manag 1993; 24.

Moritz P: Innovative nursing practice models and patient outcomes. Nurs Outlook 1991; 39(3):111–114.

Ricciardi E and Kuch AW: Improving patient outcomes: The role of the clinical nurse specialist in quality assurance. J Nurs Care Qual 1992; 6(2):46–50.

SIX

PLANNING: NURSING INTERVENTIONS AND DOCUMENTATION

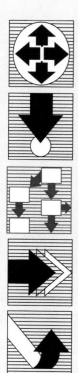

OBJECTIVES

After reading this chapter, you will be able to:

1. Define the essential characteristics of nursing interventions.
2. Differentiate between interdependent and independent nursing interventions.
3. List the characteristics of nursing interventions.
4. Identify the role of critical thinking in the development of the plan of care.
5. Document the plan of care.
6. Describe the characteristics of the plan of care.
7. Describe four types of care plans.

INTRODUCTION

The stages of the planning phase of the nursing process are (1) setting priorities, (2) developing outcomes, (3) designing nursing interventions, and (4) documentation. The first two stages were addressed in the previous chapter. Once priorities have been established and outcomes developed, the next stages of planning begin.

    The third stage of planning involves writing nursing interventions that describe how the nurse will help the client to achieve the proposed outcomes.

These interventions are based on (1) the information obtained during the assessment interview and (2) the nurse's subsequent interactions with the client and family. The final phase—documentation—involves communicating the written plan of care to other members of the nursing staff. The plan of care is designed to share information about the client's significant health care needs, the outcomes identified by the nurse, and the planned interventions. Ideally, the plan of care is written by a registered nurse following the first contact with the client, is readily available, and contains current information. As computer technology becomes more widespread in health care, nurses will have increased access to the power of the computer for developing plans of care. This chapter will address these last two stages of the planning phase: developing nursing interventions and documenting the plan of care.

DEVELOPING
NURSING INTER-
VENTIONS
Definition

STAGE 3: DEVELOPING NURSING INTERVENTIONS

Definition

Nursing interventions are specific strategies designed to assist the client in achieving outcomes. They are based on the related factor(s) identified in the nursing diagnostic statement. Therefore, nursing interventions define the activities required to eliminate the factors contributing to the human response.

Example. "Hopelessness related to communication barriers." Communication barriers are the factors contributing to the human response of hopelessness. The nursing interventions in this case would focus on developing alternate methods of communication with the client.

Nursing Interven-
tions versus
Physician's Orders

Nursing Interventions versus Physician's Orders

Nursing interventions focus on the activities required to promote, maintain, or restore the client's health. In contrast, physician's orders usually focus on the activities involved in diagnosing and treating the client's medical condition. These orders are delegated to nurses and other health care personnel. Nursing interventions may also be delegated to others such as unlicensed personnel. For example, the nursing intervention of "record intake and output" may be carried out by a nursing assistant, the client, and the family. Physician's orders are written on an order sheet or entered into a computer terminal. Nursing interventions may also be entered into a computer, or documented on the Kardex and the plan of care. Physician's orders often include administration of medication, diagnostic tests, dietery requirements, and treatments. Nurses order teaching, treatments, preventive measures, assessments, consultations with other nursing personnel, and so on.

Types of Nursing Interventions

Nursing interventions may be categorized as interdependent or independent.

Interdependent Interventions

Interdependent interventions describe the activities that the nurse carries out in cooperation with other health care team members. The interventions may involve collaboration with social workers, dietitians, therapists, technicians, and physicians, and may add details as to how physician-initiated orders are to be carried out.

Example.   Matthew Barnicle is a client who is in kidney failure. The medical order states "restrict fluids to 580 ml PO plus 720 ml 5% dextrose in 45% sodium chloride solution IV every 24 hours." To define how this will be achieved, you and the dietitian calculate the amount of fluid Matthew may receive each shift. The nursing interventions are as follows:

1. Administer IV fluids at 30 ml/hr (total of 240 ml per shift) via IV pump
2. PO fluid intake:

    7:30 AM–3:30 PM: Total of 315 ml PO
       240 ml on dietary trays
       75 ml for medications

    3:30–11:30 PM: Total of 195 ml PO
       120 ml on dietary tray
       75 ml for medications

    11:30 PM–7:30 AM: Total of 80 ml PO for medications

  In this example, you and the dietitian collaborate to individualize the plan of care. This joint effort adds detail as to how the physician's order is to be carried out.

Independent Interventions

Independent interventions are the activities that may be performed by the nurse without a physician's order. The type of activities that nurses may order independently are defined by nursing diagnoses. They are the responses that nurses are licensed to treat by virtue of their education and experience.

Example.   Jason Lance is a 16-year-old adolescent who fell down a ravine and suffered a fractured hip. He has been discharged to home but must remain on bedrest for three weeks. Because of his physical limitations and Jason's complaints of boredom, as the home health nurse you recognize that he is experiencing a diversional activity deficit and write the following nursing diagnosis, outcome, and interventions:

Nursing Interventions versus
Physician's Orders
Types
Interdependent
Independent

NURSING DIAGNOSIS
Fluid volume excess related to compromised regulatory mechanisms secondary to kidney failure
OUTCOME
Receives no more than 1300 ml per day

NURSING DIAGNOSIS	OUTCOME	INTERVENTIONS
Diversional activity deficit related to social isolation	Within one week there will be a decrease in complaints of boredom	1. Explore with Jason activities of interest to him and how they can be worked into a time schedule 2. Collaborate with mom to explore possibility of scheduling friends/visitors on a daily basis

DEVELOPING NURSING INTER-VENTIONS

Definition

Nursing Interventions versus Physician's Orders

Types

Characteristics

ANA Measurement Criteria Standard IV-1 (Standard of Care): The plan is individualized to the client's condition or needs.

Characteristics of Interventions

The planning phase of the nursing process is addressed by the American Nurses' Association's Standards of Care (Fig. 6-1). Both outcomes and interventions are established in the planning phase. Figure 6-1 presents the criteria for the plan of care, which includes the nursing diagnosis, outcomes, and interventions. For the purposes of explaining interventions, the major points in Figure 6-1 will be discussed. Before documenting the plan of care, you should determine whether the interventions meet these criteria.

The Plan Is Individualized

The selection of nursing diagnoses, outcomes and interventions is based on your knowledge of the client. The plan of care should incorporate specific interventions that will address the client's needs.

One purpose of nursing interventions is to communicate how the client's care differs from that of another with a similar nursing or medical diagnosis. When developing interventions, choose approaches that will address the client's specific physical and emotional needs. The following are guidelines that should be used in the development of individualized nursing interventions:

1. Focus on the related factor(s) of the nursing diagnosis.
2. Consider client and family strengths and weaknesses.
3. Take into account the urgency and severity of the situation.

The Plan Is Individualized by Focusing on the Related Factor. The nursing diagnosis provides a basis for establishing individualized nursing interventions. As explained previously, an actual nursing diagnosis usually has two parts: the human response and the related/risk factor(s). The related/risk factor(s) specifies the origin of the human response and provides direction for specific nursing interventions. The nurse's knowledge of the client and the problem directs the formulation of individualized nursing interventions.

STANDARD IV. PLANNING
The Nurse Develops a Plan of Care That Prescribes Interventions to Attain Expected Outcomes

---

Measurement Criteria

1. The plan is individualized to the client's condition or needs.
2. The plan is developed with the client, significant others and health care providers, when appropriate.
3. The plan reflects current nursing practice.
4. The plan is documented.
5. The plan provides for continuity of care.

FIGURE 6-1   ANA Standard IV: Planning.

(Reprinted with permission from Standards of Clinical Nursing Practice. Washington, DC: American Nurses' Association, 1991.)

Example.   Betsey Moehlich is a 17-year-old hospitalized following a motorcycle accident. She is in skeletal traction for a fractured left leg.

Dona Vessels, an 84-year-old, is a resident of a nursing home. She is thin, slightly dehydrated, and is confined to bed.

Both clients have the nursing diagnosis "high risk for impaired skin integrity related to immobility" and the outcome "no evidence of skin breakdown while on bedrest." Note that although the nursing diagnosis and outcome are the same for both clients, the nursing interventions are individualized:

NURSING INTERVENTIONS

BETSEY	**DONA**
1. Apply foam mattress to bed	1. Apply air mattress to bed
2. Encourage client to use trapeze to change position	2. Assist client to change position q2h (see turning schedule); include prone position at least once per shift

---

The Plan Focuses on the Client's Strengths and Weaknesses.   When developing individualized nursing interventions, the strengths and weaknesses of the client and the family must be considered. The client's assets should be identified and utilized in planning care. Strengths may include motivation, intelligence, a supportive family, education, and economic resources.

NURSING DIAGNOSIS
Knowledge deficit (angina management)
OUTCOME
Within one week verbalizes pathology and management of angina

Example. Erin Mirabelli is a 52-year-old with new-onset angina. Erin is highly motivated and self-disciplined. She returned to college when her children were grown and graduated with a degree in biology. She is currently employed as a laboratory technician in industry. She maintains an active schedule, including aerobics and swimming.

The nurse practitioner decides to utilize Erin's strengths in planning her education on management of angina. Erin is provided with self-learning packages on the fundamentals of pathology and management of angina. She is also identified as a good candidate for smoking cessation classes.

The client's weaknesses or deficits should also be identified. The absence of motivation, intelligence, family support, economic resources, or education may act as a deterrent to achieving identified outcomes. Other deficits might include chronic illness, debilitation, depression, social withdrawal, or a language barrier.

In the following situation, the nurse considered the client's physical deficits when planning care.

NURSING DIAGNOSIS
Impaired physical mobility related to weakness and visual deficit
OUTCOME
Ambulates independently within one week

Example. Pepe Villanueva is a 76-year-old man who had abdominal surgery last week. He is admitted to a rehabilitation facility to improve his strength prior to returning home. The physician's orders include "Ambulate TID." The nurse explains to Pepe that the usual procedure was to ambulate mid-morning, mid-afternoon, and after dinner. Pepe said, "I have trouble seeing at night. I don't want to walk in the hall after dinner." The nursing intervention is modified on the basis of Pepe's visual deficit to read "Ambulate TID 9 AM, 1 PM, and 5 PM."

In this case, the nurse develops nursing interventions based on an assessment of Pepe's physical limitations.

The plan is individualized by focusing on:
The related factor
The client's strengths and weaknesses
The severity and urgency of the client's condition

The Plan Is Individualized by Focusing on the Severity and Urgency of the Client's Condition. At times, the severity or urgency of the client's problem may influence the nursing intervention. This occurs when the altered human response may result in harm to the client or to others.

NURSING DIAGNOSIS
High risk for violence: directed at others related to

Example. Michael York, an elderly client, has an adverse reaction to a sleeping medication. He becomes confused and violent when you attempt to reorient him. This situation requires immediate independent intervention. You implement the following individualized nursing orders:

☐ Safely protect the client in bed with a jacket restraint

☐ Assign a nursing assistant to stay in the room until the client is reoriented

☐ Inform the physician of the change in the client's behavior and obtain an order for restraints

☐ Coordinate family availability to sit with patient until confusion subsides

The interventions are developed with the client, significant others, and health care providers, when appropriate.

The Plan Is Developed with Others

Client Input. After nursing diagnoses are established, outcomes are formulated with the client's input. The involvement of the client in outcome development increases the potential for individualization of nursing interventions. Likewise, after nursing interventions are formulated, they are reviewed with the client. Frequently, clients will participate more actively in their care if their ideas have been solicited. Many clients, as consumers, are demanding a greater say in discussions about health care and are assuming a more active role in making these decisions.

Example. Ida Gold, an 85-year-old woman, was recently discharged from the hospital after a total knee replacement. She is being cared for at home by a private duty nurse. She complains of being tired from having inadequate amounts of sleep. The private duty nurse explores the reasons for her fatigue and determines that Ida is having trouble sleeping because she is experiencing pain in her knee at night. Ida agrees to take a warm bath in the evening to increase comfort level, followed by pain medication at bedtime.

Significant Others' Input. In many situations the contributions of family members is essential. This is particularly helpful when the client is unable to express preferences or make suggestions because of changes in level of consciousness, language barriers, communication deficits, or other reasons.

Example. Phil Gordon, a 42-year-old HIV-positive man was brought to the hospital by his companion, Henry Chase. Phil was unable to speak coherently because of his illness. Henry explains that because of the opportunistic infection in his mouth and esophagus, Phil was experiencing pain upon swallowing. He explains that at home Phil was able to tolerate chocolate ice cream and frozen yogurt. It seemed to soothe the soreness in his mouth. You include this information on the plan of care.

Input of Other Health Care Providers. The ideas of other health care professionals may be helpful when developing nursing interventions. A different perspective or someone else's experiences with a client can be useful in problem-solving and determining interventions that are specific to the client.

Example. When you enter Samuel Davis' room with his 9 AM medications, he says, "I'm sick of taking these things. I'm not sure why I need all these pills. All I had was a little indigestion." At the nursing station one of your nursing colleagues says, "I had the same problem yesterday. He seems to be denying his myocardial infarction. Maybe a consultation with the cardiac

---

adverse reaction to sleeping medication
OUTCOME
Does not injure self or others throughout hospitalization

ANA Measurement Criteria Standard IV-2 (Standard of Care): The plan is developed with the client, significant others, and health care providers, when appropriate.

NURSING DIAGNOSIS
Sleep pattern disturbance related to nocturnal knee pain as evidenced by reports of fatigue
OUTCOME
Sleeps at least six hours a night without interruption

NURSING DIAGNOSIS
Impaired swallowing related to irritated and painful oropharyngeal cavity
OUTCOME
Swallows at least 1000 ml of fluid every 24 hours

Interventions are developed with the input of
Clients
Significant others
Health care providers

NURSING DIAGNOSIS

Ineffective denial related to perceived impact of heart disease

OUTCOME

By the time of discharge acknowledges occurrence of MI

clinical specialist could give us some idea on how to work through this denial with Mr. Davis."

Together, you and the cardiac clinical specialist come up with the following interventions:

1. Encourage Mr. Davis to discuss his feelings
2. Gently confront him with knowledge that he had an MI
3. Enlist the support of physician in helping the client come to terms with the MI
4. Begin cardiac rehabilitation phase I
5. Stress importance of taking medications to prevent recurrence of symptoms

You may also utilize the assistance of other health care providers in the development of the nursing care plan. These may include licensed practical nurses, aides, and members of other disciplines, such as social or rehabilitative services.

Example. Glenn Weiser, a 57-year-old man, is being followed up at home by the visiting nurse. He is aphasic as a result of a stroke. His sister manages his daily care and verbalizes her frustration over Glenn's inability to communicate his needs. The nurse discusses the problem with the speech therapist, who recommends the use of a picture board. This enables the client to point to the things he needs and decreases the frustration of the client and his sister.

In addition to participating in the development of the plan, other health care providers may be utilized in its implementation. However, the responsibility and accountability for the initiation of the care plan rest with the registered nurse.

ANA Measurement-Criteria Standard IV-3 (Standard of Care): The plan reflects current nursing practice.

The Plan Reflects Current Nursing Practice

You are expected to follow current standards of care by providing care that is based on acceptable practice. Your interventions should be up to date and include the findings of research studies. The American Nurses' Association's Standards of Care stress nurses' responsibility to use interventions that have been substantiated by research and to participate in research activities (Fig. 6-2).

Characteristics of interventions

Individualized

Developed with input of client, significant other, and health care provider

Nursing Interventions Are Based on a Scientific Rationale

This rationale is developed from your knowledge base, which includes natural and behavioral sciences and the humanities. Each nursing intervention should be supported by scientific principles. The following examples demonstrate nursing interventions and associated scientific principles.

STANDARD VII. RESEARCH

The Nurse Uses Research Findings in Practice

Measurement Criteria

1. The nurse uses interventions substantiated by research as appropriate to the individual's position, education and practice environment.

2. The nurse participates in research activities as appropriate to the individual's position, education and practice environment. Such activities may include

    Identification of clinical problems suitable for nursing research

    Participation in data collection

    Participation in a unit, organization, or community research committee or program

    Sharing of research activities with others

    Conducting research

    Critiquing research for application to practice

    Using research findings in the development of policies, procedures and guidelines for client care

---

FIGURE 6-2   ANA Standard VII: Research.

(Reprinted with permission from Standards of Clinical Nursing Practice. Washington, DC: American Nurses' Association, 1991.)

Examples

NURSING INTERVENTION	SCIENTIFIC PRINCIPLE
1. Encourage client to identify hazards in his home	1. Elderly clients are at greater risk for injuries and falls
2. Teach client to rotate insulin injection sites	2. Repeated use of the same site may cause fibrosis, scarring, and decreased insulin absorption
3. Increase fluids to 2500 ml daily: 7 AM–3 PM 1300 ml 3 PM–11 PM 800 ml 11 PM–7 AM 400 ml	3. Adequate fluid intake is necessary to maintain normal stool consistency and kidney function

ANA Measurement Criteria Standard IV-3 (Standard of Care): The plan reflects current nursing practice. *Based on scientific rationale*

Although scientific principles are generally not included in the written nursing intervention, the nurse must have a thorough understanding of the rationale for nursing actions. This allows modification of the nursing intervention, if necessary, without violating the principles on which it is based. Occasionally the principles may be incorporated into the nursing intervention for clarification or explanation.

Example. "Encourage client to feed self starting 1/15/90 to promote independence."

The Plan Provides for Continuity of Care

Nursing interventions should not be in conflict with the therapeutic approaches of other members of the health care team. When nurses and other professionals are working at cross-purposes, confusion and frustration result. It is important that members of various disciplines communicate their goals and define approaches to achieve those goals. Any differences of opinion need to be resolved to promote consistency in care.

Example. Kathy Smith works as an office nurse for a family practice physician. Eric Baker, a 12-year-old with numerous allergies, has been receiving allergy injections for three years. Up to this point, Eric's mother has been responsible for the injections. Kathy believes that Eric, who is very bright, is ready to learn how to inject himself. When Kathy prepares her materials to begin teaching, the physician objects. "He's too young to learn how to give himself injections. I don't want him to be taught that yet."

The physician and the nurse disagree in this situation. It is important that they resolve this conflict to promote a consistent approach to Eric's case.

CRITICAL THINKING AND PLANNING

Once the nursing diagnoses have been established, you will identify the outcomes and make decisions on how to achieve the outcomes and promote, maintain, or restore the client's health. The identification of achievable outcomes and successful nursing interventions depends on your ability to use critical thinking. Critical thinking, which incorporates hypothesizing and brainstorming, is useful in the development of outcomes and the identification of possible interventions. As you analyze information and form conclusions about which outcomes are reasonable and the interventions that may be most effective for the client, you use your logical reasoning abilities.

Hypothesizing

As part of critical thinking, you hypothesize when predicting that certain outcomes are feasible and the interventions are appropriate to reach the desired outcome. The previous chapter described how to formulate appropriate outcomes. As part of planning, you will consider nursing interventions that

---

Characteristics of interventions

Individualized

Developed with input of client, significant other, and health care provider

ANA Measurement Criteria Standard IV-3 (Standard of Care): The plan reflects current nursing practice.

Based on scientific rationale

ANA Measurement Criteria Standard IV-5 (Standard of Care): The plan provides for continuity of care.

DEVELOPING NURSING INTERVENTIONS

Definition

Nursing Interventions versus Physician's Orders

Types

Characteristics

CRITICAL THINKING AND PLANNING

Hypothesizing

(1) have been successful in the past in solving a particular problem and (2) are likely to be effective based on the client's knowledge, skills, or resources. Hypothesizing allows you to apply scientific principles, devote creative approaches to problem-solving, and facilitate the delivery of individualized care.

Example.   Leona Rakoski is a 50-year-old woman who was told yesterday that her cancer is progressing at such a rapid rate that very little can be done to slow its course. Today she has put her call light on every 15 minutes to make requests for water, to adjust her pillow, and so on. Because you are caring for five other clients, you cannot always spend the time with Leona that she is requesting. You would like to achieve the outcome of Leona feeling less anxious. Based on the knowledge of Leona's needs, you develop the following plan:

1. Once an hour you will stop by Leona's room to see if she wants anything.

2. You will set aside some time to discuss her feelings about her condition.

3. Leona's plan of care will describe these interventions so that other nurses caring for Leona will use the same approach.

Brainstorming

Brainstorming is a group technique utilizing critical thinking that is used to generate ideas from more than one person. The purpose of this approach is to stimulate creative alternatives. An atmosphere of freedom and openness must be created for effective brainstorming to take place. Brainstorming can be done with the interdisciplinary team or among nursing staff. It may occur informally between two health care professionals, during a care planning session, or during interdisciplinary care conferences. After all possible alternatives are developed, judge each in terms of its feasibility and probability of success. You will then choose those that are most appropriate for the client.

Example.   Sean O'Malley is a 7-year-old boy who is experiencing an acute flare-up of his leukemia. He has become withdrawn and refuses to go to the playroom, or talk to his roommate or his family. As the nurse assigned to Sean, you schedule a care conference to discuss Sean's needs. Those who attend include the chaplain, the pediatric clinical specialist, Sean's physician, the social worker, and you. The group considers several interventions and decides to ask a boy who Sean knows to come speak to him. This boy has leukemia also, has achieved a long remission, and is known for his positive outlook. Your group believes that Sean may be willing to talk to him about his fears.

Selection of Interventions

Nurses use critical thinking when developing the plan of care. The process of critically thinking through the alternatives involves asking questions and

NURSING DIAGNOSIS
Fear related to concern about deterioration in condition as evidenced by frequent requests for attention
OUTCOME
Demonstrates less fear within one week

CRITICAL THINKING AND PLANNING
Hypothesizing
Brainstorming

NURSING DIAGNOSIS
Social isolation related to feelings of anger and despair as evidenced by withdrawal
OUTCOME
Verbalizes feelings to person of choice within three days

testing your assumptions. Current clinical practice as described in the nursing literature (articles, textbooks, and so on) should be referred to when developing the plan of care. In the following example, the literature on pain assessment and control provides useful guidance when caring for a postoperative patient.

Example.   Maria Rosselli is a 30-year-old mother of a 2-year-old and has had lung surgery. In Chapter 5 you learned that Maria has the nursing diagnosis of "pain related to inflammatory process secondary to effects of surgery" and the outcome of "verbalizes relief of discomfort within 30 minutes after receiving comfort measures." When planning Maria's care, you recognize that you need to ask a number of questions:

1. What is the issue? First, you are concerned with maintaining an acceptable comfort level for Maria. Your focus will therefore be on the comfort measures that are likely to be most effective.

2. What information do I need and how can I obtain it? You will need to know what medications have been ordered for pain for Maria, and the other techniques that you can use to reduce her pain. Medication orders will be entered into her chart. You know, based on the findings of experts in postoperative pain control, that analgesics such as morphine are likely to be most effective in relieving postoperative pain, at least initially.

3. Are my data valid? The information about the medications ordered for pain is valid. You can rely on the findings of experts in pain management.

4. What do the data mean? In evaluating the data you recognize that:
    a. Some clients fear overmedication and are reluctant to ask for pain medication for that reason.
    b. Anxiety and activity can increase pain.
    c. Maria's description of the severity of her pain is the most reliable indicator of the nature of her pain. Maria could be in pain but still smile or laugh.
    d. Current standards recommend administering analgesics such as morphine every four hours by the clock in the immediate few days after surgery, and then switching to a prn schedule.

5. Based on the facts, what should I do? When planning Maria's care, you develop these interventions based on your critical thinking:
    a. Assess Maria's pain level every three hours. Use a pain scale of 0 to 10, with 10 being highest.
    b. Medicate Maria for pain one half hour prior to getting her out of bed.
    c. Reassure Maria that she will receive the appropriate amount of pain medication.
    d. If Maria indicates an interest, teach her distraction and relaxation techniques.
    e. Position Maria with her head elevated, on her side, with a pillow behind her back and between her knees, and one to hug.

6. Are there other questions I should ask?
   a. Has Maria been taught how to use distraction and relaxation techniques? (These are useful to supplement the effects of analgesics.)
   b. When is Maria going to be getting out of bed? She will be able to tolerate the discomfort of moving if she receives morphine before getting out of bed.
   c. What position of comfort will be best for Maria?

7. Is this the best way to deal with the issue? If the above strategies do not work, you will speak with the pain management team for additional ideas.

STAGE 4: DOCUMENTATION OF THE PLAN

ANA Measurement Criteria Standard IV-4 (Standard of Care): The plan is documented.

The fourth and final stage of the planning phase is recording the nursing diagnoses, outcomes, and interventions in an organized fashion. This is accomplished through documentation of the plan of care.

Definition

The plan of care is a method of communicating important information about the client. The format of the plan assists you in processing the information gathered during the assessment and diagnostic phases. The plan acts as a receiving center when you use it to document the results of the planning phase. It facilitates communication by identifying pertinent information. It also provides a mechanism for the evaluation of care provided. Development of pertinent plans of care require you to have assessment, diagnostic, critical thinking, and communication skills.

Purposes

The plan of care serves as a blueprint for directing nursing activities toward the fulfillment of the client's health needs. It provides a mechanism for the provision of consistent and coordinated care and is utilized as a communication tool among nurses and other members of the health care team. Furthermore, it provides a guideline for documentation on the nurse's notes and in the evaluation of the effectiveness of care delivered.

DOCUMENTA-
TION OF
THE PLAN
Definition
Purposes
Characteristics

Characteristics

Regardless of the setting in which they are written, plans of care have certain desirable characteristics. They are:

- written by a registered nurse.
- initiated following the first contact with the client.
- readily available.
- current.

Written by a Registered Nurse

The American Nurses' Association, and many nurse practice acts, have addressed the development of plans of care. They have defined the role of the registered nurse as including responsibility for the initiation of the plan of care. Based on educational preparation, the registered nurse is the person most qualified to complete this function.

Initiated Following First Contact

The plan of care is most effective when it is initiated after the nurse's first contact with the client. Immediately after obtaining the data base, begin to document actual, high-risk, or wellness nursing diagnoses, outcomes, and interventions. A partially developed plan will help you and others to focus on the client's needs. Additional interaction with the client may result in further development and refinement of the plan of care.

The nurse who obtains the data base has the most information about the client. Therefore, it is more likely that this nurse will be able to develop a comprehensive plan. Occasionally a complete data base may not be collected because of time constraints, condition of the client, or the initiation of treatment modalities. In this situation you may

- develop a preliminary plan based on the available information.
- gather the missing data during subsequent contacts with the client.
- refine the preliminary plan.
- delegate the responsibility for obtaining the missing data and refining the preliminary plan to another registered nurse.

The trend toward decreasing length of stay for hospitalized clients emphasizes the importance of initiating the plan of care on the first contact with the client. By identifying the client's needs at the time of admission, the nurse promotes efficient and coordinated intrahospital and postdischarge care.

Readily Available

The plan of care should be readily available to all personnel involved in the care of the client. It may be located on the client's medical record, at the bedside, or in a centralized location. Ready access to the plan facilitates the usefulness and its value as a communication tool.

6-1   TEST YOURSELF
Critical Thinking and Planning

One of Ted Alexander's postoperative nursing diagnoses is "Impaired physical mobility r/t pain, effects of medication and prolonged bedrest." The outcome is "During the postop period maintains muscle strength and range of motion at prehospitalization level."

Use the critical thinking format presented below in order to develop a plan of care for Ted.

1. What is the issue?

2. What information do I need and how can I obtain it?

3. Are my data valid?

4. What do the data mean?

5. Based on the facts what should I do?

6. Are there other questions I should ask?

7. Is this the best way to deal with the issue?

Critical Thinking and Planning: Answers

1. What is the issue?

   The issue is maintaining Ted's mobility despite the fact that he is in pain and has grown weak from lying in bed for approximately one week.

2. What information do I need and how can I get it?

INFORMATION TO BE OBTAINED	METHODS OF OBTAINING INFORMATION
A. Level of mobility of joints and strength prior to his illness	A. Should be in initial assessment
B. Present level of mobility and strength	B. Can reassess patient
C. Are there any positioning limitations?	C. Chart/Kardex/computer Consult with physician
D. Is Ted capable and willing to cooperate with efforts to maintain mobility?	D. Talk to Ted
E. When can he get OOB?	E. Chart/consult with physician
F. What type of pain medication is he on?	F. Chart
G. Is the pain medication effective?	G. Need to assess Ted's level of comfort

3. Are my data valid?

   Yes, I have reviewed the chart and I have made my own assessment.

4. What do the data mean?

   ■ The data I obtain will give me insight into writing nursing interventions.

   ■ It is important to have baseline data regarding strength and mobility of joints because it is desirable to maintain the prehospitalization level and I need a standard by which to judge progress.

   ■ In terms of prioritizing care, I know that Ted's level of comfort must be maintained before he can cooperate with any efforts to maintain mobility.

   ■ Therefore, knowing the type of pain medication he is on and its effectiveness is important.

Continued.

6-1 TEST YOURSELF
Critical Thinking and Planning: Answers–cont'd.

5. Based on the facts what should I do?

A. Assess and record baseline function of joint and level of strength.

B. Maintain correct body alignment when positioning in bed.

C. Passive ROM exercise of joints every three hours when awake.

D. Interest Ted in range of motion (ROM) exercises and have him do them independently when able to cooperate.

E. Assist OOB in chair as tolerated when OK with the surgeon.

F. Assess Ted's pain level every three hours. Use pain scale of 0 to 10 with 10 being the highest.

G. Give pain medication one-half hour prior to getting OOB.

6. Are there other questions I should ask?

A. Are there any special equipment or invasive devices that would impair Ted's mobility?

B. Is Ted cooperative? How enthusiastic is Ted in cooperating? What is his level of motivation?

7. Is this the best way to deal with the issue?
Initially yes. If I find out that Ted is not making progress or needs more intensive intervention, I will request a physical therapy consult.

Current

Because the plan is the blueprint for directing the client's care, it must contain current information. Therefore, it is essential that all components of the plan be updated frequently. Nursing diagnoses, outcomes, and interventions that are no longer valid are either eliminated or revised. The method of updating the plan of care varies with the type of nursing care plan format utilized and the agency policy. This is addressed more fully in Chapter 9.

Characteristics
Written by a registered nurse
Initiation following first contact
Readily available
Current Components

Example. Elaine Conner is a hospitalized client whose IV infusion infiltrated three days ago. The nurse makes a diagnosis of "pain related to edema in right forearm." The nursing interventions include "warm soaks via heating pad for ½ hour, TID at 10 AM, 4 PM, and 10 PM." Today when a different nurse attempts to apply the soaks as ordered, Elaine informs her that they were discontinued yesterday.

As a result of an outdated care plan, the nurse's time was not utilized effectively. Furthermore, the client may lose confidence in the nurse's ability to deliver appropriate care.

Components

The plan of care may be structured in several ways, depending on the system in use in the agency. However, it usually consists of three components:

1. Nursing diagnoses
2. Outcomes
3. Nursing interventions

Interventions should be

Dated and signed

Include precise action verbs and modifiers

Include who, what, where, when, how, and how often

Documentation of Nursing Interventions

Guidelines for documenting nursing diagnoses and outcomes are presented in earlier chapters. The techniques for documentation of nursing interventions are described in this section.

Nursing interventions provide the health care team with a blueprint for reaching established outcomes and resolving the altered human response. A set of nursing interventions should be written to accomplish each outcome. To be effective, they must be written as clearly and concisely as possible. To avoid confusion or repetition of activities, interventions should describe who will implement them, if other than the nurse. When nursing interventions are dependent on previous activities, they should be numbered to designate sequence. All interventions should consist of

- signature and date.
- precise action verb and modifiers.
- specification of "who, what, where, when, how, and how often."

1. Nursing Interventions Should Be Dated and Signed

All interventions should be dated to identify when they were written. The signature is included to reflect the nurse's personal and legal accountability and also allows co-workers to seek clarification if needed and to provide feedback.

2. Nursing Interventions Should Include Precise Action Verbs and List Specific Activities to Achieve the Desired Outcomes

All nursing interventions should clearly communicate the expected activities. Employing action verbs is useful in defining the specific actions. Verbs that are not precise create confusion for the care-giver. For example, if the intervention is "teach colostomy care," you could (1) demonstrate the steps used in applying a colostomy pouch; (2) identify the equipment required in colostomy care; (3) provide printed instructions and discuss their content with the client; or (4) ask the client to perform a return demonstration. In this example, the verb "teach" is not precise. A more specific verb would give clearer directions to the nurse.

3. Nursing Interventions Should Define Who, What, Where, When, How, and How Often Identified Activities Will Take Place

Specifications of "who, what, where, when, how, and how often" are necessary to make the nursing order meaningful. For example, to follow the order "irrigate wound vigorously," your co-workers need to know

- which wound—perhaps the client has more than one.
- who will irrigate—the nurse, client, or family?
- when to irrigate—prior to physical therapy? Once a day? Each time the dressing is changed?
- how to irrigate—vigorously by pouring the solution? Using a bulb syringe? With normal saline, peroxide, Betadine (providone-iodine) or antibiotic solution?

Putting all of this together, the nursing interventions may read

"4/29   Irrigate lower abdominal incision at 8 AM, 2 PM, and 10 PM.
Using a bulb syringe, irrigate vigorously with neomycin solution, followed by normal saline.
Demonstrate wound irrigation technique to client and family members.
Replace dressing with two gauze sponges and one 8×8 in pad.
Use paper tape (client's skin is very sensitive)."

Also include the duration of time, when indicated. For example, "OOB [out of bed] in chair for 30 minutes TID."

The Kardex

The plan is frequently supplemented by the use of a Kardex. This form usually consists of a checklist of frequently ordered medical and nursing functions (Fig.

The plan is documented
Definition
Purposes

UNION HOSPITAL　　**PATIENT CARE KARDEX**

ROOM NO.	NAME		AGE	PHYSICIAN		RELIGION

NEXT OF KIN		RELATIONSHIP	HOME PHONE	BUSINESS PHONE	SAC OF SICK

ADMITTING DIAGNOSIS:　　IV THERAPY

PAST MEDICAL HISTORY:

SURGERY/DATE:

ALLERGIES:

DIET	ACTIVITY	BATH	VITAL SIGNS
	AMBULATE	SELF	TPR
	ASSIST	SHOWER　TUB	B/P
FEED　ASSIST	CHAIR	ASSIST	NEURO
TUBE FEED	BRP	COMPLETE	WGT
	CBR	SITZBATH	
FLUIDS	TURN　ROM	SPECIAL SKIN CARE:	
RESTRICT　ENCOURAGE	TEDS		
I & O	GERI CHAIR		

TOILET/OUTPUT	SAFETY	RESPIRATORY	PHYSICAL THERAPY
COMMODE	SIDE RAILS	CHEST P.T.	
FOLEY　SIZE	TRAPEZE	HHN	
DATE INSERTED	FOOT BOARD	INCENT. SPIR	
DUE TO VOID	EGGCRATE	O2 THERAPY	
S & A'S	RESTRAINTS	RESPIRATOR	
GUAIAC	PRECAUTIONS	**SUCTIONING**	**DAILY LAB**
OSTOMY CARE	−SEIZURE	NASOPHARYNGEAL	
INCONTINENT	−SUICIDE	TRACH	
		N/G	
		CHEST TUBE	**PATIENT TEACHING**

TREATMENTS:

	PATIENT TEACHING
	CORONARY
	DIABETIC
	PRE OP
	POST OP
	ONCOLOGY
	OSTOMY
	MEDICATION
	DIET
	SOCIAL SERVICE

9/89 MBF　201610

FIGURE 6-3　A sample of a Kardex.

(Courtesy of Union Hospital, Union, NJ.)

6-3). Diagnostic studies and treatment may be recorded on the Kardex in specific areas. The nursing implications associated with these modalities are defined in the plan of care.

Example. Lawrence Sammut is scheduled for a cardiac catheterization tomorrow afternoon. You place the order on the Kardex, discuss the upcoming procedure with the client and family, and develop the plan of care.

NURSING DIAGNOSIS	OUTCOME	INTERVENTIONS
Ineffective individual/family coping related to misconceptions about procedure, probable outcome	Prior to procedure, accurately describes procedure, risks	1. Allow client/family to further discuss procedure 2. Review the procedure again in detail in AM 3. Have client/family explain their understanding of the procedure

Types of Care Plans

There are several different types of care plans in use. Those that are most common include individually constructed, standardized, computerized, and multidisciplinary plans.

Individually Constructed

Plans written from scratch are documented on forms that are divided into columns with the usual headings of Nursing Diagnoses, Outcomes, and Interventions.

Advantages. The individually written plan enables the documentation of the nursing diagnoses, outcomes, and interventions that are most pertinent to a particular client. No extraneous or inapplicable information is included in the care plan.

Disadvantages. Development and documentation of this type of care plan is time-consuming.

Standardized

Standardized care plans have been introduced into several types of agencies to facilitate the preparation and use of care plans. Standardized care plans consist of actual, high-risk, or wellness nursing diagnoses, outcomes, and interventions that are printed in a care plan format. The plans of care may be organized according to the client's medical diagnosis (Fig. 6-4) or nursing diagnosis (Fig.

Characteristics
Components
Documentation
of nursing interventions
The Kardex

Documentation
of the Plan
Definition
Purposes
Characteristics
Components
Documentation
of nursing interventions
The Kardex
Types

CARE OF THE PATIENT ON TELEMETRY		K. Giquinto 3/92
NURSING DIAGNOSIS	**PATIENT OUTCOMES**	**NURSING INTERVENTIONS**

STANDARD OF CARE: The patient can expect to be hemodynamically stable.

TELEMETRY INITIATED: _____
TELEMETRY DISCONTINUED: _____

Altered cardiac output related to a dysrhythmia	Patient's cardiac rhythm will be sufficient to support functional systems.	1. VS q4 hr and PRN. During nights VS 12 MN & 6 A.M. VS q ____ due to an ↑ in patient acuity. 2. Document 6 sec rhythm strip at the beginning of each shift and PRN. 3. Analyze PR and QRS interval and regularity at the beginning of each shift. 4. Nurse will sign strip after rhythm analysis is completed. 5. Strip analysis will be documented on flowsheet. 6. Assess breath sounds q ____ hr. 7. Maintain O_2 at ____ 1/min. 8. If dysrhythmia occurs, treat according to PCU Protocol. **NOTIFY PHYSICIAN.** 9. Monitor lab work and report abnormal results to physician.

FIGURE 6-4 Sample of a standardized care for a patient on telemetry.

(Courtesy of Mercer Medical Center, Trenton, NJ.)

6-5). Individualization is possible through the use of blank spaces, as illustrated in Figure 6-5. The nurse may cross off items that do not apply to the client or add additional nursing diagnoses, outcomes, and interventions. The care plans may be developed by the nursing staff of a particular agency or may be derived from the literature. Standardized care plans have been published in articles or books. Figure 6-5 is a standardized plan for the client with pain.

Standardized care plans may be used in one of two ways: (1) they may be placed in a centrally located area and referred to by nurses when developing handwritten individually constructed care plans, or (2) they may be placed directly on the Kardex or chart, dated, and signed.

Advantages.   The advantages of standardized care plans include the following:

6-2   TEST YOURSELF

Identification of Correctly and Incorrectly Written Interventions

The following is a list of interventions. Decide whether each intervention is written correctly or incorrectly. If written incorrectly, identify the guideline violated.

GUIDELINES

1. Nursing interventions should be dated and signed.
2. Nursing interventions should include precise action verbs and list specific activities to achieve the desired outcomes.
3. Nursing interventions should define where, when, who, how, and how often identified activities will take place.
4. Nursing interventions should be individualized to the client.

CORRECT   INCORRECT   GUIDELINE

9/12 P. Dolds, RN	**1.** Make client comfortable
8/7 T. Call, RN	**2.** OOB in chair for ½ hour BID
5/19 S. Snell, RN	**3.** Teach about diabetes management
8/29 B. Jackson, RN	**4.** No evidence of signs of infection
8/17 D. White, RN	**5.** Force fluids
3/2 C. Wilson, RN	**6.** Teach client to do ten ankle pumps q1h while awake
	7. Hickman catheter care daily at 10 AM
1/6 B. Walker, RN	**8.** Provide preferred fluids

6-2 TEST YOURSELF
Identification of Correctly and Incorrectly Written Interventions: Answers

		CORRECT	INCORRECT	GUIDELINE
9/12 P. Dolds, RN	**1.** Make client comfortable		✔	2,4
8/7 T. Call, RN	**2.** OOB in chair for ½ hour BID	✔		
5/19 S. Snell, RN	**3.** Teach about diabetes management		✔	2
8/29 B. Jackson, RN	**4.** No evidence of signs of infection		✔	This is an outcome
7/17 D. White, RN	**5.** Force fluids		✔	3
3/2 C. Wilson, RN	**6.** Teach client to do ten ankle pumps q1h while awake	✔		
	7. Hickman catheter care daily at 10 AM		✔	1
1/6 B. Walker, RN	**8.** Provide preferred fluids		✔	4

1. They are usually developed by clinical experts who have researched the literature carefully. They are useful in educating nurses who are not familiar with a certain medical or nursing diagnosis.

2. They reduce the amount of time spent in writing plans. This increases the efficiency of nursing care planning.

3. They provide information specific to a particular client and require less time to complete. Additionally, because they outline the expected nursing care, they enhance the quality of the delivery and documentation of care.

Disadvantages.   Using standardized care plans can be limiting because it is rare that all of the client's specific problems will be addressed by one

6-3 TEST YOURSELF

Revision of Incorrectly Written Nursing Interventions

The following interventions in Test Yourself 6-2 were incorrectly written. Revise each one so that it is correctly stated.

9/12 P. Dolds, RN	**1.** Make client comfortable
5/19 S. Snell, RN	**3.** Teach about diabetes management
8/29 B. Jackson, RN	**4.** No evidence of signs of infection
7/17 D. White, RN	**5.** Force fluids
	7. Hickman catheter care daily at 10 AM
1/6 B. Walker, RN	**8.** Provide pre-ferred fluids

6-3 TEST YOURSELF
Revision of Incorrectly Written Nursing Interventions: Answers

9/12 P. Dolds, RN	1. Make client comfortable	9/12 P. Dolds, RN	Position on left side with two pillows
5/19 S. Snell, RN	3. Teach about diabetes management	5/19 S. Snell, RN	Teach correct foot care
8/29 B. Jackson, RN	4. No evidence of signs of infection	8/29 B. Jackson, RN	Maintain sterility of urinary drainage system
7/17 D. White, RN	5. Force fluids	7/17 D. White, RN	Administer 3000 ml/24 hr: 7-3 2000 ml 3-11 500 ml 11-7 500 ml
	7. Hickman catheter care daily at 10 AM	4/9 D. Como, RN	Hickman catheter care daily at 10 AM
1/6 B. Walker, RN	8. Provide preferred fluids	1/6 B. Walker, RN	Provide preferred fluids. Client likes cola and juice

standardized care plan. If the care plan is not appropriately individualized it will not be specific to the client's needs.

Types
Individually Constructed
Standardized
Computerized

Computerized

The basic elements of care plan systems—nursing diagnoses, outcomes, and interventions—are also present in computer-generated plans. The plan of care may be prepared at a terminal in the client's room or in a central location. Once data are validated and entered, a printed version may be generated daily, on each shift, or on demand (Fig. 6-6). There are a number of mechanisms by which care plans are generated. Three commonly used systems are (1) standardized

Acute Pain

Pain related to effects of surgery, effects of ischemia, inflammatory process, effects of trauma, effects of invasive procedures, and prolonged immobility

Outcomes

Reports pain promptly when experiencing it
Verbalizes decreased pain within 30 minutes following initiation of comfort measures

Interventions

1. Help client identify pain relief measures that have been helpful in the past.
2. Explore with client feelings and attitudes related to use of pain medication and fear of addiction.
3. Instruct client/family:
   - ☐ to report pain promptly
   - ☐ to describe using 0–10 scale
   - ☐ regarding prescribed regimen for pain relief
   - ☐ to evaluate and report effectiveness of interventions
4. Assess for pain using verbal and nonverbal messages q_____ including location, quality, intensity, duration, precipitating/aggravating/relieving factors, and associated symptoms.
5. Explain source of pain/discomfort if known
6. Collaborate with physician to establish a pain control regimen:
   - ☐ Medications
   - ☐ Use of hot/cold application
   - ☐ Patient controlled analgesia
   - ☐ TENS
7. Provide therapeutic comfort measures based on appropriateness and client willingness/desire
   - ☐ Position change (specify position of comfort) _____
   _____
   - ☐ Back rub/massage
   - ☐ Relaxation techniques and guided imagery
   - ☐ Diversional activities (specify) _____
   - ☐ Alteration in environment (specify) _____
8. Reassure and support client/family during episodes of pain.
9. Provide quiet environment and organize care to promote periods of uninterrupted rest.
10. Medicate prior to activities to promote participation.
11. Assess and document findings and effectiveness of interventions.

FIGURE 6-5   Sample of a standardized care plan based on the nursing diagnosis of pain.

6-4 TEST YOURSELF
Development of Nursing Interventions

Develop correctly written nursing interventions for each nursing diagnosis and outcome presented in the following case studies. Use the guidelines listed in Test Yourself 6-2 to correctly phrase the interventions.

Case 1. Cassie Tilton is an 88-year-old woman transferred to your unit from a skilled nursing facility. Her history reveals a "flu-like" syndrome for the past five days with persistent vomiting and diarrhea. Her vital signs are: B/P 108/56, P 112, R 24, and temperature 101.4. Her mucous membranes are dry and skin turgor is decreased. She indicates that she feels weak, tired, and thirsty.

NURSING DIAGNOSIS	OUTCOMES	INTERVENTIONS
Fluid volume deficit related to vomiting and diarrhea	Within 48 hours: moist mucous membranes, vital signs within normal limits for client, intake greater than output	

Case 2. Chip Ireland is a 35-year-old businessman admitted to the outpatient surgicenter for a tonsillectomy. He indicates he has had recurrent tonsillitis for the past three years. Postoperatively he complains of being thirsty and requests a cold drink. You observe that he has difficulty swallowing and coughs up the water. He states, "my throat is too sore; it feels like it is swollen." Upon examination, you note the presence of redness and edema in the operative area.

NURSING DIAGNOSIS	OUTCOME	INTERVENTIONS
Impaired swallowing related to edema and effects of surgery	By the time of discharge (from surgicenter) demonstrates ability to swallow at least 240 ml fluid	

Continued.

6-4 TEST YOURSELF

Development of Nursing Interventions–cont'd.

Case 3. Emily Fantin is an 86-year-old woman who calls the office nurse and requests free samples of laxatives. She complains, "I've spent so much money on laxatives at the drug store; I take them twice a day so that my bowels will move three times a day. My mother always told me to take laxatives to keep myself regular. By the way, do you have any sample enemas?" Upon further questioning you find out that Emily lives alone and does her own cooking. She eats mostly frozen dinners or prepared foods with few fruits and vegetables. In addition, she shops at a local convenience store with a limited supply of fresh produce. She relies on Metamucil daily, and Ex Lax and Milk of Magnesia approximately four times a week. She states that she gets very little exercise.

NURSING DIAGNOSIS	OUTCOME	INTERVENTIONS
Perceived constipation related to long-standing family health beliefs	Within two months verbalizes satisfaction with one bowel movement every one to two days	

plans based on the medical diagnosis, (2) standardized plans based on the nursing diagnosis, and (3) individually constructed plans.

Medical Diagnoses.   In these sytems, the computer provides the nurse with nursing diagnoses, outcomes, and nursing interventions commonly associated with the medical diagnoses. These are very similar to the printed standardized care plans discussed earlier. The nurse who is formulating the plan selects the appropriate items from the standardized data base. Additional diagnoses, outcomes, and interventions may be entered to reflect other concerns of the client.

Nursing Diagnoses.   Other computerized systems are more directly associated with the specific nursing diagnoses identified at the time of the detailed nursing assessment. The computer lists each diagnosis, and the nurse defines outcomes and nursing interventions by selecting from a menu of appropriate choices. The nurse may add other specific outcomes and interventions for an individual client, if appropriate.

6-4   TEST YOURSELF

Development of Nursing Interventions: Answers

Case 1. Cassie Tilton

NURSING DIAGNOSIS	OUTCOMES	INTERVENTIONS
Fluid volume deficit related to vomiting and diarrhea	Within 48 hours: moist mucous membranes, vital signs within normal limits for client, intake greater than output	1. Monitor and document vital signs and mental status every four hours for 24 hours 2. Assess and document frequency, color, and amount of emesis and diarrhea 3. Assess skin turgor, dryness, and mucous membranes every four hours for 24 hours, then every eight hours if vomiting and diarrhea have subsided 4. Monitor urine color and specific gravity every eight hours 5. Monitor intake and output every eight hours 6. Encourage PO fluid intake as tolerated; provide 1500 ml per 24 hours: 7–3: 700 ml, 3–11: 600 ml, 11–7: 200 ml 7. Offer small amounts of fluids taken slowly 8. Instruct client to inform nursing staff if thirsty

Continued.

6-4 TEST YOURSELF
Development of Nursing Interventions: Answers–cont'd.

NURSING DIAGNOSIS	OUTCOMES	INTERVENTIONS
		9. Maintain IV fluids as ordered
		10. Administer and evaluate the effectiveness of medications ordered to control vomiting and diarrhea
		11. Monitor serum electrolyte value and report abnormalities

Case 2. Chip Ireland

NURSING DIAGNOSIS	OUTCOME	INTERVENTIONS
Impaired swallowing related to edema and effects of surgery	By the time of discharge (from surgi-center) demonstrates ability to swallow at least 240 ml fluid	1. Apply ice collar to neck per physician's order
		2. Administer and evaluate effectiveness of pain medication
		3. Offer ice chips and gradually increase to sips of cold water and bland juice
		4. Continue to assess edema every 15 minutes for one hour
		5. Instruct client to notify nurse of breathing difficulty or increased swelling

Continued.

6-4 TEST YOURSELF

Development of Nursing Interventions: Answers–cont'd.

Case 3. Emily Fantin

NURSING DIAGNOSIS	OUTCOME	INTERVENTIONS
Perceived constipation related to long-standing family health beliefs	Within two months verbalizes satisfaction with one bowel movement every one to two days	1. Discuss misconceptions regarding need for defecation two times a day 2. Provide information regarding hazards of relying on laxatives 3. Discuss with client benefits of increasing physical activity. Devise and supervise exercise plan (specify) 4. Assess daily fluid intake. Suggest at least 2000 ml per day 5. Explore use of hot water, coffee, tea, or lemon juice in early AM, and substituting natural bulk and fiber from fruits and vegetables of choice for laxatives 6. Explore alternatives to shopping at the convenience store such as neighbors, delivery service, or Meals on Wheels

Display Care Plan Screen

NURSE'S VIEW	DISPLAY CARE PLAN	09/12/00 14:51
NOR1/141-A	BLOOM, VALERIE S	PT#: 302291
SUR	DR. APPLETON	ADM DATE: 09/10/00

STD CARE PLAN: INEFFECTIVE BREATHING PATTERNS

? (D) INEFFECTIVE BREATHING PATTERNS
?   (EO) PT WILL GAIN KNOWLEDGE FOR SELF CARE
?   (I) DISCUSS CAUSE OF INEFFECTIVE BREATHING
?   (I) DISCUSS MEDICATION TREATMENT FOR HOME USE
?   (I) DISCUSS PLAN FOR FOLLOW UP CARE
?   (EO) PT WILL MAINTAIN ADEQUATE VENTILATION
?   (I) ASSESS RESPIRATORY STATUS
?   (I) ASSESS USE OF ACCESSORY MUSCLES
?   (I) AUSCULTATE BREATH SOUNDS
?   (I) DOCUMENT COLOR/CONSISTENCY AND AMOUNT OF
                         SECRETIONS
?   (I) ENCOURAGE PT TO COUGH AND DEEP BREATHE
?   (I) ENCOURAGE PURSED LIP BREATHING

!(PF14) RETURN TO NV MENU		!(PF6) ACCEPT SELECT ITEMS
!(PF15) RETURN TO STANDARDS	! SAVE	!(PF7) ADD NURS DX
! NEXT PAGE		! LAST PAGE

FIGURE 6-6   Sample of a computerized care plan.

(Courtesy of SMS, Malvern, PA.)

Individually Constructed. In these systems, the nurse develops the care plan in a fashion similar to that used in a manual individualized plan. You are not prompted to focus on specific diagnoses but use a menu to select those diagnoses, outcomes, and interventions that apply to the individual client. Additional outcomes or interventions not identified in the menu may also be added when necessary.

Most computerized care-planning systems facilitate frequent updating of the plan. The nurse identifies problems that have been resolved, and they are eliminated from the plan. Other options may include (1) revision of diagnoses, outcomes, and interventions to reflect the changing status of the client, and (2) addition of new diagnoses, outcomes, and interventions. Printed care plans, which are a permanent part of the medical record, document the client's progress as reflected by the changing plan of care.

More sophisticated programs compare the client's data with a list of defining characteristics for specific nursing diagnoses. If the client's data match the defining characteristics, the program will display the nursing diagnosis. You have the option of choosing the displayed diagnosis or rejecting it and selecting another. If the displayed diagnosis is accepted, the system will present expected outcomes and interventions that would be applicable. You choose the appropriate outcomes and interventions or enter the individualized ones.

Advantages. The advantages of computerized care plans include the following:

1. Computerized care plans increase the potential for accurate and thorough documentation of the delivery of care. The computer identifies specific nursing approaches listed on the plan and prompts the nurse to document the outcome of the intervention. This process also encourages frequent review of the plan as well as modification, when appropriate.
2. Preparation of a computer-generated care plan from a standardized plan takes less time than handwriting an individualized care plan.
3. The computerized plan can be designed to determine the staffing needs of the unit.
4. Plans that are prepared on a printer are easy to read.
5. Automated care-planning consistently uses a systematic method to develop care plans, thereby decreasing the possibility of error.
6. Utilizing computer-assisted planning permits the identification of common nursing diagnoses for research and planning purposes.

Disadvantages. Along with the many advantages, some disadvantages do exist and include the following:

1. Adequate numbers of computers must be available to the nursing staff. If sufficient hardware is not available because of cost or space considerations, the care-planning process will become more difficult.
2. Errors that occur in computerized nursing care plans may be harder to detect. Nurses have a tendency to lend more credence to computer printouts than they would to handwritten records.
3. The computer may develop a care plan that may be logically consistent but is not applicable to a client.

Types
Individually
Constructed
Standardized
Computerized
Multidisciplinary

Multidisciplinary Care Plans

In long-term care, rehabilitation, psychiatric, and drug and alcohol detoxification units, it is common for the care plan to include the contributions of other disciplines in addition to nursing. These plans may be structured to identify the client's problem (rather than using only nursing diagnosis terminology), outcomes, and interventions. Typically the plans are developed and revised in multidisciplinary team conferences. As appropriate, the client or significant other is present to offer contributions and to validate the acceptability of the plan of care.

Critical paths are a new form of multidisciplinary plan of care that emerged in the late 1980s (Fig. 6-7). The critical path is a structured document that defines the outcomes and interventions for each day of the hospitalization. These documents are a tool used in case management, which is described in Chapter 8. Case management is a method of organizing and directing the client through a hospitalization by identifying a critical path that should be followed. For example, there may be a critical path for a client who has had a total hip replacement. This plan will suggest tests, diet, treatments, consults, activity, teaching, and discharge planning that should be performed each day. In some settings the nursing diagnosis and daily outcomes are included on the critical path. This document serves as a multidisciplinary plan of care.

Advantages

1. The care of the client is strengthened by the communication that occurs when several disciplines share their perceptions.
2. Critical paths have resulted in cost savings and increased satisfaction of clients and health care professionals.

Disadvantages

1. The development of critical paths is time-consuming because it is typically done by a multidisciplinary team who must achieve agreement.
2. There is some resistance to critical paths. They are called "cookbook medicine" by those who fear that individualization of care is lost in this system.

SUMMARY

The development of nursing interventions is the third stage of the planning phase of the nursing process. Nursing interventions define the activities that assist the client in achieving desired outcomes.

Nursing interventions are developed through a scientific approach and include date, signature, precise action verbs, specific aspects of interventions, and modifications in standard therapy. The registered nurse is responsible and accountable for the development of nursing interventions.

The fourth stage of the planning phase consists of documentation of the plan. Care plans may be individualized, standardized, computerized, or multidisciplinary. Much time is wasted when care plans are not developed. New forms of plans of care are expected to emerge as health care delivery continues to change.

Multidisciplinary Plan

MD Review _____   Pt./S.O. Review _____   Date: _____

CAREGIVER INTERVENTIONS

	Date: OR	M	U	N/A	Date: (POD #1)	M	U	N/A	Date: (POD #2)	M	U	N/A
			Day 1				Day 2				Day 3	
Assessments/ Consults	Anesthesia. Respiratory.				Social Service prn.							
Tests	Labs–CBC, Bun, Creat, lytes.				Labs–CBC, BUN, Creat, lytes.				Labs–CBC, BUN, Creat, lytes. Possible Urine C&S.			
Treatments	Foley with CBI. Hand irrigate with toomey prn. TEDs.				D/C CBI, foley at drainage, hand irrigate foley prn.				Foley at drainage, hand irrigate prn clots.			
Medications	IV fluids, antibiotics, stool softeners, PRN-pain med.				IV, Hep loc, prn pain med, stool softener, consider changing antibiotics to po.				D/C IV, laxative prn, po antibiotics.			
Nutrition	Regular diet.				Regular diet as tolerated. Encourage increase po fluids.				Encourage po fluids.			
Safety/Activity	Bedrest.				OOB with assistance in a.m. → independent in p.m.				OOB.			
Teaching	Pre-op and post-op teaching				Post-op activity, diet, bowel habits.				Review Activity, limitations and need for fluids.			
Discharge Conclusion	Assess home environment.				Begin D/C teaching. Social Service if needed.				Discharge teaching.			

OUTCOME STATEMENTS

PROBLEM/FOCUS	Date: OR	M	U	N/A	Date: (POD #1)	M	U	N/A	Date: (POD #3)	M	U	N/A
			Day 1				Day 2				Day 3	
Hemodynamics (fluid volume)	Pt will maintain stable vital signs, adequate I&O and labs WNL.				Pt will have urine less than punch color and without clots. Vital signs are stable. Pt has equal I&O. Labs within normal limits.				Pt will have pink urine without clots and urine output greater than 30 cc/hr.			
Infection	Pt will not be febrile.				Pt will not have a temp and will tolerate ambulation in hallway x 2.				Pt will not be febrile and ambulate ad lib.			
Pairs	Pt expresses relief of pain. Maintains comfort level. Pain is assessed and appropriate pain med given. Foley potency is maintained.				Pt will verbalize satisfaction with pain control.				Pt will verbalize satisfaction with pain control.			
Nutrition	Pt will tolerate regular diet and increase fluids po ad lib.				Pt will tolerate diet and maintain t in po fluids. Pt will have a patent foley.				Pt will tolerate diet and t fluids ad lib.			
Elimination	Pt will not strain to have bowel movement. Pt will have a patent foley.				Pt receiving stool softeners and will not strain to have BM.				Pt will have foley patent without clots. Maintains adequate bowel function with stool softener and laxative prn.			
Knowledge	Pt verbalizes undersatanding of pre-op and post-op teaching.				Pt has understanding of signs/symptoms that should be reported, abd pain, chills, dribbling around foley, rectal pressure, nauses/vomiting. Pt begins D/C teaching and understands.				Pt verbalizes understanding of reportable signs/symptoms. Pt understands D/C teaching and verbalizes and questions/concerns.			

FIGURE 6-7   Portion of a critical path.
(Courtesy of Princeton Medical Center, Princeton, NJ.)

BIBLIOGRAPHY

Alicea K: Why was Lois so demanding? Nursing 93 1993 August; 44–45.

Brider P: Who killed the nursing plan? Am J Nurs 1991 May; 35–39.

Chana CH: Documenting the nursing process: a perioperative nursing care plan, AORN J 1992 May; 55(5), 1231–1233.

Clinical Practice Guideline: Acute Pain Management: Operative or Medical Procedures and Trauma, Rockville, MD: US Department of Health and Human Services, 1992.

Crummer MB and Carter V: Critical pathways—the pivotal tool. J Cardiovasc Nurs 1993; 7(4):30–37.

Holzemer WL: Computer-supported versus manually generated nursing care plans, Computers in Nursing 1992; 10(1):19–24.

Larabee J et al: Developing and implementing computer-generated nursing care plans. J Nurs Care Qual 1992; 6(2):56.

Maves M: Mutual goal setting. In Bulacheck G and McCloskey J (eds): Nursing interventions: Essential Nursing Treatments, 2nd ed. Philadelphia, WB Saunders, 1992.

McWilliams G: Care planning: a team effort. Nurs Manag 1992 March, 67.

Smook K: Evaluation of a computerized nursing care planning system in two small hospitals. Nurs Pract 1992; 5(2):8–11.

Turner SJ: Nursing process, nursing diagnosis and care plans in a clinical setting. J Nurs Staff Develop 1991; 7(5):239–243.

Worthy MK and Siegrist-Mueller L: Integrating a "plan of care" into documentation systems. Nurs Manag 1992; 23(10):68–70.

SEVEN

IMPLEMENTATION

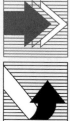

OBJECTIVES

After reading this chapter, you will be able to:

1. Describe the stages of implementation.
2. Define the preparation that is necessary prior to implementation.
3. Identify six major types of interventions.
4. Describe typical interventions for each of the nine human response patterns.
5. Appropriately utilize a variety of documentation formats.

Implementation is the initiation of the nursing care plan to achieve specific outcomes. The implementation phase begins after the plan of care has been developed and focuses on the initiation of those nursing interventions that assist the client to accomplish desired outcomes. Specific nursing interventions are implemented to modify the factors contributing to the client's problem.

Nurses implement plans of care in a variety of health care environments. Throughout this text we have used examples of nurses practicing in different settings such as hospitals, homes, long-term care facilities, schools, clinics, doctors' offices, and so on. Regardless of the setting, the nursing process is used to provide care to clients. The American Nurses' Association (ANA) has defined three criteria that describe the standard that addresses implementation (Fig. 7-1). This chapter will cover these three measurement criteria through a discussion of the implementation phase of the nursing process.

STAGE 1: PREPARATION

Implementation is accomplished in three stages: (1) preparation, (2) intervention, and (3) documentation.

The first stage of the implementation phase requires you to prepare for the initiation of nursing interventions. This preparation involves a series of activities, each of which requires the use of critical thinking:

STANDARD V. IMPLEMENTATION
The Nurse Implements the Interventions
Identified in the Plan of Care

Measurement Criteria

1. Interventions are consistent with the established plan of care.
2. Interventions are implemented in a safe and appropriate manner.
3. Interventions are documented.

FIGURE 7-1 ANA Standard V: Implementation.

(Reprinted with permission from *Standards of Clinical Nursing Practice*. Washington, DC: 1991.) American Nurses' Association.

1. Reviewing the nursing interventions to be sure they are consistent with the established plan of care.

2. Analyzing the nursing knowledge and skills required.

3. Recognizing the potential complications associated with specific nursing activities.

4. Providing necessary resources.

5. Preparing a safe environment conducive to the types of activities required.

Reviewing the Interventions

Prior to providing care, review the plan of care. This allows you to determine if the interventions are appropriate for the client and are consistent with the interventions of other health care professionals. If you notice discrepancies you will have an opportunity to seek clarification on unclear interventions and to be sure you are not working at cross purposes with other professionals. Reviewing the interventions is also important because you may encounter unexpected changes in the client's condition or concerns that will alter your plan.

STAGE 1: PREPA-RATION

Reviewing the Interventions

ANA Measurement Criteria Standard V-1 (Standard of Care): Interventions are consistent with the established plan of care.

Analyzing Knowledge and Skills Required

After reviewing the interventions in the plan of care, you should identify the level of knowledge and types of skills required for implementation. Determine if you have the needed knowledge and can perform the skills or the resources you will require to provide the care.

STAGE 1: PREPA-RATION

Reviewing the Interventions

Analyzing Knowledge and Skills Required

Example. You are assigned to a diabetic client, Edith Bleakley. The plan of care calls for observing the client's ability to test her blood sugar accurately with a glucometer. Although you have been shown how to use a glucometer, you have not had the opportunity to use it yourself within the last six months. You therefore recognize the need to review the procedure before you can observe Mrs. Bleakley's technique. The steps you might take to refresh your own knowledge include asking the diabetic clinical specialist or head nurse for help, reviewing the procedure manual, or checking the instructions in the lid of the glucometer's carrying case. After you check the instructions in the case, you feel confident that you can adequately observe Mrs. Bleakley's technique.

As the example illustrates, when you determine that you do not have the required knowledge or skills, it is your professional responsibility to seek out help in order to proceed with giving care. In instances where you lack the knowledge base and cannot obtain the knowledge that you need, you are obligated to report this situation to the person in charge of the unit, who can then either provide the assistance or assign the responsibility to another nurse.

Recognizing Potential Complications

The initiation of certain nursing procedures may involve potential risks to the client. You need to be aware of the most common complications associated with the activities specified in the client's nursing interventions. This allows you to initiate preventive approaches that decrease the risk to the client.

Example. Pat Ponticello is a 35-year-old woman who is three days postop following an abdominal hysterectomy. Her urinary catheter has been removed and nursing interventions include "ambulate to bathroom twice each shift; utilize nursing measures to encourage voiding—e.g., running water; check for bladder distention q4h (10 AM, 2 PM, 6 PM, etc.); catheterize q8h prn."

In this clinical example, both bladder distention and catheterization pose a risk for the client. Distention may result in a bladder without good muscle tone, while infection may be associated with catheter insertion. Based on this knowledge, you palpate and percuss the abdomen carefully to identify the presence of distention. Should catheterization be necessary, you utilize meticulous sterile technique to avoid the introduction of organisms at the time of insertion.

Providing Necessary Resources

When preparing to initiate nursing interventions, a number of concerns about resources should be addressed. These include time, personnel, and equipment. The appropriate use of resources is mandatory in today's cost-conscious environment (Figure 7-2).

Time

There are a variety of time considerations that affect the nurse's ability to implement the plan. Select the appropriate time for the initiation of specific interventions first, and be willing to modify your plans as warranted by the situation.

ANA Measurement Criteria Standard VIII-1 (Standard of Professional Performance): The nurse evaluates factors related to safety, effectiveness and cost when two or more practice options would result in the same expedient client outcome.

Example. James Boardman is a 56-year-old who is receiving intravenous antibiotics for an infected wound. The medication is ordered every eight hours. When selecting administration times, you choose 6 AM, 2 PM, and 10 PM rather than 2 AM, 10 AM, and 6 PM.

In this situation, your choice avoids disruption of the client's sleep at 2 AM. This allows Mr. Boardman to conserve the energy required for the healing process.

Be sure to allow adequate time for completion of the nursing interventions. A thorough understanding of the actions necessary to implement the nursing interventions will allow you to anticipate the time required. Careful organization will prevent the problems associated with hasty implementation.

STANDARD VIII. RESOURCE UTILIZATION
The Nurse Considers Factors Related to Safety, Effectiveness and Cost in Planning and Delivering Client Care

Measurement Criteria

1. The nurse evaluates factors related to safety, effectiveness and cost when two or more practice options would result in the same expected client outcome.
2. The nurse assigns tasks or delegates care based on the needs of the client and the knowledge and skill of the provider selected.
3. The nurse assists the client and significant others in identifying and securing appropriate services to address health related needs.

FIGURE 7-2   ANA Standard VIII: Resource Utilization.

(Reprinted with permission from *Standards of Clinical Nursing Practice*. Washington, DC: 1991.) American Nurses' Association

Personnel

The nurse should evaluate the availability of sufficient numbers of personnel to implement the intervention.

Example.   Henry Smithson is a 27-year-old athlete who is recovering from chest surgery. He is 6 ft tall and weighs 255 lb. In preparing to ambulate this client for the first time, you anticipate the need for assistance by at least one additional staff member. This will prevent injury to the client or to you during the ambulation process.

Equipment

Another consideration when preparing to implement nursing interventions is the identification and procurement of necessary supplies. Again, you must have a thorough understanding of the identified nursing action. This allows you to identify the required equipment. Be aware of the types of equipment readily available within an agency and in the community. Utilize the assistive device that is most useful, at the least cost, and yet acceptable to the client.

Example.   In preparing to insert a nasogastric tube, you recognize that you will need a variety of equipment. These supplies include a nasogastric tube, lubricant, ice, tape, gloves, an irrigation tray, intermittent suction device, glass of water, and a straw.

The nurse's inability to anticipate the need for the equipment may result in inefficient performance of the procedure. Therefore, you should determine in advance what you will need and provide the supplies necessary to ensure that the intervention is accomplished in an efficient and timely fashion.

STAGE 1: PREPA-RATION
Reviewing the Interventions
Analyzing Knowledge and Skills Required
Recognizing Potential Complications
Providing Necessary Resources
Preparing a Conducive and Safe Environment
Comfort
Safety

Preparing a Conducive and Safe Environment

Successful implementation of nursing interventions requires an environment in which the client feels comfortable and safe. Chapter 2 described a number of approaches designed to create a **therapeutic** environment in which clients and nurses can work toward resolving the factors that are contributing to the presence of unhealthful responses in the client.

Comfort

The creation of a **comfortable** environment involves consideration of both physical and psychosocial components. Physical concerns include the immediate environment (e.g., room and space), privacy, noise, odor, lighting, and temperature.

Example.   Ed Kearney is a 78-year-old man who had cataract surgery three days ago. Following discharge from the same day surgery unit, he is being managed by his family at home with the assistance of a visiting nurse. Mr. Kearney requires a daily change of his eye patch and administration of medication. Before removing the dressing, you ensure the client's comfort by pulling the shades and darkening the room to avoid the pain associated with exposure to light.

Be sure to consider psychosocial concerns when preparing to implement nursing actions. These frequently require the use of interpersonal skills to provide an environment in which clients are comfortable in expressing their needs, fears, feelings, concerns, and frustrations.

Example.   Valerie Lezan is a 10-year-old girl who fractured her leg. As the nurse in the emergency department, you begin to help Valerie remove her blouse. She says, "Please don't do that. I don't want you to look at my chest." You hand Valerie a gown and say, "I will stand outside your curtain while you change."

In this situation you demonstrate respect for Valerie's need for privacy. Management of psychosocial concerns usually involves both verbal and nonverbal communication skills, including interviewing, counseling, listening, and demonstrating.

The caring environment is therapeutic for the client. You can demonstrate concern by the nonverbal components of behavior: tone of voice, touch, and eye contact. You also convey compassion by such actions as treating the client with respect and courtesy, by listening, and by being helpful.

Nursing interventions that help to demonstrate caring include the following:

- Notify client's family when client returns from recovery room.
- Help client to identify support groups in the community.
- Encourage client to verbalize feelings about loss of spouse.

Safety

A number of factors must be considered when you attempt to create a safe environment. These include the client's age, degree of mobility, sensory deficits, and level of consciousness or orientation.

Those clients who are particularly at risk for injury include infants and children and those who are elderly, debilitated, or under anesthesia. There are numerous nursing actions designed to create a safe environment for these individuals. Common nursing interventions designed to maintain safety are listed in Box 7-1.

The infant and toddler may be unable to communicate sensations such as pain or burning. Additionally, young children tend to explore their environment and the objects in it. Therefore, in preparing to initiate procedures, you must ensure that special consideration is given to the child's safety.

Example. Kevin Chen is a 4-year-old admitted to pediatrics with a diagnosis of septicemia. Kevin requires intravenous therapy and a cooling mattress to control his high temperature. In managing Kevin's care, you are careful to ensure that his IV line is securely taped to reduce the possibility that he will pull it out. The control clamp is also placed out of Kevin's reach to prevent him from inadvertently increasing the infusion rate. When preparing to place Kevin on the cooling mattress you make sure that the mattress is padded to avoid skin injury from contact with the cold mattress.

Developmental changes associated with aging also require you to prepare a safe environment for the elderly client. Decreased muscle strength and reflex speed prevent the older individual from recovering lost balance. Aging may also be accompanied by decreased visual and hearing acuity.

Degree of Mobility. The client's degree of mobility may be affected by disease or trauma, external restrictions such as traction or casts, or the need to conserve energy or equilibrium.

Example. John Cambria is a 28-year-old man admitted to the hospital for lumbar strain. His physician has ordered bedrest, with bathroom privileges for bowel movement only. In anticipating the care of Mr. Cambria, you are careful to place necessary supplies, such as water and the call bell, within his reach. This helps the client to avoid moving or reaching incorrectly, reducing the potential for further back strain. You also instruct him to call for assistance when getting out of bed to avoid the potential for injury associated with a sudden drop in blood pressure after long periods of bedrest.

ANA Measurement Criteria Standard V-2 (Standard of Care): Interventions are implemented in a safe and appropriate manner.

Preparing a Conducive and Safe Environment
Comfort
Safety
Degree of Mobility
Sensory Deficits

BOX 7-1
Interventions Designed to Protect Clients from Injury

Frail Elderly

- Place bedside table within reach (for client on bedrest).
- Instruct client on potential hazards in the home, such as throw rugs.
- Keep night light on in hospital room after dark.
- Keep side rails elevated at night.
- Help client into tub, checking bath water temperature carefully.

Anesthetized Client

- Monitor vital signs every 15 minutes.
- Keep side rails up at all times.
- Observe for evidence of vomiting.

Child

Teach parents to:

- child-proof the house.
- keep rail of crib up at all times.
- place safety net over top of crib.
- avoid leaving dangerous objects within reach of crib.
- keep syrup of ipecac available.

Sensory Deficits. The client who has decreased perception in sight, hearing, smell, taste, or touch may be at risk for injury. You should adapt the environment to protect the client's safety.

Example. Gladys Goldstein is a 26-year-old quadriplegic who has developed an inflammation on her left thigh. She is seen in the outpatient clinic by a nurse practitioner. Her treatment orders include warm soaks to her left thigh four times a day for 20 minutes.

In this clinical example, because Gladys has no feeling in her legs, you will attempt to ensure that the hazards of the treatment are reduced. This may be accomplished by instructing Gladys and her husband to check the temperature of the heating pad and to set a timer to avoid the possibility of burns associated with prolonged application of heat.

Clients with visual deficits may be encouraged to wear corrective lenses. Remind the client with a hearing deficit to wear a hearing aid if available. In addition, touch the client to attract attention, approach from the client's good side, or be sure to be seen by the client before attempting to communicate or initiate other interventions.

Level of Consciousness/Orientation. Clients who have decreased levels of consciousness or who are disoriented often require special attention or interventions to promote safety. Clients may be lethargic, stuporous, confused, or disoriented. These responses require adjustment of the environment to prevent injury.

Example. Tyrone Magee is a 54-year-old man who is recovering from a cerebral concussion. He is frequently disoriented and is found wandering in the hall looking for his dog. You reorient him and return him to his room. In addition, you put the bed in the lowest position, arrange the room so that he will not fall, and keep a light on in his room at night.

Preparing a Conducive and Safe Environment
Comfort
Safety
Degree of mobility
Sensory deficits
Level of consciousness/ orientation

STAGE 2: INTERVENTION

The focus of the implementation phase is the initiation of nursing interventions designed to meet the client's physical or emotional needs. Your approach may involve the initiation of independent and interdependent actions. The interventions designed to meet the client's physical and emotional needs are numerous and varied, depending on individual, specific problems.

Generally, implementation of nursing care fits into one of six categories:

1. Supporting strengths.
2. Assisting with activities of daily living.
3. Supervising the work of other members of the nursing staff.
4. Communicating with other members of the health care team.
5. Teaching.
6. Providing care to achieve the client's outcomes.

Supporting Strengths

In contrast to the physician's focus on diagnosing and treating disease, the nurse views the client as a whole being. We examine the client's strengths, problems, and relationships with others. As you may recall from Chapter 1, nursing theorists have given us their definitions of nursing. Some specifically emphasize the nurse's role in supporting strengths. For example, Virginia Henderson defines nursing as "assisting the individual, sick or well, in the performance of those activities contributing to health or its recovery . . . ." Myra Levine says,

STAGE 2: INTERVENTION
Supporting Strengths

"Nursing is a human interaction whose goal is the promotion of wholeness for all people, well or sick." As nurses have increasingly recognized our responsibility to promote health as well as address problems, we have included more interventions in our practice that emphasize supporting strengths. Examples are provided throughout this book to illustrate how we identify and support strengths.

NURSING DIAGNOSIS
Health-seeking behaviors
NURSING DIAGNOSIS
Family coping, potential for growth

The client's strengths may include

- a high educational level.
- a motivation to learn or change behavior.
- a close supportive family.
- an employer who is willing to provide time off to attend health care appointments or encourages wellness behaviors by creating a running path on the company's property.
- excellent health care insurance.
- the capacity to cope with severe stress (or the ability to be a "survivor").
- freedom from addictions to eating, smoking, alcohol, or drugs.
- adequate financial resources.

In the previous chapter you read about Erin Mirabelli, who is 52 years old, and was recently diagnosed as having angina. Erin is a highly motivated and self-disciplined woman. She worked her way through college and graduated with a degree in biology and is currently employed as a laboratory technician in industry. She maintains an active schedule, including aerobics and swimming.

In this example Erin's strengths included motivation, self-discipline, the capacity for hard work, a college education, being employed, and maintaining her physical fitness. When teaching Erin about angina, the nurse practitioner would capitalize on Erin's strengths. Teaching would be geared to Erin's level of knowledge. In addition, if Erin becomes discouraged after finding out how much she needs to learn about angina, you could remind Erin about all that she had to learn in order to get a degree in biology. Erin could be helped to keep this new challenge in perspective.

Supporting strengths can consist of several types of interventions. These may include

- helping the client identify existing strengths.
- praising the client's efforts to learn new skills or accept new responsibilities.
- helping the client accept a new role by pointing out that there is no growth without some type of change.

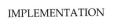

- reminding the client of the previously demonstrated ability to cope with crises or weather personal storms.

Assisting with Activities of Daily Living

Bathing, toileting, grooming, dressing, eating, and walking are considered activities of daily living. Many clients require nursing care because some problem is interfering with their ability to care for themselves. During the performance of activities of daily living you have an opportunity to carry out other aspects of the nursing process. You can

- assess for new problems.
- collect data about existing difficulties.
- assess the client's strengths.
- discuss your findings with the client and plan on how to proceed.
- evaluate the effectiveness of the interventions.

Figure 7-3 illustrates how the process of administering medications is more than "pushing pills."

Supervising the Work of Other Members of the Nursing Staff

As the head of the nursing team, the registered nurse is legally responsible for the delivery of nursing care. You delegate care to the appropriate people, using your knowledge of the needs of the client and the capabilities of the staff member. Throughout this book we have emphasized the need to individualize care based on the unique needs of the client. The more accurately you identify the needs of the client, the greater the likelihood that you will implement effective care.

Example. As you prepare the assignment for the shift on the rehabilitation unit on which you work, you stop when you come to Ram Sambashivan's name. Ram is a bright, 18-year-old Indian boy who was in a motor vehicle accident. He is now a paraplegic, and a very angry one at that. You believe that Ram needs to be able to ventilate his feelings to a safe, supportive person. You assign him to Mary Thomas, an Indian female nurse known for her calm manner. As you enter Ram's room later in the shift, you find Ram and Mary deep in conversation. Mary shares with you that Ram has been discussing how the accident has shattered his life, and is grieving the loss of his independence. You are pleased that Ram has opened up to Mary and that

---

STAGE 2: INTER-VENTION

Supporting Strengths

Assisting with Activities of Daily Living

STAGE 2: INTER-VENTION

Supporting Strengths

Assisting with Activities of Daily Living

Supervising the Work of Others

ANA Measurement Criteria Standard VIII-2 (Standard of Professional Performance): The nurse assigns tasks or delegates care based on the needs of the client and the knowledge and skills of the provider selected.

Example

Are nurses simply 'pill pushers'? When you administer medication you could do the following:

1. Attend to the client's safety needs by being sure the client's identification bracelet is on, the siderails are up, if applicable, and the client's personal items are within reach

2. Assess the client by monitoring an apical pulse or taking a blood pressure prior to giving the medication

3. Make pertinent observations about the client's status, including listening to breath sounds, noting the appearance of the skin, the IV site, the urinary output, and so on

4. Instruct the client on the medication you are administering, including actions and side effects

5. Evaluate the interactions between the client and the visitors who are in the room, noting any signs of strong relationships or evidence of problems

6. Provide a cupful of liquid to use to swallow the pills to encourage adequate intake

7. Adjust the lighting or pull a curtain between beds to promote comfort and privacy

8. Answer the client's questions and take action based on the identification of new nursing diagnoses

As you can see, medication administration is more than "pill pushing"!

FIGURE 7-3 Are nurses simply pill pushers?

Mary has been effectively using her communication skills to establish a rapport with Ram.

In the above example, care was delegated based on the needs of the client and the capabilities of the individual nurse. Also consider the needs of the client in relation to the use of licensed and nonlicensed staff. Ask yourself if the client's needs are best filled by a registered nurse, a licensed practical nurse, or a nursing assistant.

The ANA has issued a position paper on the use of unlicensed assistive personnel, such as nursing assistants (Fig. 7-4). It defines the responsibilities of the registered nurse as including the determination of the scope of nursing practice, the supervision of others, and the retention or accountability for the delivery of nursing care, and provides some strong words of caution about the involvement of unlicensed personnel in these areas.

American Nurses Association Position Paper on Registered Nurse Utilization of Unlicensed Assistive Personnel

Summary

The American Nurses Association (ANA) recognizes that unlicensed assistive personnel provide support services to the RN which are required for the registered nurse to provide nursing care in the health care settings of today.

The current changes in the health care environment have and will continue to alter the scope of nursing practice and its relationship to the activities delegated to unlicensed assistive personnel (UAP). The concern is that, in virtually all health care settings, UAP are inappropriately performing functions which are within the legal practice of nursing. This is a violation of the state nursing practice act and is a threat to public safety. Today, it is the nurse who must have a clear definition of what constitutes the scope of practice with the reconfiguration of practice settings, delivery sites and staff composition. Professional guidelines must be established to support the nurse in working effectively and collaboratively with other health care professionals and administrators in developing appropriate roles, job descriptions and responsibilities for UAP.

The purpose of this position statement is to delineate ANA's beliefs about the utilization of unlicensed assistive personnel in assisting the provision of direct and indirect patient care under the direction of the registered nurse.

FIGURE 7-4   Introduction to ANA Position Statement on Registered Nurse Utilization of Unlicensed Assistive Personnel.

(Reprinted with permission of American Nurses' Association, Washington, DC.)

Communicating with Other Members of the Health Care Team

The registered nurse is responsible for coordinating the patient's care to ensure continuity and an organized approach to resolving the client's problems. The ANA has defined the nurse's responsibilities for collaborating with the client, significant others, and other health care providers to ensure continuity of care (Fig. 7-5). You may communicate with others at discharge planning conferences, during the change of shift report, by making phone calls to other health care personnel, or in informal discussions. Discharge planning conferences are an opportunity for a multidisciplinary group to sit down to discuss a client's problems and make plans for continuing care. Nurses communicate much

STAGE 2: INTER-VENTION
Supporting Strengths
Assisting with Activities of Daily Living
Supervising the Work of Others
Communicating with Others in the Health Care Team

ANA Measurement Criteria Standard VI-1 (Standard of Professional Practice): The nurse communicates with the client, significant others, and health care providers regarding client care and nursing's role in the provision of care.

STANDARD VI. COLLABORATION

The Nurse Collaborates with the Client, Significant Others and Health Care Providers in Providing Client Care

Measurement Criteria

1. The nurse communicates with the client, significant others and health care providers regarding client care and nursing's role in the provision of care.

2. The nurse consults with health care providers for client care, as needed.

3. The nurse makes referrals, including provisions for continuity of care, as needed.

FIGURE 7-5   ANA Standard VI: Collaboration.

(Reprinted with permission from *Standards of Clinical Nursing Practice.* Washington, DC: 1991.) American Nurses' Association.

valuable information through the change of shift report that will influence the care of the client on the following shift (Fig. 7-6).

Informal discussions occur between nurses and other members of the health care team in which data, impressions, plans, strategies, and goals are shared. Phone calls to other health care personnel are used to convey information, obtain physician's orders, schedule tests, and so on.

NURSING DIAGNOSIS

Dressing self-care deficit related to mobility limitations secondary to hip surgery

OUTCOME

Dresses self using adaptive equipment prior to discharge

Example. Zack Cronin is an elderly client recently transferred to an extended care facility after a total hip replacement. He often verbalizes frustration over his inability to put on his shoes. Nursing interventions for Mr. Cronin include "teach client to put on his shoes." When you discuss this goal with the occupational therapist, he suggests that you use a long-handled shoehorn.

Communication with other health care personnel can be problematic and difficult for new nurses. A recent study by the Virginia Hospital Association showed that while schools of nursing focus on teaching nursing tasks, hospitals increasingly expect registered nurses to think critically, work in an interdisciplinary team, resolve conflicts, and communicate (Eubanks, 1992). New graduates are often uncertain about when to call physicians about changes in the client's condition. Figure 7-7 lists two common situations that develop on adult medical surgical units with suggestions on what information to obtain before contacting the physician. It stresses the need to have all of the data readily available before you make the call. Each phone call should be followed by documentation in the client's medical record. The documentation should include the information you shared with the physician and actions you took

---

What to Say During Change of Shift Report

1. Background information about the client, such as name, age, name of doctor, medical diagnosis, room number, code status (If there is a Do Not Resuscitate Order)

2. Description of the client's condition, including significant data only, and any changes in status that occurred on your shift

3. Actions that you took in response to changes in the client's status, including any calls that were made to physicians. Mention any calls that have not been returned so that the next nurse can follow up on this.

4. Any unusual events that occurred during the shift, such as incidents like falls, medication errors

5. Important information not on the kardex that the next nurse will need to know to plan care, such as when the next dressing change is due

---

FIGURE 7-6   What to say during change of shift report.

based on the physician's response, as well as an evaluation of the effectiveness of the intervention.

 7-1   TEST YOURSELF
Change of Shift Report

Listen to a change of shift report on a nursing unit. How does it compare with the guidelines in Figure 7-6? If the report consisted of different information see if you can determine why there were differences.

Teaching

The teaching-learning process for the client includes the acquisition of new knowledge, attitudes, and skills and related changes in behavior. The nursing interventions involved in the teaching-learning process include the following:

■ Assess the client's learning needs.

STAGE 2:
Supporting Strengths
Assisting with Activities of Daily Living
Supervising the Work of Others
Communicating with Others in the Health Care Team
Teaching

What to do if . . . .

The client has not voided in a long period of time (usually 8 hours or more)

1. Palpate the abdomen to see if the bladder is distended.
2. Determine how much fluid the client has taken in during the last 8 hours.
3. Find out if the client has had a catheter removed in the last 8 hours.
4. Ask the client if he or she is uncomfortable.
5. Run water in the sink.
6. If the client is capable and allowed out of bed, ask if the client would like to try to urinate in the bathroom.
7. If the client is unsuccessful in voiding, determine if there is an order to catheterize the client prn. If there is, catheterize the client.
8. If there is no order, call the physician and report the presence of distention and discomfort.

The client complains of chest pain

1. Take the vital signs and obtain a clear description of the pain.
2. Unless contraindicated, elevate the head of the bed to reduce the effort of breathing.
3. If the client does not have oxygen on, bring oxygen equipment to the bedside.
4. Inform the client that you are calling the physician and a cardiogram will probably be ordered.
5. Review the medication record to determine if the client is receiving cardiac medications, and if there is an order for prn nitroglycerine.
6. Administer a dose of nitroglycerine if ordered.
7. Call the physician and be prepared to describe the client's status.

FIGURE 7-7   Clinical decision-making: What to do if . . . .

(Modified from Lang A: Who to Call and When. Mercer Medical Center, Trenton, NJ.)

- Determine the client's readiness to learn.
- Identify the factors that influence the client's ability to learn.
- Develop outcomes that are realistic.
- Determine the strategies needed to help the client and family to achieve desired outcomes.

- Present the content in an understandable fashion using appropriate resources.
- Evaluate the client's understanding of the content.
- Modify the plan as required.

Assess Learning Needs

Gather data to evaluate the client's individual learning needs. Clients should be encouraged to identify the needs they perceive as important. These needs may be evidenced by direct questions, such as "What happens when they do an ultrasound?" "Why can't I eat after midnight when I'm going for surgery tomorrow?" "How do I get dressed with this cast on?"

Learning needs may also be identified by observing the client's condition or behavior. For instance, the visiting nurse notes that the skin around Mr. Conover's colostomy stoma is red and excoriated. The nurse questions the client and determines that he has not been using a skin barrier because it is "too expensive." The school nurse observes that Maria Brown does not wash her hands before leaving the bathroom. These situations demonstrate indirect identification of client learning needs.

At times, clients may directly identify their learning needs by requesting information to promote, maintain, or restore their health.

Example.   Rorie Parrella is a 30-year-old who had a biopsy for a benign breast mass. When you question the client regarding her ability to do breast self-examination, she indicates that she is not sure how to do it but would like to learn.

Your intervention, which consists of teaching breast self-examination, will help the client to maintain her health by early detection of additional masses.

Determine the Client's Readiness to Learn

One of the cardinal principles of teaching is that the client has to be motivated and receptive in order to learn. If you find out that the final exam is worth 75 percent of your grade, you will ordinarily be more motivated to learn the material than if you are told that there will be no test on the content. A client is usually motivated to learn information that is perceived to be important and directly applicable to his or her situation. Physical and emotional factors can interfere with learning, and must be addressed before learning can take place.

Example.   You work in a drug and alcohol rehabilitation program as a nurse practitioner. Geraldo Torres has been court mandated to attend the program after being arrested for drunk driving. At the second educational session you detect the smell of alcohol from Geraldo and note that he is inattentive. You recognize that Geraldo is not ready to learn at this point.

Teaching
Assess Learning Needs

NURSING DIAGNOSIS
Health-seeking behaviors

Assess Learning Needs
Determine Readiness to Learn

Assess Learning
Needs

Determine Readi-
ness to Learn

*Identify Factors
that Influence
Learning Ability*

Identify Factors Influencing Ability to Learn

There are a number of factors that affect the client's ability to learn, including pre-existing knowledge, level of education, age, perceived locus of control, state of health, and lifestyle.

Clients' current *level of knowledge*, including their misconceptions and misinformation, frequently affects their ability to learn. Some knowledge is prerequisite for additional learning. For example, clients who need to change a sterile dressing may encounter great difficulty if they do not know the basics of good hand-washing.

Level of education frequently defines clients' knowledge of health and disease. If the information presented is above that level, the client may be unable to learn. The reverse may also be true. If information is presented at a level significantly below the client's level of education, the client might feel insulted and therefore fail to learn the material.

Age also affects ability to learn. The very young child may have difficulty in grasping concepts unless they are presented in very concrete terms. Some elderly clients may have ingrained ideas of "myths" that affect their ability to accept new changes. Additionally, they may have physiological deficits that interfere with their ability to learn (e.g., vision or hearing problems).

Not all clients desire information. Some prefer to delegate the responsibility for promoting, maintaining, or restoring their health to family members or health care personnel. Others in a state of denial may refuse to acknowledge the need to learn about their illness. Therefore, it is very difficult for these clients to learn effectively.

The client's perceptions about *locus of control* will also affect readiness to learn. Locus of control is defined as the belief in one's ability to control reinforcements or results. If an individual perceives that results come from outside forces, such as luck, fate, or powerful others, this person is said to have an *external* control orientation. An individual with an *internal* control orientation perceives that the outcomes of one's own behavior are contingent upon one's own behavior and abilities (Bigbee, 1983). A client who has an internal control orientation will be more likely to be motivated to learn than individuals who believe that fate is in charge of their health status.

The client must be *physically and emotionally prepared* for the teaching-learning experience. Plan to use interventions directed toward relief of pain, fear, anxiety, or fatigue before attempting to involve the client in learning activities. The state of health of the client may affect ability to learn. The client with a critical illness, severe debilitation, or sensory-perception deficits may be unable to process or absorb information. This may also be the case for clients with terminal disease, since they may lack motivation or ability.

The client's *lifestyle* may affect ability to learn. This is particularly pertinent when considering low socioeconomic groups and people of certain cultures. The client's learning problem may be associated with deficits in the types of experiences that make learning a desirable outcome. The client may not be stimulated in his or her culture to learn content perceived to be unnecessary or unimportant. Certain personality types—e.g., dependent or irresponsible persons—may also have inherent motivational problems.

Develop Realistic and Attainable Outcomes

The learning outcomes for each client involve knowledge, attitudes, and skills. For example, you may be required to teach the client who needs an ostomy so that the client will be able to

- describe how the surgery has altered the gastrointestinal tract (knowledge).
- explain how the ostomy will affect the client's relationship with spouse (attitude).
- list types of equipment necessary to manage the ostomy (knowledge).
- cleanse the stomal area and apply a pouch (skill).
- irrigate the ostomy (skill).
- express confidence in the ability to manage the ostomy (attitude).

Outcomes must be realistic. The involvement of the client in outcome decisions helps to ensure that they will be realistic.

Example. For the client with an ostomy described above, the nurse may write this outcome: "correctly irrigates ostomy and applies pouch prior to discharge." This goal may be unrealistic for a variety of reasons: (1) the client may be discharged before the skill has been mastered, (2) the client may be unwilling or unable to perform irrigation or application of the pouch, or (3) the client may not require irrigation.

Determine Teaching Strategies

The teaching strategies you utilize should be individualized to the client's needs and the type of outcome desired. Knowledge outcomes frequently require the mastery of facts and concepts. These are most effectively taught by using written materials and audiovisual aids reinforced by discussion. For example, when teaching the structure and function of the heart, you may use a booklet and a model of the heart.

Skill outcomes, such as self-injection or taking blood pressure, are more likely to be achieved if the client is exposed to demonstration, discussion, practice, and reinforcement. Attitudes about self-care and health maintenance are more difficult to influence and to measure. However, discussion, role modeling, and problem-solving experience help the client to gain insight and accept new attitudes.

You may choose a variety of approaches, depending on the client's needs, the goal of teaching, the environment, available resources, time, and so on.

Assess Learning Needs
Determine Readiness to Learn
Identify Factors that Influence Learning Ability
Develop Realistic Outcomes

Assess Learning Needs
Determine Readiness to Learn
Identify Factors that Influence Learning Ability
Develop Realistic Outcomes
Determine Teaching Strategies

Individual or group instruction may be used to accomplish the learning outcomes.

Present Content

Identify the specific strategies and resources required to accomplish individual learning outcomes. Teaching methods previously described, when presented at the client's level of understanding, increase the possibility that new knowledge, skills, or attitudes will be acquired by the client. The pace of the program should be consistent with the client's ability to learn and should build on the client's previous knowledge. Learning is also facilitated when the nurse is a warm, accepting individual who encourages the active participation of the client. Retention is increased when (1) a number of the senses are involved in the learning process, (2) written material is not too technical for the client's reading level, (3) facts and skills are repeated, (4) the learner has the opportunity to apply the information, and (5) immediate feedback is provided.

Regardless of the strategy utilized in the teaching process, the interaction between the nurse and the client will affect the amount of learning that occurs. Supplemental teaching materials often enhance the client's ability to absorb content. Audiovisual aids, such as transparencies, films, filmstrips, slides, and audiotapes, may assist in the learning process. Models, posters, programmed instruction, and other printed materials appropriate to the reading level of the client may be utilized in specific instances. Review and evaluate these materials before using them. The materials selected should be appropriate, purposeful, and consistent with the goals of the teaching program. Additional resources should include sufficient time and personnel to ensure that the client receives timely pertinent information. Presentation of the content is followed by evaluation of the client's comprehension of the information, and modification of the teaching plan as needed. This will be discussed further in Chapter 9.

Providing Care to Achieve the Client's Outcomes

The implementation phase builds on the assessment, diagnosis, and planning phases of the nursing process. The initial detailed assessment was covered in Chapter 2. The assessment process utilized during the implementation phase is ongoing and involves the nurse's ability to collect and process data before, during, and after the initiation of nursing interventions. For example, before getting a postoperative client out of bed, the nurse observes that he is short of breath and slightly diaphoretic. Based on these findings, the nurse assesses the client's vital signs and chooses to defer his ambulation at that time.

The client's physical and emotional needs are identified in the assessment phase of the nursing process. A nursing diagnosis and outcomes are formulated, and individualized nursing interventions are written. During the implementation phase, the nurse initiates these interventions to achieve the client's outcome.

Human Response Patterns

STAGE 1:
PREPARATION
STAGE 2:
INTERVENTION
Human response patterns

The following subsections discuss the type of interventions used based upon the North American Nursing Diagnosis Association taxonomy. In this section, a definition is provided for each pattern. The focus for nursing interventions associated with each pattern is described and illustrated with examples. Interventions are directed toward identifying usual patterns, detecting specific related factors, developing preventive or corrective approaches to alleviate the related factor, and providing client education.

Exchanging

Definition. Human response pattern involving mutual giving and receiving.

The implementation of nursing interventions for the Exchanging pattern may be directed toward (1) identification of unhealthy patterns through assessment, (2) determination of the factors precipitating their potential or actual occurrence, (3) identification of available resources, (4) provision of specific education, and (5) implementation of corrective or preventive approaches.

Example. Constance Sohodski is a 40-year-old woman who works as a computer operator. She tells the industrial nurse, "I'm so embarrassed. Since I've gained all this weight, every time I cough or sneeze I leak urine. If this gets worse I'm going to start getting wet spots on the back of my dresses. What should I do?"

The focus of interventions for this client with stress incontinence would include (1) advising client to see her urologist for an examination, (2) instructing her on the use of Kegel pelvic floor exercises, (3) encouraging her to urinate at frequent intervals to avoid a full bladder, and (4) suggesting the use of sanitary pads or adult diapers.

NURSING DIAGNOSIS
Stress incontinence related to obesity
OUTCOME
Identifies method to remain dry within one week

Communicating

Definition. Human response pattern involving the sending of messages.

The focus of nursing interventions is to identify related factors for the communication deficit and to design strategies to facilitate communication.

Example. Gerhardt Woerner has had surgery on his larynx and is unable to speak. The nurse provides him with a pen and paper and a poster of common objects and words. When Gerhardt is unable to write his messages because of fatigue, he uses the poster to communicate his needs.

In this example the nurse provides two methods for the client to use to specify his needs. The nurse also ensures that Gerhardt's call bell is always within reach, since he is unable to verbally call for help.

NURSING DIAGNOSIS
Impaired verbal communication related to effects of surgery
OUTCOME
Communicates needs nonverbally within 24 hours

NURSING
DIAGNOSIS

Altered parenting
related to pro-
longed separa-
tion from son as
evidenced by
frustration

OUTCOME

Verbalizes positive
statements
regarding parenting
abilities within
one week

Relating

Definition. Human response pattern involving establishment of bonds.

The implementation of nursing interventions may be directed toward (1) assisting the client to clarify perceptions about roles, (2) identifying barriers to performance of one's role, (3) identifying resources to alleviate the related/risk factors, and (4) providing specific education.

Example. Tony Angeli is a navy submarine officer who is frequently at sea for prolonged periods of time. Therefore, his interactions with his youngest son, age 8 months, have been minimal. He verbalizes his frustration and feelings of parental failure in a conversation with the clinic nurse.

Here, the nurse's interventions focus on counseling to assist the father in achieving a more positive feeling about his parental skills.

NURSING
DIAGNOSIS

Spiritual distress
related to
disruption in usual
religious patterns

OUTCOME

Within two days
identifies methods
of practicing reli-
gious beliefs while
hospitalized

Valuing

Definition. Human response pattern involving the assignment of relative worth.

Nursing interventions will be focused on (1) identifying the specific value or belief pattern involved, (2) determining particular sources of conflict, when appropriate, (3) obtaining available resources to facilitate the practice of religious beliefs or the resolution of conflicts, and (4) providing information regarding health management to assist the client in making informed choices regarding continued health practices.

Example. Maria Bucellato is an 82-year-old woman who is hospitalized after falling on the ice and fracturing her hip. She says to the nurse, "I just don't know what I am going to do. I go to Mass at my church every Sunday. It doesn't feel right to miss church."

The nurse's interventions for this client would include arranging for the priest to visit the client. Additionally, the nurse would investigate the possibility of utilizing the hospital's closed-circuit television system for showing a videotape of Sunday Mass.

NURSING
DIAGNOSIS

Ineffective indi-
vidual coping
related to sensory
overload secondary
to prolonged
ICU stay

OUTCOME

Verbalizes three
strategies to cope
with sensory over-
load

Choosing

Definition. Human response pattern involving the selection of alternatives.

The implementation of nursing interventions may be directed toward (1) assisting the client to identify personal patterns of response to individual or family stress, (2) identifying the sources of stress for the client as an individual, (3) developing positive coping strategies to avoid distress, (4) providing education regarding identified variables and the use of relaxation, and (5) obtaining additional resources when required.

Example. Paul West is an elderly client hospitalized in an intensive care unit. He has been in the unit for one week and suddenly begins screaming that he can't take it anymore. He complains that all the noises are "driving me crazy,

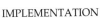

I never get any rest, and I'm tired of all this fussing and these newfangled machines."

This is a classic response to the sensory overload associated with critical care areas. In this situation, utilize interpersonal skills to assist the client in identifying alternative coping strategies. The use of relaxation techniques may be particularly beneficial if accompanied by a reduction in environmental stimulation. Adjusting the times when care is provided might allow Paul to obtain longer rest periods.

Moving

Definition.   Human response pattern involving activity.

The nursing interventions are directed toward (1) identifying usual patterns and related factors, (2) implementing preventive, supportive, or therapeutic approaches to increase the amount of rest the client receives, (3) providing specific education, and (4) providing adaptive devices to assist with self-care.

Example.   Mabel Miller is a 92-year-old with rheumatoid arthritis who has been a resident at a long-term care facility for several years. She is presently experiencing an acute flare-up of her arthritis that is interfering with her ability to wash herself.

Nursing interventions are designed to provide pain relief through application of heat for stiffness and cold compresses for swollen joints. The nurse contacts Mabel's doctor to request appropriate medication to control the symptoms. In addition, the nurse provides adaptive devices, including a long-handled toothbrush, comb, and mitten washcloth.

NURSING DIAGNOSIS
Bathing/hygiene self-care deficit related to joint stiffness
OUTCOME
Bathes self with assistance when pain free

Perceiving

Definition.   Human response pattern involving the reception of information.

The focus of nursing interventions includes (1) assisting the client to define the perception of self, (2) identification of related factors, (3) referral to available resources, and (4) helping the client to develop problem-solving skills to deal with the effects of change, loss, or threat.

Example.   Laurie Bower is a 10-year-old girl who visits you in the school nurse's office frequently with vague physical complaints. Your approach has been to investigate each complaint and to reassure Laurie. During these conversations, you learn that Laurie feels awkward because she is 5 in taller than all of her friends, including the boys in her class. She has also begun to menstruate and is afraid that others will find out and make fun of her.

You recognize that this client's self-image has been affected by rapid body changes associated with puberty. Nursing approaches will focus on continuing your trusting relationship and helping Laurie to deal with rapid physical changes. In addition, you will help Laurie practice behaviors that will help her deal with peer pressure.

NURSING DIAGNOSIS
Body image disturbance related to effects of puberty
OUTCOME
Verbalizes one positive statement about self daily

NURSING DIAGNOSIS

Altered thought processes related to unfamiliar environment

OUTCOME

Oriented to time, place, and person within 48 hours

Knowing

Definition. Human response pattern involving the meaning associated with information.

The implementation of nursing interventions may be directed toward (1) identifying the barriers to education, (2) providing specific educational resources, (3) determining the source of the client's deficits in perception, and (4) obtaining additional resources when required.

Example. Bill McCandless is a 75-year-old man admitted to a long-term care facility. He states on admission, "Where did my mother go? Has she finished shopping? When am I going to school? If I am late the principal will cane me."

The nurse recognizes that some of Bill's confusion may be related to being placed in a new environment. The nurse provides familiar objects (if available), presents information to Bill in a slow concise manner, and uses the calendar and clock in his room to orient him to time.

Feeling

Definition. Human response pattern involving the subjective awareness of information.

The focus of nursing interventions includes (1) identifying unhealthful patterns, (2) referral to available resources, (3) helping client to clarify responses to traumatic events, and (4) identifying positive strategies to cope with loss.

NURSING DIAGNOSIS

Rape trauma syndrome

OUTCOME

Identifies positive feelings about self within one month

Example. Chris Sopko is a 17-year-old runaway seen in the community health clinic with symptoms of depression, withdrawal, and sleep disturbances. He tells the nurse that he was raped by a homosexual four months ago. He describes feelings of guilt and disgust and indicates that this was probably his punishment for running away. Additionally, he is fearful that he may have contracted AIDS through the experience.

The nurse's interventions in this case are directed toward providing psychological support to this traumatized client. The therapeutic relationship should be maintained, and the nurse should reassure the client, help him to resolve his guilt feelings, and help him to develop a realistic plan for the future. Additional counseling, therapy, and testing for AIDS may be necessary.

STAGE 1: PREPARATION

STAGE 2: IMPLEMENTATION

Critical Thinking and Implementation

CRITICAL THINKING AND IMPLEMENTATION

Critical thinking is an inherent part of implementation. The nurse who uses critical thinking to implement nursing care is constantly anticipating problems, revising the approach to care based on the client's responses, and problem solving to overcome obstacles.

Example. As you recall from previous chapters, Maria Rosselli is a 30-year-old woman who had lung surgery yesterday. Because Maria has had lung surgery she is at risk for respiratory complications. Therefore you initiated the nursing diagnosis of "high risk for ineffective airway clearance related to pooling of secretions." You are also aware that although coughing and deep breathing are effective interventions to prevent collection of fluid in the lungs, these maneuvers can be painful to a postoperative patient. As you planned your care, you recognized that your interventions may be based on the following assumptions:

1. It is appropriate to assess the patient before instructing her to cough and deep breathe.

2. It is easier to perform coughing and deep breathing when a client has minimal or no pain.

3. Although Maria may have been taught how to cough and deep breathe before surgery, her anxiety level might have interfered with her learning.

As you prepared to give Maria care, you asked yourself these questions:

1. When did Maria last have pain medication?

2. What is her pain level now on a scale of 1 to 10 with 10 being highest?

3. Has Maria been taught how to cough and deep breathe?

When you enter the room, you find Maria lying in bed with her hands clenched into fists. Her eyes are closed and she is frowning. You infer that she is in pain. To validate this conclusion you ask her, "On a scale of 1 to 10 with 10 highest, how is your pain now?" She replies, "I'm not in pain but I am worried about my 2-year-old daughter, who is having a hard time figuring out why I am not home with her." You realize that this may be a good time to discuss Maria's concerns, and then to proceed with your plan to help her cough and deep breathe.

Based on Maria's response, you develop the nursing diagnosis of "fear related to effects of separation from child." Fear is the appropriate diagnosis, rather than anxiety, since Maria is able to identify the source of her concerns. Review the definitions of Anxiety and Fear in the Appendix if you are unclear on the differences between these two diagnoses.

Applying the critical thinking model to this example, you asked yourself:

1. *What is the issue?*
In this case, the issue was whether Maria was in pain and how that would affect your plan to help her cough and deep breathe.

2. *What information do I need and how can I obtain it?*
Are my data valid? The simplest way to determine if Maria is in pain is

NURSING DIAGNOSIS
High risk for ineffective airway clearance related to pooling of secretions

OUTCOME
Clear breath sounds throughout hospitalization

NURSING DIAGNOSIS
Fear related to effects of separation from child as evidenced by expression of concerns

OUTCOME
Describes less fear within two days

to ask her. Asking the client if she is in pain should provide valid data because she is in the best position to answer this question.

3. *What do the data mean?*
Maria provides the information that she is not in pain, but is anxious. This information will change your immediate intention to help her cough and deep breathe.

4. **Based on the facts, what should I do?**
You decide to address Maria's anxiety by giving her an opportunity to discuss her concerns about her child.

5. *Are there other questions I should ask?*
As you explore with Maria the implications of her hospitalization, you inquire about the relationship of Maria's child with her father and the possibility of the child being brought to the hospital during visiting hours.

6. *Is this the best way to deal with the issue?*
You have established a relationship with Maria. She is comfortable talking with you. If this were not the case, you may find another person who will be able to discuss her anxiety. You recognize that until Maria can talk about her concerns, she will be unable to cooperate with coughing and deep breathing. You have encouraged her to verbalize her fears, identify strategies to deal with her fear, and explore options to have the child brought to the hospital for a visit.

The use of critical thinking enables you to determine if the planned interventions are still appropriate or if the plan of care needs to be modified.

STAGE 1: PREPA-
RATION
STAGE 2: IMPLE-
MENTATION
STAGE 3: DOCU-
MENTATION

ANA Measurement
Criteria Standard
V-3 (Standard of
Care): Interventions
are documented

STAGE 3: DOCU-
MENTATION
Types of Documen-
tation Systems
Narrative Charting

STAGE 3: DOCUMENTATION

The implementation of nursing interventions must be followed by complete and accurate documentation of the events occurring in this stage of the nursing process. There are five major types of systems of record-keeping utilized in the documentation of client care. They are (1) narrative charting, (2) problem-oriented (SOAP) charting, (3) Focus® charting (4) charting by exception, and (5) computerized records. Each of these systems will be explored in this section.

Narrative Charting

Narrative charting, the traditional charting system, continues to be utilized by a number of institutions and agencies. In this system, information is recorded chronologically within specific time periods. The medical record is divided into sections according to the source of the data. Each discipline records information on a separate section, e.g., nurses' notes, physician progress notes, physical therapy notes, respiratory therapy notes, and social service notes.

7-2 TEST YOURSELF
Critical Thinking and Implementation

In the previous chapter critical thinking was used to design a plan of care for Ted Alexander regarding his risk of immobility. One of the interventions suggested was to get Ted OOB (out of bed) for as long as tolerated. The surgeon has ordered Ted OOB in a chair for the first time today. You have been assigned to Ted. It is your first day back after a three-day vacation. Ted is a new client to you.

Use the critical-thinking format presented below in order to implement the intervention of getting Ted OOB.

1. What is the issue?

2. What information do I need and how can I obtain it?

3. What do the data mean?

4. Based on the facts, what should I do?

5. Are there other questions I should ask?

6. Is this the best way to deal with the issue?

7-2 TEST YOURSELF

Critical Thinking and Implementation: Answers

1. What is the issue?

The issue involves getting Ted out of bed safely and successfully.

2. What information do I need and how can I obtain it?

COLUMN I	COLUMN II
A. How long has Ted been in bed?	**A.** Check chart
B. What is his level of strength at this time?	**B.** Assess strength Look at progress notes
C. Is he comfortable? When was the last time he had pain medication? How does the pain medication affect his mentation?	**C.** Assess Ted Check medication Kardex Review chart Consult other staff members
D. How big is Ted, what is his height and weight?	**D.** Check chart
E. How does Ted feel about getting OOB? What are his concerns? —pain —trauma to his incision —passing out How is his motivation?	**E.** Need to discuss with Ted
F. What invasive equipment does Ted have that will need to be moved/protected in the process of getting him OOB?	**F.** Assess environment
G. What type of chair will he be most comfortable in? Wheelchair? Lounge chair? Upright chair?	**G.** Need to draw on your experience May ask Ted
H. What resources are available on your unit today?	**H.** Check unit to see how many chairs you have How many staff members are available to help

Continued.

7-2 TEST YOURSELF

Critical Thinking and Implementation: Answers–cont'd.

COLUMN I	COLUMN II
I. Does he need to be lifted OOB or can he stand and pivot? How much can he do himself?	**I.** Talk to Ted Draw on own clinical experience
J. How many people might it take to get Ted OOB?	**J.** Base on your experience Ask opinion of co-workers
K. On which side of the bed should Ted get out?	**K.** Assess where invasive equipment is located, size of room, furniture arrangement
L. What is the best time to get Ted OOB so it does not interfere with any other activities?	**L.** Review Kardex for any other tests ordered

3. What do the data mean?
The answers I obtain to these questions will give me a clear direction on how to proceed with getting Ted OOB.

4. Based on the facts, what should I do?
Proceed with getting Ted OOB. Document how it was done so that there is continuity of care.

5. Are there other questions I should ask?
Has Ted been taught to splint and support his incision to protect it from disturbing the suture line?

6. Is this the best way to deal with the issues?
Yes. By answering these questions, I have been able to come up with an organized approach to getting Ted OOB. This will ensure his safety and security.

The frequency of documentation in a narrative system is dependent on the client's condition. In an acute-care setting, notes may be documented as frequently as every few minutes for a critically ill client. More commonly, the nurse documents observations over the course of the shift and includes assessment data, implementation of nursing and medical orders, and the client's response to nursing or medical interventions. In other settings, such as nursing homes, community health centers, or physicians' offices, findings may be documented less frequently: daily, weekly, monthly, or less often, as indicated by institutional policy or client contact.

A sample of a narrative note is shown in Figure 7-8. Narrative notes may be combined with additional forms such as flowsheets, patient teaching forms, discharge summaries, and the like.

Advantages

- Ready access to the location of the forms and subsequent documentation of each discipline.

- As the oldest method of charting, it is the most familiar to nurses.

- It does not require organizing the entries according to subject, but rather is organized based on the time.

Disadvantages

- Fragmentation of the documentation of the client's care according to the provider.

- Scattered documentation of teaching when accomplished by many disciplines, e.g., nursing, nutrition, respiratory therapy.

- Narrative notes are not organized into topics, making it difficult to retrieve data about a particular problem.

- Tendency for lengthy charting that often duplicates information given on flowsheets.

Problem-Oriented (SOAP) Records

The problem-oriented system of documentation parallels the nursing process. Both include data collection, identification of client responses (nursing diagnoses), development and implementation of the plan of care, and evaluation of outcome achievement. In this system, information focuses on the client's problems (diagnoses) and is integrated and recorded by all disciplines, utilizing a consistent format. This facilitates multidisciplinary recording utilizing the same data base and progress notes. Therefore, data are more accessible and focus on the client's individual needs.

There are two major components of a problem-oriented record: (1) the problem list and (2) the progress notes.

Problem List

The problem list is a cumulative listing of actual or potential client problems that may require intervention to improve the client's health or well-being. Problems may be identified independently by specific health care providers or collaboratively in client care conferences. The problem list is usually on the front of the chart and serves as the index or table of contents to the medical record. It

G-013

HAMILTON HOSPITAL
NURSES NOTES

(Patient Identifying Data)

DATE	HOUR	OBSERVATIONS AND REMARKS	SIGNATURE
12/27/85	7:30 AM	Client alert, oriented and responsive to verbal and tactile stimuli. No complaints of pain or discomfort at this time. I.V. infusing via #18 angio in left forearm. Hypoactive bowel sounds in R & L upper quadrants only. Breath sounds clear bilaterally. Coughing and deep breathing independently. Turns with minimal assistance.	
	8:00 AM	Tolerated 450 cc clear liquids @ breakfast	
	8:15 AM	Assisted with partial bath. I.V. dsgs. changed - no evidence of redness, swelling @ site. Anti-embolism stockings removed and reapplied. Abdominal dressing changed - no redness, swelling noted	
	8:45 AM	C/o incisional pain - medicated c̄ Demerol 100 mg. I.M	
	9:15 AM	Sleeping @ intervals with no C/o pain	
	11:45 AM	Foley catheter drained 300 cc clear amber urine - removed per M.D. order - encouraged to force fluids p.o.	
	12 noon	Tolerated 500 cc clear liquids for lunch - expelling flatus @ this time	
	1:50 pm	C/o incisional pain - medicated c̄ Demerol 100 mg. I.M	
	2:15 pm	Voided 450 cc amber urine - C/o burning on urination - encouraged to continue forcing fluids	
	3:00 pm	Sleeping @ present	Janet M. Ypek RN

FIGURE 7-8 Narrative note.

(Courtesy of Hamilton Hospital, Trenton, NJ.)

includes the diagnoses of nursing, medicine, and other disciplines. Each problem on the list is designated by number. This number reflects the sequence in which the problems have been identified, rather than their priority or intensity.

Although the number remains fixed, the status of each problem is

Problem List

NO.	PROBLEM	DATE ENTERED	DATE RESOLVED
1	Cholecystitis	1963	1963
2	Pneumonia	1972	1972
3	Fractured left hip	12/2/94	
4	Pain	12/2/94	
5	Impaired physical mobility	12/2/94	
6	High risk for trauma	12/2/94	

FIGURE 7-9   Problem list.

dynamic. It may be active, in the process of resolution, or inactive. Signs or symptoms may appear as components of the problem list to indicate the need for further investigation. If the client's condition improves and the sign or symptom subsides, it is eliminated from the problem list. If it persists, a diagnostic label is formulated, and it becomes an active component of the problem list. When a problem is resolved, the date is entered; however, the number assigned to the problem is not used to identify subsequent problems. In Figure 7-9, problems 1 and 2 have been resolved, while 3, 4, 5, and 6 are active.

Progress Notes

The second component of the problem-oriented system comprises the progress notes. These are designed to document the client's response to the plan. Integrated progress notes include entries from all disciplines. Evaluation of the information documented in these notes assists in measuring the client's progress toward outcome attainment. This also allows the evaluator to modify the plan accordingly. The frequency of the recording of progress notes may vary depending on the setting or specific institutional policies. They may be done hourly, once each shift, daily, monthly, or only when significant changes occur.

The format for progress notes in this system is specific and structured. The acronym SOAP was used when problem-oriented records were first developed. The letters represent *S*ubjective data, *O*bjective data, *A*ssessment, and *P*lan. *Subjective* data include the client's feelings, symptoms, and concerns, e.g., fears about the outcome of diagnostic studies. Frequently the client's words or a summary of the conversation is documented in the subjective data. *Objective* data consist of the findings gathered through assessment. These data consist of the defining characteristics of the nursing diagnosis. *Assessment* includes the nurse's interpretation of the subjective and objective data. Some nurses include the nursing diagnosis in this section of the note. The *plan* consists of the steps that will be taken to assist the client with the resolution of the problem.

SOAPIE or SOAPIER are common variations of the original SOAP format.

Soapie Progress Notes

DATE/TIME
8:30

PROBLEM
6

NOTES

S --- "I'm going to have to watch myself when I go home. I don't want to hurt myself again."

O --- Tense, wringing hands, expressed concern about hurting self.

A --- Aware of the relationship between hazards in the home and occurrence of injuries. Motivated to avoid harm to self.

P --- Encouraged to reorganize and correct hazards in home environment.

I --- Discussed home environment with client to identify hazards.

E --- Identified loose rug at top of stairs as hazardous. Plans to request home hazard survey by visiting nurse prior to discharge.

FIGURE 7-10   SOAPIE note.

The I stands for the interventions performed to alleviate problems. The E is used to evaluate the effectiveness of the interventions in achieving the outcome. The R or revision documents any changes in the nursing interventions based on the evaluation of the client's response.

Figure 7-10 is a sample of a SOAPIE note. The problem number refers to the list of problems kept in the chart.

It is not necessary to include each component of the format in every set of progress notes. For example, there may be no subjective data if the client is unable to communicate. Therefore, no entries would be included in the S area.

Advantages

- Quality care is facilitated because the entire health care team focuses on the same identified problems.
- All disciplines involved in the care of the client have rapid access to data reflecting the plan of care.
- The collaboration of all health care team members is encouraged because multidisciplinary findings are readily available.
- Learning is increased because each discipline identifies and observes what others have done.

- Evaluation of the quality of care is easily performed and deficiencies more clearly identified.
- Research is facilitated because records tend to be more accurate and complete.

Disadvantages

- The education of a variety of disciplines in the utilization of the system may be lengthy and costly.
- Members of some disciplines may resist the utilization of an integrated system.
- If care is fragmented and nonindividualized, documentation will not resolve these problems.
- It is sometimes difficult to determine what information belongs in each component of the SOAPIE note.
- Some nurses find the use of the problem list to record nursing diagnoses to be redundant with the nursing care plan.

STAGE 3: DOCU-
MENTATION

Types of Documen-
tation Systems

Narrative Charting

Problem-Oriented
or SOAP

Focus

Focus® Charting

Focus® charting is a method of organizing information on the nurse's notes that includes three components:

1. The use of a focus to label the nursing progress note
2. Organization of the progress note into the categories of data, action, and response
3. Flowsheets for documenting data.

Focus notes are used to

- "expand on the data recorded on a flowsheet to record an unusual or unexpected event.
- document patient response to medical or nursing care or teaching.
- document the discharge plan.
- describe the status of the patient at the time of transfer from one nursing unit to another or at the time of discharge to fully describe the needs of the patient" (Lampe, 1988).

Focus Column

The phrases placed in the focus column may include signs or symptoms, client concerns or behavior, short phrases from a nursing diagnosis, acute changes in the client's condition or significant events. The focus does not necessarily have to describe an actual problem. The focus of the note may be directed toward identifying potential problems or strengthening the client's health status.

Examples

Signs or symptoms	Dizziness
	Irregular pulse
	Vomiting
Client concerns or behavior	Withdrawn
	Anxiety about discharge
	Home care needs
Phrases from nursing diagnosis	Impaired mobility
	High risk for aspiration
	Effective breast-feeding
Acute changes in condition	Seizure
	Cardiac arrest
Significant event	Return from surgery
	Fall
	Blood transfusion

Nursing Progress Notes

The progress notes are organized into three categories:

Data: Subjective or objective data that are related to the focus of the note.
Action: Nursing interventions that have been implemented.
Response: Evaluation of the effectiveness of the interventions in addressing the focus.

Not every note will contain each category of information. For example, additional time may be needed before the nurse is able to evaluate the effectiveness of the interventions. Figure 7-11 shows an example of a Focus® note.

Advantages

- The format of Focus® charting organizes information into two distinct columns.
- Use of key words in the focus column makes it easy to locate content on a specific aspect of patient care.
- The Data, Action, Response (DAR) format provides a complete concise description of each focus of care.
- Including subjective and objective data in the same section eliminates the need to distinguish between these types of data.

DATE/TIME	FOCUS	NOTES
6/19 8:00 AM	Constipation (phrase from nursing diagnosis)	D: Client states she has not had a B.M. for three days.
8:30 AM		A: MD informed of client's constipation. Laxative administered as ordered.
12:00 PM	Fever (sign or symptom)	D: Temperature 102.
		A: Tylenol administered.
		Client encouraged to increase intake of fluids to 2000 cc until 9:00 PM. Advised to stay in bed and call for help if she wants to get out of bed since fever may make her dizzy.
1:00 PM	Fever	R: Temperature now 101.2°F
		Client following instructions to increase fluid intake. Has consumed 400 cc so far.
		J. Long RN _____
4:00 PM	Concern about discharge (client concern or behavior)	D: Client states, "I was planning to go home tomorrow. How can I go home if I have this fever?"
		A: Encouraged to talk about her feelings. Explained need to be sure fever has disappeared before she is ready to go home.
		R: Client states, "I guess you are right. I'd be even more disappointed if I went home and had to come back to the hospital."
8:15 PM	Fall (Significant event)	D: Roommate put on light and said client was lying on floor. Upon entering room client was found lying on floor in feces. Stated the laxative worked. Denies pain in legs, hips, head.
		A: Assisted to bed. House physician notified and examined client. Instructed client to remain in bed and use call light when wishing to get out of bed.
		R: Client verbalized understanding of instructions.
		J. Reynolds RN _____

FIGURE 7-11 FOCUS® charting note.

Disadvantages

■ Some of the data that are described in the note may be redundant with the data recorded on the flowsheets.

Charting by Exception

Charting by exception (CBE) is a documentation system that was developed by staff nurses in an effort to streamline charting and reduce the amount of time spent on documentation.

Nursing/Physician Order Flowsheets are used to document assessment findings and nursing interventions for a 24-hour period (Fig. 7-12). The column labeled Nursing Diagnoses is used to refer to a nursing diagnosis by number, a physician order (DO), or an incidental order (IO). An incidental order is a nursing intervention that does not require the formulation of nursing diagnosis

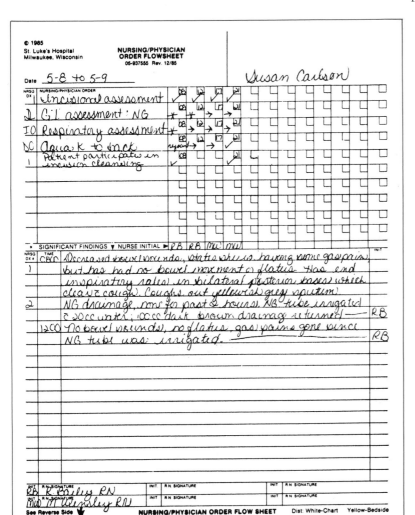

FIGURE 7-12   Nursing physician order flowsheet.

(Courtesy of Delmar Publishers, Inc.)

or is an interdependent nursing intervention specific to a protocol or use of medical equipment.

The time when the nurse completes the intervention is indicated in the upper right hand corner of each square. Symbols used in each block include:

✔ A checkmark to indicate that there were no significant findings. (Normal findings are identified in Fig. 7-13.)

* An asterisk to refer the nurse to the "See Significant Findings" section of the flowsheet.

GUIDELINES FOR USE OF THE NURSING/PHYSICIAN ORDER FLOW SHEET

1. Indicate the Nursing Diagnosis which relates to the nursing order in the far left hand column of the category boxes. If the order is a physician order, indicate "D.O." ("Doctor Order") instead of the nursing diagnosis number.

2. Indicate the nursing or physician order. If the nursing order includes an assessment to be completed, use the following protocol:

   a. "NEUROLOGICAL ASSESSMENT" will include orientation, pupils, movement, sensation, quality of speech/swallowing & memory.

   b. "CARDIOVASCULAR ASSESSMENT" will include apical pulse, neck veins, CRT, peripheral pulses, edema, & calf tenderness.

   c. "RESPIRATORY ASSESSMENT" will include respiratory characteristics, breath sounds, cough, sputum, color of nailbeds/mucous membranes, & CRT.

   d. "GASTROINTESTINAL ASSESSMENT" will include abdominal appearance, bowel sounds, palpation, diet tolerance & stools.

   e. "URINARY ASSESSMENT" will include voiding patterns, bladder distention, & urine characteristics.

   f. "INTEGUMENTARY ASSESSMENT" will include skin color, skin temperature, skin integrity & condition of mucous membranes.

   g. "MUSCULOSKELETAL ASSESSMENT" will include joint swelling, tenderness, limitations in ROM, muscle strength & condition of surrounding tissue.

   h. "NEUROVASCULAR ASSESSMENT" will include color, temperature, movement, CRT, peripheral pulses, edema & patient description of sensation to affected extremity.

   i. "SURGICAL DRESSING/INCISIONAL ASSESSMENT" will include condition of surgical dressing and/or color, temperature, tenderness of surrounding tissue, condition of sutures staples/steri-strips, approximation of wound edges, & presence of any drainage.

   j. "PAIN ASSESSMENT" will include patient description, location, duration, intensity, radiation, precipitating factors, & alleviating factors.

   OR

   Specify exactly which parts of assessment should be completed.

3. Top of sheet should be dated. Time should be indicated in the small box in upper right hand corner of each category box.

4. Upon carrying out an order that has no significant findings, a " ✓ " in the appropriate category box is sufficient to indicate it was done. If the order includes an assessment, the following parameters will be considered a negative assessment and constitute the use of a "✓":

   a. "NEUROLOGICAL ASSESSMENT" - Alert & oriented to person, place, & time. Behavior appropriate to situation. Pupils equal & reactive to light. Active ROM of all extremities with symmetry of strength. No paresthesia. Verbalization clear & understandable. Swallowing without coughing and choking on liquids & solids. Memory intact.

   b. "CARDIOVASCULAR ASSESSMENT" - Regular apical pulse. S 1 & S 2 audible. Neck veins flat at 45 degrees. CRT < 3 sec. Peripheral pulses palpable. No edema. No calf tenderness.

   c. "RESPIRATORY ASSESSMENT" - Respirations 10-20/min. at rest. Respirations quiet & regular. Breath sounds vesicular through both lung fields, bronchial over major airways, with no adventitious sounds. Sputum clear. Nailbeds & mucous membranes pink. CRT < 3 sec.

   d. "GASTROINTESTINAL ASSESSMENT" - Abdomen soft. Bowel sounds active (5-34/min.). No pain with palpation. Tolerates prescribed diet without nausea & vomiting. Having BMs within own normal pattern & consistency.

   e. "URINARY ASSESSMENT" - Able to empty bladder without dysuria. Bladder not distended after voiding. Urine clear & yellow to amber.

   f. "INTEGUMENTARY ASSESSMENT" - Skin color within patient's norm. Skin warm and intact. Mucous membranes moist.

   g. "MUSCULOSKELETAL ASSESSMENT" - Absence of joint swelling & tenderness. Normal ROM of all joints. No muscle weakness. Surrounding tissues show no evidence of inflammation, nodules, nail changes, ulcerations, or rashes.

   h. "NEUROVASCULAR ASSESSMENT" - Affected extremity is pink, warm, & movable within patient's average ROM. CRT < 3 sec. Peripheral pulses palpable. No edema. Sensation intact without numbness or paresthesia.

   i. "SURGICAL DRESSING/INCISIONAL ASSESSMENT" - Dressing dry & intact. No evidence of redness, increased temperature, or tenderness in surrounding tissue. Sutures/staples/steri-strips intact. Wound edges well-approximated. No drainage present.

   j. "PAIN ASSESSMENT" - If medication alone relieves pain & expected outcome is met, documentation on the Medication Profile is sufficient. No specific problem need be identified in the Nurses' Notes or Flow Sheet.

5. Upon carrying out an order that has significant findings, an asterisk is entered in the appropriate box. An asterisk " * " in the category box indicates to "See Significant Findings Section".

6. If status remains unchanged from previous asterisk entry, current entry may be indicated with an " → "

7. If an order no longer needs to be carried out, the next unused category box in that row should indicate "order D/Ced", and a line should be drawn through the remaining boxes. Any unused rows can be left blank.

8. Each Flow Sheet is used for 24 hours.

FIGURE 7-13   Guidelines for the nursing physician order flowsheet.

(Courtesy of Delmar Publishers, Inc.)

→ An arrow to indicate that significant findings remain unchanged from the previous assessment.

Nursing Progress Notes are written in the SOAP or SOAPIER format to document the initial care plan and its revision as well as completion of orders that cannot be documented with checkmarks, such as psychosocial assessments.

Forms kept at the bedside include the Nursing/Physician Order Flowsheet, the Patient Teaching Record, the Graphic Record, and the Patient Discharge Note.

Advantages

- Trends and changes in the client's status are easily detected through the specially designed flowsheets.
- Normal physical findings are concisely documented.
- Printed guidelines are available on the back of forms to increase the consistency of their use.
- Data are recorded immediately on bedside forms and are always available for review.

Disadvantages

- Implementation of CBE requires a major change in an agency's documentation system, affecting large numbers of forms.

Computerized Records

Computerized progress notes may be documented by using several approaches. Data entry may be accomplished by touch screen, light pen, bar code, voice, keyboard, mouse, or other device. The progress notes may be structured or open-ended. The components of a progress note may be simple statements (such as "completed" or "not completed") or more detailed descriptions of care. Another method builds the progress notes by selection of data from displays. This allows documentation of current data and the addition of new findings. The nurse chooses from structured screens. These screens contain significant symptoms and physical findings that serve as a guideline for additional assessment and nursing management. Some programs permit the notes to be sorted and printed out in chronological order (Fig. 7-14) or by category of nursing diagnosis.

A number of additional screens may be used to document nursing interventions, such as administration of medications. The nurse initials those medications given to the client either on the screen or on a worksheet generated by the program.

Advantages

- Documentation of nursing interventions using computers results in completely legible notes.
- Many studies have shown that after the initial period of learning, using the computer to document takes less time than using manual systems.
- Nurses' notes can be printed at the end of the shift and used during change of shift report.
- The client's computer record can be used by several people at the same time.

NURSING NOTES REPORT

11/30/1991 07:00 -- 11/30/1991 13:00   **page 1 (end)**

Printed in chronological order, for all categories.

Room: 208W   **SMITH, MARY**   Acct: 85746738   MR: 98345789   Admit: 11/17/91

DATE	TIME	CATEGORY	NURSE	NOTES/VITAL/I&O
11/30/91	07:19	RESP - RHYTHM/SOU	BGM, RN	RHYTHM: regular, labored PATTERN: periods of SOB SITE: bilateral SOUNDS: diminished, course crackles
	07:19	RESP - COUGH	BGM, RN	COUGH: productive
	07:24	RESP - COUGH	BGM, RN	SPUTUM: sm amount, clear, white, sent to lab
	07:24	RESP - INTERVENTI	BGM, RN	INTERVENTIONS: HOB elevated 30 degrees, o2 per 30% mask, breathing treatment q 2 hr
	07:27	ADL - HYGIEN/COMF	BGM, RN	HYGIENE: bath, w assist, oral care, skin care, completed
	07:28	DIET - DIET/APPET	BGM, RN	DIET: soft APPETITE: decreased, pt ate 50% FED BY: self
	10:02	PSCH - FEELING	BGM, RN	BEHAVIOR: cooperative, anxious VERBALIZATION OF: anxiety, related to illness
	10:02	PSCH - RELATING	BGM, RN	RELATIONSHIPS: family supportive
	10:05	ADL - ACTIVITY	BGM, RN	ACTIVITY: BRP, tol poor, c/o SOB, instructed to call for assist, not get up without help, siderails up
	12:47	DIET - DIET/APPET	BGM, RN	APPETITE: unchanged, pt ate 50%; tol fairs
	12:51	IV - OBSERVATION	BGM, RN	SITE: rt forearm OBS: no redness DSG: changed
	12:52	RESP - RHYTHM/SOU	BGM, RN	PATTERN: no c/o SOB SITE: bilateral SOUNDS: diminished, fine crackles

Vital Signs:

11/30/91	07:30	VITAL SIGNS	BGM, RN	TEMP(c)loc: 91.8(33.2)o HR: 90 RESP: 20 SYS/DIAS 130/70 MAP: 90
	10:09	VITAL SIGNS	BGM, RN	TEMP(c)loc: *****(*****) HR: *** RESP: 18 SYS/DIAS ***/**
	12:57	VITAL SIGNS	BGM, RN	TEMP(c)loc: 99.0(37.2)o HR: 88 RESP: 20 SYS/DIAS 126/80 MAP: 95

Intake & Output:

11/30/91	07:29	INTAKE/OUTPUT	BGM, RN	IN: PO . . . . . . 150 IV #1 200
				OUT: URINE . . . 200
	12:54	INTAKE/OUTPUT	BGM, RN	IN: PO . . . . 50 IV #1 150
				OUT: URINE . . . 100

Nurses Signatures:

BGM-BARB MILLER RN

Room: 208W   **SMITH, MARY**   Acct: 85746738   MR: 98345789   Admit: 11/17/91

NSU1   VITALNET System v4.4c-PRE. Printed: Sat 11/30/91 - 13:00:18   (c)1984 thru 1991 CRITIKON, INC

FIGURE 7-14   Nursing notes report.

(Reprinted with permission of Critikon, Boulder, CO.)

7-3 TEST YOURSELF
Documentation of Implementation

Charles Stewart is a 67-year-old man who was admitted to the hospital two days ago with a diagnosis of stomach cancer. The following is a segment of his care plan.

NURSING DIAGNOSIS	OUTCOME	INTERVENTION
Altered nutrition: less than body requirements related to decreased oral intake	Loses no more than 5 pounds throughout hospitalization	1. Provide small frequent meals at 8 AM, 1 PM, 4 PM, 6 PM 2. Supplemental feeding: Ensure 90 ml at 11 AM and 9 PM 3. Assess likes/dislikes 4. Encourage food from home if permitted 5. Obtain dietary consult (date: 7/5) 6. Monitor food intake 7. Weigh daily at 8 AM

While you are caring for Mr. Stewart, he shares the following information with you. "I don't like strawberry Ensure, although the other flavors are all right. What I'd really like would be some of my wife's lasagna." When Mr. Stewart's trays were observed after each meal, you noted that he consumed all of his breakfast, two thirds of his lunch, and 45 ml of Ensure at 11 AM. His weight at 8 AM was 148 lb, which constitutes a loss of 3 pounds since admission. Therefore you suggest to Mr. Stewart's physician that a consultation with a dietitian be obtained. She agrees, and the dietitian visits at 1:30 PM. When Mrs. Stewart visits at 2:00 she agrees to bring in some lasagna for her husband.

Based on the information provided above, document the implementation of this segment of the plan of care using source-oriented, SOAPIE, and Focus® charting.

7-3 TEST YOURSELF
Documentation of Implementation: Answers

SOURCE-ORIENTED NOTE

DATE	TIME	FOCUS	NURSES' NOTES
7/5/91	8 AM		Discussed dietary preferences with client—indicates that he wants "my wife's lasagna or bread pudding." Weight 148 lb this AM. Consumed entire breakfast
	10:00 AM		Dr. Klein visited—discussed weight loss—dietary consult order requested and received
	11:00 AM		Consumed ½ Ensure feeding. Client indicates that "I don't like strawberry Ensure although the other flavors are all right"
	1 PM		Consumed ⅔ of lunch
	1:30 PM		Visited by dietitian—will make changes in diet and discontinue strawberry Ensure
	2:00 PM		Wife visited—agreed to bring in lasagna
			Janet York-Blasser, RN

SOAPIE NOTE

DATE	TIME	FOCUS	NURSES' NOTES
7/5/91	8 AM		S: "I don't like strawberry Ensure. I'd like some of my wife's lasagna." O: Weight 148 lb. Consumed all of his breakfast
	11 AM		Drank 45 ml of Ensure

Continued.

7-3 TEST YOURSELF

Documentation of Implementation: Answers–cont'd.

SOAPIE NOTE

DATE	TIME	FOCUS	NURSES' NOTES
	12 PM		Ate ⅔ of his lunch. *A:* Significant weight loss of 3 pounds since admission probably related to decreased caloric consumption
	12:30 PM		*P:* Request order for dietary consult
			I: Received order for dietary consult. Notified dietary department
			E: Visited by dietitian
			E: Visited by wife, who agreed to bring in lasagna
			Janet York-Blasser, RN

FOCUS® NOTE

DATE	TIME	FOCUS	NURSES' NOTES
7/5/91	12:00 PM	Altered nutrition	*Data:* Dislikes strawberry Ensure, wishes to have wife's lasagna. Ate all of breakfast and ⅔ of lunch, plus 45 ml of Ensure. Has lost 3 pounds since admission
			Action: Requested a dietary consult
			Response: Order obtained for dietary consult
	1:30 PM		Visited by dietitian
	2:00 PM		Wife agreed to bring in lasagna
			Janet-York-Blasser, RN

Disadvantages

- Frequent printing of notes and reports can result in thick medical records, creating more paper rather than less.

- Documentation of nursing notes using computers requires a large investment of time and money. Software and hardware are expensive and the time spent to teach staff is extensive.

- Maintaining confidentiality of information in a computerized record can be more difficult. Although access to records can be restricted through passwords, many people fear that confidentiality and security of records is difficult to maintain.

SUMMARY

Implementation is the phase of the nursing process that involves the initiation of the nursing care plan. The goal of implementation is the achievement of outcomes. The implementation phase is divided into three stages: preparation, interventions, and documentation. Preparation includes reviewing anticipated nursing actions, analyzing the nursing knowledge and skills required, and recognizing the potential complications associated with specific nursing orders. Preparation also involves determining and providing necessary resources and preparing an environment conducive to the types of interventions required. The client's physical and emotional needs may be divided into nine human response patterns. (While each has an infinite variety of interventions associated with it, assessment, planning, and teaching are common approaches.) The nurse uses critical thinking throughout implementation to identify problems and effectively resolve them.

Documentation, the last stage, may utilize a variety of charting formats. The traditional ones include narrative and problem-oriented charting. Focus® charting, charting by exception, and computerized records are increasingly being used to replace the more traditional and cumbersome charting formats of the past.

REFERENCES

Bigbee J: Locus of control and the obese adolescent: a pilot study. In Chinn O (ed): Advances in Nursing Theory Development. Rockville, MD: Aspen, 1983.

Eubanks P: Survey shows gaps in competencies of new RNs. Hospitals 1992; December; 5:49–50.

Lampe S: Focus Charting. Minneapolis: Creative Nursing Management, 1988.

BIBLIOGRAPHY

Barry C and Gibbons L: Information systems technology: Barriers and challenges to implementation. J Nurs Admin 1990 February; 40–42.

Bialorucki T and Blaine M: Protecting patient confidentiality in the pursuit of the ultimate computerized information system. J Nurs Care Qual 1992; 7(1):53.

Cline A: Streamlined documentation through exceptional charting. Nurs Manag 1989 February; 62–64.

Collins H: Legal risks of computer charting. RN 1990 May; 81–86.

Dixon E and Park R: Do patients understand written health information? Nurs Outlook (6):278–281.

Gross D and Andrea J: Development of a nursing process-based documentation system. J Emerg Nurs 1991; 17(3):173–6.

Hampton D: Implementing a managed care framework through care maps. J Nurs Admin 1993, 23(5):21–27.

Iyer P and Camp N: Nursing Documentation: A Nursing Process Approach, 2nd ed. St. Louis: Mosby–Yearbook, 1994.

Iyer P: Preventing falls in the elderly. Southern California Nurs Rev 1988 October; 14–16.

Kerr S: A comparison of four nursing documentation systems. J Nurs Staff Develop. 1992 January/February; 26–31.

Lampe S and Hitchcock A: Documenting nursing diagnosis using focus charting. In Mclane A (ed): Classification of Nursing Diagnosis: Proceedings of the Seventh Conference. St. Louis: CV Mosby, 1987, 337–387.

Lucatorto M and others: Documentation: A focus for cost savings. J Nurs Admin 1991: 21(3):32–35.

Lumsdon K: Computerized patient records gain converts. Hospitals 1993; April 5, 44.

Masson V: Nursing the charts. Nurs Outlook 1990: 38(4):196.

Murphy J and Burke L: Charting by exception. Nursing 90 1990 May; 65–67.

EIGHT

IMPLEMENTATION: NURSING CARE DELIVERY SYSTEMS

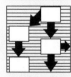
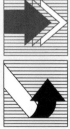

OBJECTIVES

At the completion of this chapter, you will be able to:

1. Identify the advantages and disadvantages of the major methods of organizing the delivery of care.
2. Recognize the most common delivery systems.
3. Analyze how care is delivered in each of the major nursing care delivery systems.

INTRODUCTION

Regardless of the type of setting in which nurses practice, one of five major models is utilized for implementing nursing care. These five approaches are (1) functional nursing, (2) team nursing, (3) primary nursing and its variations, (4) case management, and (5) patient-focused care. Their differences lie primarily in the systems used to organize and carry out the types of activities necessary to satisfy client needs. Nursing care may be accomplished by using individual models in their pure form or by adapting one or more methods. The choice of the practice model is affected by a number of factors, including the types of nursing staff that are available, the costs of delivering care, the philosophy of the agency, and so on. Long-term care facilities, for example, usually have large numbers of nursing assistants deliver the majority of physical care. Licensed practical nurses and registered nurses oversee their care and give medications and treatments. Acute-care facilities usually employ a mix of nursing assistants, licensed practical nurses, and registered nurses, with higher numbers of licensed nurses than nursing assistants.

Regulatory standards may define how many registered nurses must be employed at the agency and present at any time. Professional standards, such as the American Nurses' Association (ANA) standard on resource allocation

---

STANDARD VIII. RESOURCE UTILIZATION
The Nurse Considers Factors Related to Safety,
Effectiveness, and Cost in Planning and
Delivering Client Care

Measurement Criteria

1. The nurse evaluates factors related to safety, effectiveness, and cost when two or more practice options would result in the same expected client outcome.

2. The nurse assigns tasks or delegates care based on the needs of the client and the knowledge and skill of the provider selected.

3. The nurse assists the client and significant others in identifying and securing appropriate services to address health related needs.

FIGURE 8-1   ANA Standard VIII: Resource Utilization.

(Reprinted with permission from *Standards of Clinical Nursing Practice*, Washington, DC: American Nurses' Association, 1991.)

(Fig. 8-1), stress the need to consider safety, effectiveness, and cost factors when selecting a model of delivering nursing care or assigning staff to care for clients. The factors that should be considered include the following:

1. What type of nursing personnel are needed to **safely** deliver care? Does the client require care that should be given by a registered nurse or can a nursing assistant provide the care? For example, a registered nurse would administer IV antibiotics but a nursing assistant could make a bed. You will note that the descriptions of the nursing care delivery models describe how several levels of nursing personnel are used in each model.

2. Who is the most **effective** care-giver for the client? In order to achieve consistency in care, often the most effective care-giver is the person who has cared for the client before or is familiar with the needs of the client. For example, continuity of care is enhanced when the client is assigned to the same nurse for several days in a row. As you read the descriptions of the delivery models, look for the models that support continuity of care.

3. Who can deliver the most **cost effective** care? In many settings the registered nurse is often asked to perform a variety of non-nursing functions. Non-nursing functions include responsibilities performed by

other departments, including housekeeping, maintenance, transportation, clerical, and so on. Nurses are often asked to assume these responsibilities on the evening or night shift. Many facilities have recognized the cost associated with having registered nurses perform tasks that could be delegated to unlicensed personnel. Delivery systems have been redesigned to ensure that the registered nurse carries out the professional activities associated with the nursing process. As you learn about each model think about the costs associated with the model.

One of the challenges of today's health care environment is that inefficient models of delivering nursing care can be very difficult to change. Resistance to change must be overcome in order to move to a system that safely, efficiently delivers cost effective care.

This chapter will explore functional, team, primary nursing, case management, and patient-focused care. Each will be defined and the advantages and disadvantages of the model will be presented.

FUNCTIONAL NURSING

Definition

In the functional approach to nursing care delivery, nursing responsibilities are divided by task and performed by varying levels of nursing personnel. All care-givers are involved in the client's care, but each individual is assigned to complete selected functions, such as monitoring vital signs, administering medications, or giving treatments. The individual functions are assigned to various levels of personnel based on the complexity of the task, including the knowledge, skills, and experience required to complete them.

For example, on a nursing unit on any given day, one registered nurse may be in charge of unit management while another administers medications, and a third completes client teaching. The licensed practical nurse may be assigned to measure vital signs or bathe clients, while the nursing assistant makes beds or delivers meal trays.

In an office setting, the licensed practical nurse may take client histories, record vital signs, and perform simple treatments. The registered nurse similarly accomplishes physical assessment, administers medications, completes complex treatments, and provides education to the client.

Advantages

1. The emphasis in this model is on the efficient delivery of nursing care. Because the system allows the use of less-skilled personnel to complete

INTRODUCTION
FUNCTIONAL
NURSING
Definition

FUNCTIONAL
NURSING
Definition
Advantages
Disadvantages

many tasks, it may also be more economical. Staff members become more skilled and efficient when assigned to the same tasks on a regular basis. This may also more effectively utilize the nurse's skills and experience. Some nurses are particularly skilled at initiating intravenous therapy or administering medications and tend to be more motivated and efficient when completing those tasks than when performing treatments or teaching clients.

2. The volume of supplies and equipment required may also be decreased because fewer numbers of personnel utilize them. Consistency of task assignment may also decrease maintenance costs of equipment, because staff members become more proficient in the use of the types of equipment required to complete their specific function.

3. This method also tends to facilitate the organization of work, because assignments are clearly defined. Therefore, the overlapping of responsibilities and the associated confusion are minimized.

Disadvantages

1. The primary concern with the functional model is the fragmentation of care. Assigning a variety of personnel to specific tasks frequently becomes inefficient and impersonal. The client's care is often divided into segments, each of which must be managed by a different individual. One nurse administers medications, a second provides teaching, and a third monitors vital signs. This tends to make the client feel insecure and frustrated.

2. Continuity of care is difficult, if not impossible, because no single staff member has a complete picture of the client's needs and responses to nursing or medical interventions. This allows unnoticed gaps to occur in client care.

3. From the nurse's perspective, this type of care delivery may become monotonous. Administration of medications for weeks at a time may decrease the nurse's motivation and limit continued personal development because of reduced exposure to a variety of experiences.

4. Job satisfaction may also be diminished in a functional approach because the nurse's role in the client's recovery may not be clearly defined or perceived as valuable by the client, other staff members, or supervisory personnel.

5. Communication and decision-making may be compromised, because care-givers are focusing on individual aspects of the client's care. Frequently, the nurse manager is the only staff member who receives complete information on the client. The responsibility and accountability for decision making is focused on the manager rather than on individual staff members who actually implement the plan of care.

TEAM NURSING

Definition

Team nursing is a system of nursing care delivery in which a group of professional and nonprofessional personnel work together to deliver nursing care to a number of clients. It was designed after World War II to alleviate the problems associated with functional nursing. Team nursing is frequently utilized in nursing homes and hospital settings. Comprehensive client care is provided by the staff member under the direction of a registered nurse who is the team leader. Other team members may include registered nurses, licensed practical nurses, and nursing assistants. However, the size and composition of a team are often dependent on the setting. A nursing unit is divided into two or more teams based on the number of beds and the geography of the unit. For example, in a nursing unit consisting of a long hall, the hall would be divided in half with a team assigned to each of the halves.

The team leader is the key person in this model. Leaders must have particular knowledge and skills not only in client care procedures and techniques but also in management and decision-making strategies. The team leader has the authority and responsibility for assigning the care of a group of clients to team members. These assignments are based on client needs and the knowledge, skills, and experiences of team members. In many settings the team leader administers medications to a group of clients. Registered nurses, licensed practical nurses, and nursing assistants provide direct care for clients assigned to them. For example, a registered or licensed practical nurse would take vital signs, bathe and feed clients, and complete their treatments such as soaks or dressing changes. The team leader usually performs treatments for clients who are assigned to a nursing assistant.

The success of the team approach is dependent on effective communication. This method relies on the use of written client care assignments, timely development and revision of nursing care plans, frequent participation in client care conferences, and frequent reports and feedback among team members. (As the acuity of clients continues to increase, care conferences occur with less frequency.)

Advantages

1. Although nursing care in a team approach is divided among several staff members, it is less fragmented than in the functional method. This is a result of the extensive communication and coordination built into the system. Continuity of care is facilitated, particularly in systems where teams are constant. Therefore, team nursing is more satisfying to clients, because they are able to identify and communicate more effectively with the personnel responsible for delivering care.

2. From the nurse's perspective, the team model is more satisfying because the skills of each team member are frequently identified, recognized, and utilized. This provides the opportunity for nurses to identify their role in the client's progress along the illness-wellness continuum. The participation of team members in client care conferences such as discharge planning sessions improves the quality of decision-making and facilitates the development of individual team members. The cooperation and communication inherent in the system increase the potential for the delivery of quality nursing care.

Disadvantages

1. The team nursing model can very easily become a duplication of the functional method. For example, if team members are responsible for individual functions, such as administering medications, monitoring vital signs, or giving baths, it is difficult to differentiate this system from functional team nursing.

2. Team nursing may be less efficient than a functional system. The communication and coordination required for the success of the system are compromised if the team leader does not have skills in organization, leadership, communication, motivation, and nursing care delivery. This method can also be ineffective if staff members are not client-centered, skilled in nursing practice, and able to communicate clearly.

3. The number of personnel caring for clients is not substantially reduced in a team approach. This may not be cost effective and may dilute the quality of care provided, particularly in settings in which a large volume of non-nursing personnel provide direct care.

4. The dilution of individual responsibility and accountability may also decrease the quality of care provided.

5. Team nursing may also promote a task-oriented approach to client care.

6. The constant assignment of administration of medications to the team leader can result in a decline of medication administration skills of the registered and licensed practical nurses.

PRIMARY NURSING

Definition

Primary nursing is a system of care delivery that evolved in the 1980s in which the registered nurse is responsible and accountable for directing the care of a client or group of clients. The primary nurse develops the plan of care and ensures that the plan is implemented around the clock. In the absence of the primary nurse, the care of the client is delegated to an associate nurse, who follows the plan of care as developed by the primary nurse.

Primary nursing may be utilized in a variety of settings, including hospitals and public health agencies. Primary nursing systems emphasize

- the nurse's responsibility and accountability for management of care.
- decentralized decision-making with authority held by the primary nurse.
- the importance of accurate and complete assessment, diagnosis, and planning.
- the client's involvement in validation and goal-setting.
- the need for communication between primary nurses and other nurses, members of the health care team, and clients and their families.
- preparation for discharge through client and family teaching, identification of available resources, and referral to other systems when required.
- continuity of care by assigning the client to the primary nurse on a consistent basis.

In some settings, primary nurses select their own clients. This nurse provides direct care to a caseload, which usually does not exceed six clients. The head nurse functions as the coordinator of the unit and is a resource person for the primary nurses. The primary nurse plans and provides the care, administers medications and treatments, interacts with the physician and other health professionals, and reports on the client's status. Other levels of staff, including licensed practical nurses and nursing assistants, aid the primary nurse in the provision of care. Client care conferences, which involve primary and associate nurses as well as other members of the health care team, are sometimes utilized to discuss specific client problems and to develop strategies for resolving them.

The professional nurse functioning in a primary-care setting must have (1) a thorough knowledge of the nursing process, (2) refined communication skills, (3) the ability to perform nursing procedures identified in nursing interventions, (4) well-developed problem-solving techniques, and (5) a commitment to client-focused care.

Variations on Primary Nursing

Total Patient Care

In total patient care the nurse assigned to the client may be a registered nurse or a licensed practical nurse. In hospitals the nursing assistants are usually not assigned to clients but provide such useful services as answering call lights, offering water and snacks, transporting clients and specimens, obtaining equipment, making beds, and so on. The nurse assigned to the client administers medications, assists the client with activities of daily living, communicates with the other members of the health care team, performs treatments, and so on. In contrast to primary nursing, the nurse providing total patient care is usually not consistently the same person, but varies from day to day. This individual is responsible for ensuring that the plan is implemented during the shift, but not around the clock. Total patient care does not incorporate the roles of primary and associate nurses.

Modular Nursing

In this delivery system an attempt is made to assign the nurse to a group of clients in a district or module. A module consists of clients who are located within the same section of the nursing unit in nearby rooms. A registered nurse and often another person such as a registered nurse, licensed practical nurse, or nursing assistant are consistently assigned to the same module and care for any client admitted to a bed in the module. The registered nurse or licensed practical nurse provides total patient care for the individuals who are in the module, including giving medications. The result is a more efficient delivery of care. This system does not mandate 24-hour-a-day accountability for the care of the client, and is based on the premise that there are sufficient numbers of full-time staff nurses to allow for consistent assignment to the same module.

**PRIMARY
NURSING**
Definition
Variations
Advantages
Disadvantages

Advantages

1. The primary nursing and modular nursing methods of delivery promote consistent client care by virtue of the quality and frequency of interactions between the client and the nurse. Each primary or modular nurse is responsible for coordinating all aspects of care, including physical and emotional care, teaching, and the medical regimen.

2. This method promotes increased autonomy and responsibility in individual nursing practice. The nurse may be more satisfied because involvement in direct care is increased, and therefore the nurse's role in the client's recovery is more clearly defined. Additionally, the nurse is more accountable, because care responsibilities focus on the total care of a small number of clients rather than the partial care of many.

3. Primary nursing also provides the opportunity for professional growth. The nurse's involvement in all aspects of the client's care, particularly the decision-making component, facilitates the acquisition of new knowledge and skills. Nurses frequently believe that they are more effective in a primary system because they have a more global view of the needs of the client and family.

4. Clients are also generally more satisfied because of the increased frequency of interaction with one specific nurse who is particularly knowledgeable about them. This allows the client to identify clearly the

primary nurse and creates an atmosphere of trust and open communication.

5. Other health care providers, such as physicians, therapists, and dietitians, also appreciate the ability to interact with a nurse who is informed about the client.

6. Total patient care is a useful model when it is difficult to provide a consistent primary nurse. This happens, for example, when a unit is staffed by a number of part-time nurses or those working 12-hour shifts.

Disadvantages

1. Total patient care, modular nursing, and primary nursing require competent practitioners who can function independently when implementing the nursing process. Not all nurses are comfortable in accepting the responsibility associated with this system.

2. In some instances, primary nursing may be less economical than functional or team nursing, because this model may require a larger percentage of registered nurses. However, the abilities of the registered nurse can be spread through the use of a "nurse extender," a person working as an assistant to an experienced primary nurse. The registered nurse delegates responsibilities to the nurse extender while remaining accountable for care-planning.

CASE MANAGEMENT

Definition

Case management is the second generation of primary nursing. It evolved in the 1980s from the emphasis on decreasing length of stay and focus on achieving timely client outcomes and the need to improve the effectiveness and efficiency of health care delivery. Case management is the organization of care to achieve specific client outcomes within a time frame that is consistent with the length of stay designated by the client's diagnoses. The goals of case management include:

1. to facilitate the achievement of expected and/or standardized client outcomes.

2. to facilitate early discharge or discharge within an appropriate length of stay.

3. to promote appropriate and/or reduced utilization of resources.

4. to promote collaborative practice, coordination of care, and continuity of care.

5. to promote professional development and satisfaction of hospital-based registered nurses.

6. to direct the contributions of all care providers toward the achievement of patient outcomes (Bower, 1988).

Case managers are nurses with expertise in a particular clinical area. They may work with other similarly educated nurses in a group practice. The members of the group work in a variety of hospital units. "For example, nursing group practice members for patients with vascular disorders would include specifically identified nurses in the ambulatory care area, the general inpatient unit, the operating room, the intensive care unit, and the rehabilitation unit. Each of these nurses would be the primary nurse for the patients while they receive care in the various settings. One of the group practice members would be identified as an individual patient's case manager and would assume responsibility for the outcomes of the patient's care for the episode of illness" (Bower, 1988). The group practice works with other health care professionals to facilitate care that achieves the expected clinical outcomes within a reasonable time frame.

In another model, a facility hires a number of case managers who each specialize in a specific category of illness, such as cardiovascular medicine, orthopaedic surgery, or neurology.

Hospitals are moving to case management by hiring nurses into the case manager role or offering these positions to existing nursing personnel. Frequently case managers have backgrounds as utilization review nurses (who monitor the reason clients were admitted to the hospital and their length of stay), or were formerly team leaders, assistant head nurses, or staff nurses. These experiences prepare case managers to assume their role by providing leadership, clinical expertise, and organizational skills.

Two types of tools are used by nurses in case management: (1) A *case management plan* is a comprehensive plan of care that outlines the client's diagnoses, expected outcomes, and interventions. The plan is developed collaboratively by nurses and physicians and includes both medical and nursing interventions. (2) The *critical path* or *patient outcome timeline* is a one-page summary of the case management plan. This is also known as practice guidelines or parameters, clinical guidelines or protocol. An example was shown in Chapter 6 (Fig. 6-7).

CASE MAN-AGEMENT
Definition
Advantages
Disadvantages

Advantages

1. There is enhanced collaboration between nurses and other health care professionals, clients, and their families.

2. The critical path defines the prescribed care even if the care-giver changes or the case manager is not available.

3. The case manager is able to coordinate care more effectively by breaking down interdepartmental barriers.

4. Nurses experience increased morale, job satisfaction, and improved image as other personnel recognize them as leaders. This facilitates recruitment and retention efforts.

5. Discharge planning and client education begins earlier in the process, often prior to the hospital admission. For example, the teaching for a planned surgery may begin at the time of preadmission diagnostic testing. The assessment of the client may take place on this date, as well as the identification of individualized postoperative needs. This enables you and the client to more adequately plan for the postoperative recovery phase.

6. Achievement of client outcomes within a fiscally responsible time frame is enhanced.

7. Resources of the health care agency are utilized more efficiently, resulting in cost savings and reduction in length of stay.

8. Critical paths serve as teaching tools, especially in hospitals when new or inexperienced nurses are not familiar with the standards of care for certain client populations.

9. Clients are well informed and actively participate in their progress.

10. Case management promotes the establishment of standards of care for specific case types.

11. Part-time and agency nurses have a clearer indication of what needs to be done during the shift to move the client toward the outcomes.

12. Timely discharge of patients is facilitated.

13. Staff nurses have increased knowledge about the financial impact of the client's length of stay.

Disadvantages

1. The model requires a great deal of planning and cooperation to establish the system.

2. It may be difficult to obtain the cooperation of physicians in defining how to manage certain case types and to collaborate with nurses on a professional level. Some physicians fear that critical paths will produce cookbook medicine; others are threatened by collaboration with a case manager.

3. Some nurse managers have difficulty adjusting to this model as they give up their clinical duties and function more as managers.

4. Some staff nurses have difficulty accepting the increased accountability that is a part of being a case manager, whereas others are reluctant to give

up the coordination, client education, and discharge-planning roles to a case manager.

PATIENT-FOCUSED CARE

Definition

As a result of cost-containment pressures and the desire to improve the delivery of care, a new delivery model, patient-focused care, emerged in the early 1990s. Broadly defined, patient-focused care is "the redesign of patient care so that hospital resources and personnel are organized around patients rather than around various specialized departments" (Lumsdon, 1993). Fueled by a recognition that a health care facility is overcompartmentalized and forces the client to interact with too many people, patient-focused care is a radical restructuring of care delivery.

Principles

The principles of this model are as follows:

1. Place as many services on the nursing unit as possible to minimize the trips the client has to make for tests or services. Typically the unit will contain a pharmacy, radiology or laboratory testing equipment, and clerical personnel.

2. Cross-train health care professionals and unlicensed personnel to assume new responsibilities. These may include preparing housekeeping, laboratory, physical and respiratory therapy personnel to take part in the bedside care.

3. Intensify collaboration and communication between all levels within the organization.

4. Increase the ratio of direct client care-givers while reducing the number of people the client interacts with.

5. Redesign job descriptions and eliminate some of the departments in the hospital. For example, one hospital providing patient-focused care has a 44-bed medical surgical unit with five job classifications:
   a. **Unit representative:** performs clerical jobs, including handling medical records and answering questions about insurance.
   b. **Unit support assistant:** cleans and stocks the rooms and transports patients.
   c. **Team care specialist:** gives bedside care and comes from a variety of backgrounds, including registered nurses, licensed practical nurses, nurse aides, respiratory and physical therapists, electrocardiology technicians, radiology technicians, and admitting clerks. These indi-

viduals are able to provide bedside care, document, draw blood, do electrocardiograms, assist with discharge planning and x-rays, and provide patient education. (Some models pair a registered nurse with an unlicensed person and refer to this dyad as a *care pair*.)

   d. **Pharmacist:** prepares medications and provides patient education.

   e. **Clinical manager:** directs and supervises all unit activities; is a registered nurse with a nursing management background (Farris, 1993).

6. Often the nursing unit is redesigned with the elimination or reduction in size of the nurse's station. Smaller substations may be established. Linen, supplies, medications, and the client's medical record are moved to a cabinet inside or directly outside the client's room.

7. Patient-focused care may involve case management principles and activities, including case managers and critical paths.

The end result of all of these changes is a team of individuals who work together without the traditional department barriers. The client becomes the focus of care, instead of the organization trying to meet the needs of its departments.

Advantages

PATIENT-FOCUSED CARE
Definition
Principles
Advantages
Disadvantages

1. Clients report increased satisfaction with care because of the personalized care, the reduction in the number of interactions with personnel, and the reduction in time spent waiting for tests to be performed.

2. Hospital personnel have increased satisfaction as a result of improved efficiency and morale, autonomous problem-solving, and increased contact with clients.

3. The model promotes an efficient team of health care providers with improved communication.

4. Errors are reduced.

5. Continuity of care is increased.

6. Length of stay in the facility is reduced.

7. Cost savings have resulted from the reduction in errors and improved efficiency.

Disadvantages

1. Gaining physician acceptance of the change can be a major challenge.

2. There are high costs associated with education of personnel to assume new roles.

3. Nurses must learn to be managers of their care partner.

4. There are considerable costs associated with remodeling the nursing unit.

5. The move to patient-focused care is a radical departure from the traditional model of organizing a hospital into rigid departments. This change can be very threatening.

6. Some allied professionals fear that nurses cannot perform the same tasks as well as the allied professionals, even with training.

7. Nurses may be concerned about the blurring of the nursing role.

CASE STUDY

The following example depicts how the delivery systems might affect the care of a hypothetical client. Paul Kumar, age 56, was admitted to the hospital for major abdominal surgery. His postoperative course was uncomplicated. Depending on the type of nursing care delivery system in place, his first day after surgery may have fit one of these descriptions.

Functional Nursing

At the change of shift report the head nurse assigned everyone to a task for the day. Paul's day began when the nursing assistant woke him and all of the clients by taking their temperatures. The licensed practical nurse came by a few minutes later to take Paul's blood pressure. An hour later the medication nurse delivered his medications on the way down the hall with the medication cart. A licensed practical nurse assisted him in washing because this nurse was assigned to do baths. A registered nurse doing the treatments for the day came in after lunch to change his dressing. Paul wanted to complain to someone that he waited until 11:00 AM for his morning bath so he shared his dissatisfaction with the head nurse. The head nurse revised his plan of care to reflect his preference for an early bath. Change of shift report was given by the head nurse based on all the information provided by the staff nurses.

Team Nursing

The shift began when the head nurse placed the nurses on a team. The team leader, a registered nurse, assigned a registered nurse to take care of Paul. The registered nurse took Paul's vital signs, assisted him with his bath, and changed his dressing. Meanwhile, the team leader spent the day giving medications. When Paul complained to the team leader that he had to wait until 11:00 AM for his morning bath, the team leader explained that an emergency had caused a delay in the work schedule of his assigned nurse. The team leader made a few additions to Paul's care plan based on the registered nurse's feedback and shared these during the change of shift report.

8-1 TEST YOURSELF

Nursing Care Delivery System

When you are on the clinical unit, observe the delivery of nursing care. Answer the following questions:

1. Who makes the assignments?
2. Is the same nurse assigned to the client more than one day in a row?
3. Are there any critical paths in use on this unit?
4. What levels of personnel are providing nursing care on this unit?
5. Are nursing assistants or technicians working on this unit? If yes, what are they doing?
6. Do you see any nurses performing non-nursing tasks? What are they? Compare observations with your classmates.
7. Ask your client, "If you had a complaint about your care, who would you go to?"
8. Review the nursing care plans on the unit. Have they been developed by staff nurses or has one person done them all? Who is that person?
9. Who gives the report at the end of the shift? Who listens to report?
10. Are supplies centrally located or near every room? Does the location of the supplies have any effect on your delivery of care?
11. Does the unit have a pharmacy? If no, ask a staff nurse for an opinion on whether it would be helpful to have a pharmacy on the unit.
12. Who transports clients to other areas of the hospital? If this is the responsibility of the nurse, ask a staff nurse for an opinion on how well this system works.
13. Based on your observations, what model of nursing care is being used to deliver care?
14. Ask the head nurse and a staff nurse what model of nursing care is being used on the unit. Are their answers the same as yours? If there is a discrepancy, see if you can figure out why.

CASE STUDY
Functional Nursing
Team Nursing
Primary Nursing
Case Management
Patient-Focused
Care

Primary Nursing

At change of shift report the head nurse reviewed the assignment. Paul's primary nurse had admitted him on the morning of his surgery and was assigned to provide his care. The primary nurse took his vital signs, helped him wash, provided his medications, and changed his dressing. Paul realized that this bath was delayed until 11:00 AM because he had been told by his primary nurse that it would be more comfortable for him to bathe after pain medication had taken effect. The primary nurse made a few additions to Paul's care plan and discussed these during change of shift report. Paul's nurse gave report directly to the nurse on the evening shift who was going to be taking care of Paul.

Case Management

Paul's case manager was a registered nurse who was part of the abdominal surgical group practice. After change of shift report, the staff nurse took Paul's vital signs and administered his medications. Paul's bath and dressing change were performed by his staff nurse. During the morning the case manager and the surgeon reviewed the critical path and saw no need to make revisions in it. Paul did not complain about his bath being done at 11:00 AM because he knew his first priority was to be kept comfortable with pain medication. His critical path indicated that he was to get out of bed with assistance in the afternoon, which his case manager explained to him early in the admission. When the staff nurse gave report to the nurses on the next shift, Paul's response to ambulating to the chair was discussed. His progress on the critical path was reviewed as well.

Patient-Focused Care

After change of shift report a care pair consisting of a registered nurse and person with physical therapy training entered Paul's room. The registered nurse performed a physical assessment and took Paul's vital signs. The nurse also administered the medications that were prepared by the unit-based pharmacist. The therapist assisted Paul with his bath at 11 AM and helped him to walk in the hall. Concerned about some lung congestion, the physician ordered a chest x-ray, which was done on the nursing unit by the therapist. When the x-ray indicated the beginning of pneumonia, Paul was started on antibiotics. The purposes and side effects of the medication were explained to him by the pharmacist. At change of shift report the registered nurse explained Paul's change in condition and revised the plan of care.

SUMMARY

Functional, team, primary nursing, case management, and patient-centered care are methods of delivering nursing care. The differences among the systems are dependent on the mechanisms utilized by nurses to organize and deliver care. Each method has advantages that influence the efficiency and effectiveness of the system. In the 1990s functional nursing is the least common method of delivering nursing care. Case management is projected to be the most commonly used method of nursing care delivery, with patient-focused care gaining in acceptance.

REFERENCES

Bower K: Managed Care: Controlling Costs, Guaranteeing Outcomes. Definition 1-3, Summer, 1988a.

Bower K: Case Management: Meeting the Challenge. Definition 3-1, Winter, 1988b.

Farris, B: Converting a Unit to Patient Focused Care, Health Progress, 1993 April; 22.

Lumsdon K: Putting patients first. Hospitals 1993 5:14.

BIBLIOGRAPHY

Anderson C and Hughes E: Implementing modular nursing in a long term care facility. J Nurs Admin 1993; 23(6):29.

Brett J and Tonges M: Restructured patient care delivery: Evaluation of the ProACT™ model. Nurs Econ 1990; 8(1):36.

Brider P: The move to patient focused care. Am J Nurs 1992 September; 26.

Cassidy J: Patient-focused delivery promises to reshape hospitals. Health Progress 1992 May; 20.

Cassidy J: Patient participation. Health Progress 1992 December; 42.

Flynn A and Kilgallen M: Case management: A multidisciplinary approach to the evaluation of cost and quality standards. J Nurs Care Qual 1993; 8(1).

Glandon G, Colbert K, and Thomasma M: Nursing delivery models and RN mix: cost implications. Nurs Manag 1989 20(5):31–33.

Lumsdon K and Hagland M: Mapping care. Hospitals Health Networks 1993; 20:34.

Townsend M: Patient focused care: is it for your hospital. Nurs Manage 1993; 24(9):74.

Watson P and others: Operational restructuring: A patient focused approach. Nursing Administration Quarterly 1991 Fall; 45.

Woodyard L and Sheetz J: Critical pathway patient outcomes: The missing standard. J Nurs Care Qual 1993 8(1):51.

NINE

EVALUATION

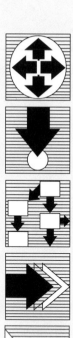

After reading this chapter, you will be able to:

1. List six questions that are used in the evaluation phase of the nursing process.
2. Document the client's achievement of outcomes on the progress notes.
3. Differentiate between quality assurance and quality improvement.
4. Utilize a systematic process for evaluating the quality of care.

INTRODUCTION

Evaluation is the final phase in the nursing process and occurs whenever the nurse interacts with the client. The American Nurses' Association (ANA) standards, the nursing process, regulatory agencies, and the nurse practice act all require that evaluation be a part of nursing practice. The ANA standard on evaluation identifies evaluation as an essential component of the nursing process (Fig. 9-1).

EVALUATION IS SYSTEMATIC AND ONGOING

Evaluation can be conducted as part of the nursing process when you compare the client's health status with the outcomes defined by the plan of care. As a

ANA Measurement Criteria Standard VI-1 (Standard of Care): Evaluation is systematic and ongoing.

STANDARD VI. EVALUATION
The Nurse Evaluates the Client's Progress Toward Attainment of Outcomes

Measurement Criteria

1. Evaluation is systematic and ongoing.
2. The client's responses to interventions are documented.
3. The effectiveness of interventions is evaluated in relation to outcomes.
4. Ongoing assessment data are used to revise diagnoses, outcomes, and the plan of care, as needed.
5. Revisions in diagnoses, outcomes, and the plan of care are documented.
6. The client, significant others, and health care providers are involved in the evaluation process, when appropriate.

FIGURE 9-1   ANA Standard VI: Planning.

(Reprinted with permission from *Standards of Clinical Nursing Practice*, American Nurses' Association, Washington, DC, 1991.)

result of this activity you determine if the care plan is appropriate, realistic, current, or in need of revision. If the client has not achieved the outcomes you will engage in problem-solving to determine how to revise the care plan.

Evaluation is accomplished by asking a series of questions:

1. Was the outcome in the plan of care achieved?
2. If not, were the outcomes appropriate?
3. Was the nursing diagnosis resolved?
4. If not, were the human responses and related factors in the nursing diagnosis accurate?
5. Were the interventions appropriate?
6. If not, does the plan of care need to be revised?

Figure 9-2 illustrates the steps of the evaluation process. Each step will be discussed in detail in this chapter.

Was the outcome achieved?

1. Was the Outcome Achieved?

After gathering data, compare the client's current health status with the outcomes identified on the plan of care.

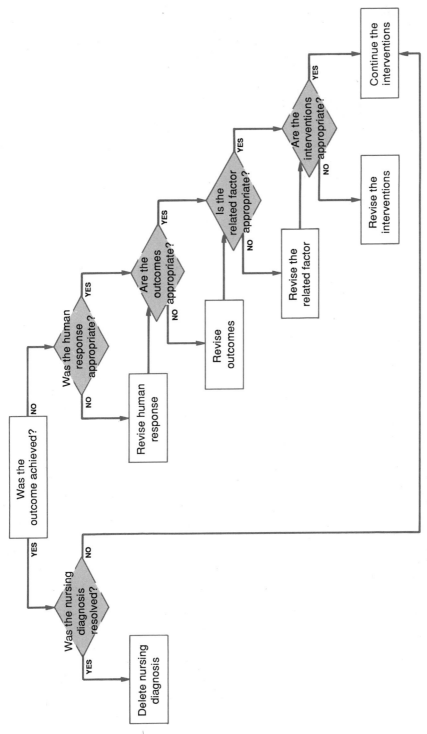

FIGURE 9-2 Diagram of the evaluation process.

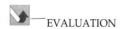

Example

NURSING DIAGNOSIS	OUTCOME
Altered skin integrity related to prolonged immobility	Throughout hospitalization, free from skin breakdown over bony prominence

To evaluate this outcome carefully inspect the client's skin, paying particular attention to the sacrum, elbows, hips, and heels. The inspection would occur as an ongoing part of care while the client is being bathed or positioned.

After gathering data about the client's health status and comparing the data with the outcome, you will make a judgment about the client's achievement of the outcome. There are two possible responses:

1. The outcome was achieved and

2. The outcome was not achieved.

The Outcome Was Achieved

Example.   Robin Johnson delivered her first child by cesarean birth two days ago. On the first day after delivery she has many questions about breast feeding. Robin expresses the fear that she will never be able to learn how to breast-feed because it seems so complicated. On the second day after delivery Robin tells the nurse, "I feel so much better about breast feeding. I'm getting the hang of it." The nurse notes that Robin is using the correct technique and congratulates her on her progress.

NURSING DIAGNOSIS	OUTCOME	EVALUATION DATA
Ineffective breast-feeding related to feelings of inadequacy and lack of knowledge	Within two days demonstrates ability to breast-feed	Observed to be using correct technique

ANA Measurement Criteria Standard VI-2 (Standard of Care): The client's responses to interventions are documented.

In this example the nurse compared the data or cue with the outcome. The judgment was made that the client had achieved the outcome. The response identified by the nursing diagnosis had been resolved because Robin was able to breast-feed successfully.

Progress notes document the client's status in relation to the desired

---

BOX 9-1

**Examples of How to Document
When the Client Achieves the Outcomes**

Area to Evaluate	Example of Evaluation Comments
Progress toward achieving outcomes	Incision shows no signs of infection
Response to prn medications	Verbalized relief of pain 45 minutes after injection of morphine
Response to change in activity	Able to walk from bed to bathroom without getting dyspneic
Response to treatments	Following Fleets enema had large amount of watery brown stool
Ability to perform activities of daily living, particularly those which may influence discharge planning	Able to move from bed to chair with assistance of one person
Response to diet or advancement of diet	Consumed all of full liquid lunch; stated she was hungry and wanted more solid food

---

outcomes. The client's responses are compared with the outcomes defined by the plan of care. Box 9-1 contains concepts typically addressed in the progress notes, together with examples of evaluative comments.

The Outcome Was Not Achieved

At times the outcome is not achieved. This may be due to a variety of reasons, including that the outcome, nursing diagnosis, or interventions were not appropriate. The evaluation of each of these components of the plan of care will be discussed next.

2. Was the Outcome Appropriate?

The outcome that you defined with the client may no longer be applicable to the client's needs. Sometimes changes in the client's circumstances or condition invalidate the outcome and require a change in the plan of care.

Was the outcome achieved?

If not, was the outcome appropriate?

Example. Linda Dote is admitted to the hospital after an argument in which her husband fractured her ribs and ruptured her spleen. On the second day after admission you helped Linda to set an outcome of being able to work out a plan to move out of her home permanently. During discussions Linda continues to say, "Part of me wants to leave him and part of me is afraid to try to make it on my own. I've never lived alone. I'm afraid I would be lonely." On the fourth day of her hospitalization, Linda's husband shows up with a dozen red roses and promises to never hit her again. Although you explain to her that this is a predictable phase in the cycle of violence, Linda is unwilling to listen. "Don't you see? He promised he wouldn't hurt me. I think he really means it this time." Recognizing that Linda was now uninterested in moving out, you give her written information on the local shelter for battered women. You say, "Linda, you may need this information some day. You will be protected at the shelter and will have a chance to think while your husband cools off." Linda replies, "I am sure I will never need this phone number but I will keep it—just in case."

NURSING DIAGNOSIS	OUTCOME	EVALUATION DATA	REVISED OUTCOME
Decisional conflict (separation from husband) related to fear of loneliness	By the time of discharge identifies a plan for alternative living arrangements	Unwilling to listen to explanation of cycle of violence Not interested in moving to a shelter	By the time of discharge is able to describe how to contact shelter

In this example you determined that Linda was not ready to achieve the outcome of planning a move out of her home. Because the nursing diagnosis was appropriate, you revised the outcome.

Was the outcome achieved?

If not, was the outcome appropriate?

Was the nursing diagnosis resolved?

3. Was the Nursing Diagnosis Resolved?

Does the nursing diagnosis describe an ongoing problem or human response, or has the response been resolved? If the nursing diagnosis has not been resolved, gather additional data to determine if the human response and related/risk factors in the nursing diagnosis were accurate.

At times the client does not achieve the outcome because the nursing diagnosis is not accurate, applicable, or appropriate. When the outcomes are not achieved first review the human response to determine if it accurately describes the client's status. This process is done by comparing the defining characteristics associated with the diagnosis with the client's symptoms. If the diagnosis is not pertinent to the client's problems, assessment skills are used to gather more data.

Was the outcome achieved?

If not, was the outcome appropriate?

Next, the related/risk factor in the nursing diagnosis is reviewed when an outcome is not achieved after the human response and outcome are evaluated to be applicable to the client. Determine if the related/risk factor is accurate in describing the cause of the human response. You can use assessment data to decide if the related/risk factor is descriptive and current.

Was the nursing diagnosis resolved?

If not, was the human response and related factor in the nursing diagnosis accurate?

Example.   Peter Greene, age 72, was admitted to the hospital a week ago with pancreatitis. He is very restless, changes position in bed frequently, and indicates anticipation of his wife's visit because she knows how to make him feel better. Although he is capable of washing himself, he tells you that he wants to wait until his wife comes in.

You put these data together and conclude that Mr. Greene's restlessness is caused by anxiety. However, when his wife arrives at 2:00, he continues to be restless. Wondering if something other than anxiety is at the root of Mr. Greene's symptoms, you begin asking him questions and assessing his physical status. When you discover that Mr. Greene had a distended bladder, he states, "Things haven't been working right since that tube came out of my bladder last night." You realize that *urinary retention* is a more specific diagnosis for Mr. Greene and contacted his doctor.

ORIGINAL PLAN OF CARE		
NURSING DIAGNOSIS	OUTCOME	EVALUATION DATA
Anxiety related to unknown cause	Verbalizes decrease in anxiety at the time of wife's visit	Restlessness
REVISED PLAN OF CARE		
NURSING DIAGNOSIS	OUTCOME	EVALUATION DATA
Urinary retention related to effects of diminished sensory impulses 2° to catheterization	Empties bladder by voiding or by catheterization within one hour	Distended bladder Difficulty voiding

In this example the original diagnosis did not accurately describe the symptoms the client was experiencing. Further assessment resulted in additional data and revision of the nursing diagnosis and plan of care.

Example.   Carla Woerner is a 19-year-old nursing student who has completed the first semester of her program. She visits the college health nurse, stating she was upset about her grades. "I feel overwhelmed by all of this studying I have to do. I feel so helpless. I always got good grades in high school. Why can't I get A's in nursing school?" The nurse encourages Carla to talk about her feelings and refers her to the academic advisor for information on study skills. Additionally, Carla is given an appointment to revisit the nurse in three weeks.

When Carla comes in for her second visit she looks tired and disheveled. She has not bathed or changed clothes in a week. "It is no use," she tells the nurse. "I'll never learn all of this stuff. My parents will be angry at me for wasting their money. I must confess I've thought about ending it all." When the nurse asks Carla about her desire to "end it all," Carla says, "My roommate has some sleeping pills. I've been wondering if it hurts to die." The nurse recognizes that Carla is at high risk for suicide and arranges for her to be seen by the staff psychiatrist within half an hour.

ORIGINAL PLAN OF CARE

NURSING DIAGNOSIS	OUTCOME	INTERVENTIONS
Situational low self-esteem related to perceived academic overload	Within three weeks makes positive statements about self and ability to complete studies	1. Refer to academic advisor for study skills review 2. Encourage to verbalize feelings 3. Set up revisit in three weeks

REVISED PLAN OF CARE

NURSING DIAGNOSIS	OUTCOME	INTERVENTION
High risk for injury: self-directed related to feelings of failure	Does not harm self while suicidal	1. Obtain immediate psychiatric attention

---

In this situation the nurse identified that Carla did not achieve the outcome of verbalizing more positive feelings about herself. Additional assessment data revealed that Carla had a plan for committing suicide and was in immediate danger. The nursing diagnosis was revised along with the outcomes and interventions.

More data are gathered and revision of the related factor and interventions occurs when the nurse determines that the related factor is not appropriate.

Example.   During Janie Howard's monthly visit to the outpatient department her blood pressure is found to be elevated. The clinic nurse concludes that Janie needs a review of the causes and treatment of high blood pressure and gives her pamphlets to read. Janie's blood pressure is still elevated during her visit the following month. While being questioned by the nurse, Janie says, "Oh, I know I need to take my pills. I just can't afford to keep refilling my prescription. Instead of taking one pill every day, I've been taking one every other day to make them last longer." At this point the nurse realizes that financial concerns are the real reason for Janie's noncompliance. Janie is given a list of discount drugstores in the area and a new prescription for a medication that would be just as effective yet less expensive.

ORIGINAL PLAN OF CARE

NURSING DIAGNOSIS	OUTCOME	INTERVENTIONS
Ineffective management of therapeutic regimen related to lack of financial resources	Takes prescribed medication daily	Educate on cause and treatment of hypertension

REVISED PLAN OF CARE

NURSING DIAGNOSIS	OUTCOME	INTERVENTIONS
Ineffective management of therapeutic regimen related to lack of financial resources	Takes prescribed medication daily	1. Contact physician for change in prescription 2. Provide client with discount drug store list

5. Were the Interventions Appropriate?

As you examine and evaluate each part of the plan of care, including the outcomes and nursing diagnoses, you will also judge the interventions. You may choose to continue the interventions after determining that they are appropriate.

Example. Floyd Kendrick is hospitalized because of widespread bone cancer. His pain is being managed with a continuous infusion of morphine. When asked about his pain, Floyd states, "The medicine keeps it under control."

Was the outcome achieved?

If not, was the outcome appropriate?

Was the nursing diagnosis resolved?

If not, was the human response and related factor in the nursing diagnosis accurate?

Are the interventions appropriate?

NURSING DIAGNOSIS	OUTCOME	INTERVENTION	EVALUATION DATA
Pain related to effects of terminal illness	While morphine infusion is present, verbalizes that he is comfortable	1. Maintain morphine infusion at ordered rates 2. Evaluate level of pain every three hours	Client states, "The medicine keeps the pain under control"

In the above example, the nurse asked Floyd about his pain level. Involvement of the client, significant others, and health care personnel in

ANA Measurement Criteria Standard VI-3 (Standard of Care): The effectiveness of the interventions is evaluated in relation to the outcomes.

ANA Measurement Criteria Standard VI-6 (Standard of Care): The client, significant others, and health care providers are involved in the evaluation process, when appropriate.

providing information about the plan of care gives you valuable data. Floyd's pain is being managed jointly by the nurses and the physician. Each will have important data to share to determine if Floyd is receiving the most effective therapy. Ultimately it is Floyd's perception about his level of comfort that will be most valid.

Revise the Interventions

When the nursing diagnosis is not resolved and the outcomes have been revised, the nurse should review the interventions specified in the plan of care and determine why they were not effective in assisting the client. Careful analysis of the approaches used may indicate alternative strategies that will assist the client in achieving the outcome.

Example.   A newly diagnosed diabetic has been taught how to inject himself with insulin. He is instructed using normal saline and an orange. A week later he is hospitalized with a blood glucose level of 680 mg/ml (normal value is 80 to 120 mg/ml). After he is stabilized, a nurse brings him a vial of insulin and asks him to demonstrate his injection technique. The client draws up the correct dosage without difficulty and then looks around, appearing confused. "I can't give this. I don't have an orange." The nurse discovers he has been injecting the orange with insulin and then eating it (Roc, 1992).

Clearly something went wrong during the initial instruction and in the evaluation of this client's understanding of the teaching provided. The interventions were revised to include reteaching insulin injection technique.

Progress notes document the client's status in relation to the desired outcomes. When the client's responses are compared with the outcomes and the client has not met the outcomes, document your evaluation. Box 9-2 illustrates how to document in these situations.

Was the outcome achieved?

If not, was the outcome appropriate?

Was the nursing diagnosis resolved?

If not, was the human response and related factor in the nursing diagnosis accurate?

Are the interventions appropriate?

Does the plan of care need to be revised?

6. Does the Plan of Care Need to Be Revised?

Evaluation of the achievement of outcomes carries the nurse through the nursing process to the revision of the plan of care. Any of the components of the plan of care may need to be revised: the nursing diagnosis, outcomes, or interventions. Additional diagnoses, outcomes, or interventions may need to be added to the plan. Many of the examples used up to this point of the chapter include information on how the nurse revised the plan of care.

For example, when the client continues to experience the symptoms associated with the diagnosis, you should consider developing additional outcomes. Some nursing diagnoses describe complex human responses in which it is appropriate to set outcomes at increasing levels of difficulty. For example, a severely dehydrated client with a nursing diagnosis of fluid volume deficit related to decreased oral intake might have an initial outcome of

---

BOX 9-2
Examples of How to Document
When the Client Does Not Achieve the Outcomes

Area to Evaluate	Example of Evaluation Comments
Progress toward achieving outcomes	Unable to identify the impact of substance-abusing behavior on his life
Response to prn medications	Has developed a pattern of requiring progressively large doses of medication of pain
Response to change in activity	Client is very reluctant to increase his activity by walking in the hall with help
Response to treatments	Unwilling to participate in group therapy
Ability to perform activities of daily living, particularly those that may influence daily living	Unable to wash herself without developing extreme shortness of breath
Response to diet or advancement of diet	Cannot tolerate an increase in her diet beyond clear fluids; complains of nausea when she tries to eat solid food

---

"consumes 3000 ml every 24 hours." As the client's condition improves the outcome may be revised to read "consumes 2000 ml every 24 hours."

Example. Linda Van Aulen has a newly inserted permanent pacemaker. After two sessions with you, Linda is able to correctly calculate her pulse rate. You explain that the next skill to be mastered involves learning to check her pacemaker over the telephone.

ANA Measurement Criteria Standard VI-5 (Standard of Care): Revisions in the diagnoses, outcomes, and the plan of care are documented.

NURSING DIAGNOSIS	ORIGINAL OUTCOME	EVALUATION DATA
Knowledge deficit (calculation of pulse, pacemaker evaluation technique)	Within two days correctly counts pulse rate	Observed to correctly calculate pulse rate

NEW OUTCOME
Demonstrates correct technique for trans telephonic pacemaker evaluation by 9/10

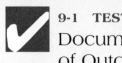
An evaluative comment is a judgment made by comparing data or cues with the outcome. Read the following case studies. Assuming the interventions you developed in Chapter 6's Test Yourself exercise were implemented, write an evaluative comment demonstrating that the outcome has been met and one demonstrating the outcome has not been met.

Case 1. Cassie Tilton is an 88-year-old woman transferred to your unit from a skilled nursing facility. Her history reveals a "flu-like" syndrome for the past five days with persistent vomiting and diarrhea. Her vital signs are: B/P 108/56, P 112, R 24, and T 101.4. Her mucous membranes are dry and skin turgor is decreased. She indicates that she feels weak, tired, and thirsty.

NURSING DIAGNOSIS	OUTCOMES
Fluid volume deficit related to vomiting and diarrhea	Within 48 hours: moist mucous membranes, vital signs within normal limits for client, intake greater than output

OUTCOME ACHIEVED

OUTCOME NOT ACHIEVED

Case 2. Chip Ireland is a 35-year-old businessman admitted to the outpatient surgicenter for a tonsillectomy. He indicates that he has had recurrent tonsillitis for the past three years. Postoperatively he complains of being thirsty and requests a cold drink. You observe that he has difficulty swallowing and coughs up the water. He states, "My throat is too sore; it feels like it is swollen." Upon examination, you note the presence of redness and edema in the operative area.

NURSING DIAGNOSIS	OUTCOME
Impaired swallowing related to edema and effects of surgery	By the time of discharge (from surgicenter) demonstrates ability to swallow at least 240 ml fluid

OUTCOME ACHIEVED

OUTCOME NOT ACHIEVED

Continued.

9-1   TEST YOURSELF
Documentation of Achievement of Outcomes–cont'd.

Case 3. Emily Fantin is an 86-year-old woman who calls the office nurse and requests free samples of laxatives. She complains, "I've spent so much money on laxatives at the drug store; I take them twice a day so that my bowels will move two times a day. My mother always told me to take laxatives to keep myself regular. By the way, do you have any sample enemas?" Upon further questioning you find out that Emily lives alone and does her own cooking. She eats mostly frozen dinners or prepared foods with few fruits and vegetables. In addition, she shops at a local convenience store with a limited supply of fresh produce. She relies on Metamucil daily, and Ex Lax and Milk of Magnesia approximately four times a week. She states that she gets very little exercise.

NURSING DIAGNOSIS	OUTCOME
Perceived constipation related to long-standing family health beliefs	Within two months verbalizes satisfaction with one bowel movement every one to two days

OUTCOME ACHIEVED
_____

OUTCOME NOT ACHIEVED
_____

When the nursing diagnosis has been resolved, the care plan is revised. This is commonly accomplished by crossing off the nursing diagnosis, outcomes, and interventions; or by placing a date in a column labeled "Date Resolved." These methods are illustrated in Figure 9-3.

EVALUATION AND THE NURSING PROCESS

Evaluation is a complex and systematic part of the nursing process. It reviews the nursing diagnosis (human response and related/risk factors and interventions). Each phase of the nursing process is linked to evaluation.

Some individuals mistakenly use the words "assess" and "evaluate"

EVALUATION IS
SYSTEMATIC
AND ONGOING
EVALUATION
AND THE NURS-
ING PROCESS

9-1   TEST YOURSELF

Documentation of Achievement of Outcomes: Answers

Case 1. Cassie Tilton

NURSING DIAGNOSIS	OUTCOMES
Fluid volume deficit related to vomiting and diarrhea	Within 48 hours: moist mucous membranes, vital signs within normal limits for client, intake greater than output

OUTCOME ACHIEVED

Client is well hydrated. Vital signs: B/P 118/80, P 78, R 18, and T 98.8. No evidence of vomiting and diarrhea, mucous membrane moist. Intake and output: 3060 ml intake and 2200 ml output.

OUTCOME NOT ACHIEVED

Still exhibits signs of dehydration. Vomited 600 ml of brownish-green fluid. No evidence of diarrhea. Unable to tolerate any PO fluids. Vital signs: B/P 110/54, P 116, R 22, T 101 rectally. Lips dry and crusted, complains of being thirsty.

Case 2. Chip Ireland

NURSING DIAGNOSIS	OUTCOME
Impaired swallowing related to edema and effects of surgery	By the time of discharge (from surgicenter) demonstrates ability to swallow at least 240 ml fluid

OUTCOME ACHIEVED

Client ready for discharge. No evidence of swelling or difficulty breathing. Drank 300 ml of ice water with minimal difficulty.

OUTCOME NOT ACHIEVED

Client still reports feeling of swelling in throat. Ice maintained to neck. Denies difficulty breathing. Refusing to sip water but is taking ice chips occasionally.

Continued.

9-1 TEST YOURSELF
Documentation of Achievement
of Outcomes: Answers–cont'd.

Case 3. Emily Fantin

NURSING DIAGNOSIS	OUTCOME
Perceived constipation related to long-standing family health beliefs	Within two months verbalizes satisfaction with one bowel movement every one to two days

OUTCOME ACHIEVED

Emily proudly reports today that she has been having one bowel movement daily. States she has not used a laxative in two weeks.

OUTCOME NOT ACHIEVED

Emily complains she has stomach bloating and increased flatus. She has been taking laxatives despite the fact that she has been having a daily bowel movement. States she needs them to help get rid of the bloated feeling.

DATE / INITIALS 9–10 KS			DATE / INITIALS 9–10 KS			
NURSING DIAGNOSIS	OUTCOME	INTERVENTIONS	NURSING DIAGNOSIS	OUTCOME	INTERVENTIONS	RESOLVED
		1. ~~Teach effective breastfeeding techniques.~~			1. Teach effective breastfeeding techniques.	9–12
~~Ineffective breastfeeding related to feelings of inadequacy~~	~~Within two days demonstrates ability to breastfeed~~	2. ~~Provide with booklet:~~ "Feeding your baby." 3. ~~Reinforce correct techniques.~~	Ineffective breastfeeding related to feelings of inadequacy	Within two days demonstrates ability to breastfeed	2. Provide with booklet: "Feeding your baby." 3. Reinforce correct techniques.	

FIGURE 9-3 Examples of how to indicate the nursing diagnosis has been resolved.

interchangeably. In the nursing process, assessment involves collecting data. Evaluation occurs when you compare the data to the outcomes and make a judgment about the client's progress. The results of this judgment may lead to the revision of the plan of care.

ANA Measurement Criteria Standard VI-4 (Standard of Care): Ongoing assessment data are used to revise diagnoses, outcomes, and the plan of care, as needed.

The nurse re*assesses* the client's responses to determine whether the outcomes have been achieved. Objective and subjective data (defining characteristics) are reviewed to ensure that the *nursing diagnoses* identified for the client are correct. Next, judgments are made about the appropriateness of the *planned* outcomes and interventions. Finally, revisions are *implemented* as necessary.

NURSING DIAGNOSIS

Pain related to inflammatory process secondary to surgery

OUTCOME

Verbalizes relief of pain within 30 minutes after comfort measures

NURSING DIAGNOSIS

High risk for ineffective airway clearance related to retained secretions

OUTCOME

Clear breath sounds throughout hospitalization

NURSING DIAGNOSIS

Fear related to effects of separation from 2-year-old as evidenced by expression of concern

OUTCOME

Describes less fear within two days

CRITICAL THINKING AND EVALUATION

Clearly, evaluation cannot take place without critical thinking. The process of making judgments is founded on the ability to critically analyze the information presented to you. As you sort through data and determine the additional facts that you need to evaluate the client's progress, you use critical thinking and analytical skills.

Example.   In previous chapters you learned about Maria Rosselli, who had lung surgery. Maria's postoperative nursing diagnoses include pain related to inflammatory process secondary to surgery, high risk for ineffective airway clearance related to retained secretions, and fear related to effects of separation from 2-year-old child as evidenced by expression of concerns.

Applying the critical thinking model to Maria, you would ask the following questions:

1. *What is the issue?*
   In the evaluation phase of the nursing process, you are interested in knowing if Maria's nursing diagnoses have been resolved.

2. *What information do I need?*
   In order to evaluate Maria's pain level you would ask:
   a. Is the dose of morphine appropriate for Maria based on her size and response to pain?
   b. Is the morphine keeping Maria comfortable?
   c. Is there any evidence that Maria is oversedated by the dose she is receiving? For example, is her respiratory rate 16 to 20? Is she able to answer questions coherently?
   To evaluate Maria's airway clearance, you would
   a. listen to her breath sounds to see if her chest is clear.
   b. determine if Maria is able to perform coughing and deep breathing.
   c. see if Maria can expectorate excessive amounts of mucus.
   Focusing on the nursing diagnosis of fear, you would
   a. determine if Maria is expressing less fear.
   b. decide if Maria's fear is interfering with her ability to recover from surgery. For example, is she able to obtain adequate rest?

3. *Are my data valid?*
   You can rely on your physical assessment skills because you have learned

to listen to breath sounds. You have accurately counted Maria's respiratory rate. The information that Maria slept all night came from the night nurse during change of shift report.

4. *What do the data mean?*
When you examine Maria, her breath sounds are clear. She has been able to arrange for her husband to bring her child to the hospital and is relieved that her daughter seems to be adjusting to her absence. However, Maria is very lethargic, has slurred speech, and has a respiratory rate of 12.

5. *Based on the facts, what should I do?*
Using your critical-thinking abilities, you evaluate possible causes for Maria's behavior. After reviewing the medications she is on, you determine that there are no drug interactions that would explain Maria's behavior. You also rule out the possibility that Maria has been drinking alcohol or taking any illicit drugs. The medication records shows that Maria has been receiving a large dose of morphine at frequent intervals. Concerned that Maria is receiving too much morphine, you contact the physician and describe Maria's behavior. The doctor reduces the dose of morphine.

6. *Is there other information I need?*
With this revision in Maria's pain management, you will be carefully observing her to determine if her pain level is kept under control with a reduction in dosage.

7. *Is this the best way to deal with the issue?*
In order to evaluate Maria, you have systematically collected data, drawn inferences from the data, taken action to protect Maria from the hazards of the narcotic she is receiving, and instituted a plan to reevaluate Maria. This reflects the essence of the nursing process.

EVALUATION OF THE QUALITY OF CARE

EVALUATION IS
SYSTEMATIC
AND ONGOING

EVALUATION
AND THE NURS-
ING PROCESS

CRITICAL THINK-
ING AND
EVALUATION

EVALUATION OF
THE QUALITY OF
CARE

Up to this point the concept of evaluation has been discussed from the perspective of the nurse who evaluates the client's achievement of outcomes. Part of the professional responsibilities of a nurse include evaluating the care given to groups of clients. Three ANA standards address our responsibility to evaluate the practice of others (Figs. 9-4 to 9-6).

Each of the measurement criteria of the ANA Quality of Care standard (Fig. 9-4) will be briefly discussed. The activities described in this standard fit into the broad category of quality assurance. Quality assurance involves systematically monitoring the quality of care and taking actions to improve the care. Quality improvement, which evolved out of quality assurance, focuses more on improving the system in which care is delivered. For example, quality assurance monitoring may evaluate how well nurses are following the policy to put the date on intravenous tubing. Quality im-

STANDARD I. QUALITY OF CARE

The Nurse Systematically Evaluates the Quality and Effectiveness of Nursing Practice

Measurement Criteria

1. The nurse participates in quality of care activities as appropriate to the individual's position, education, and practice environment. Such activities may include:

   - Identification of aspects of care important for quality monitoring.
   - Identification of indicators used to monitor quality and effectiveness of nursing care.
   - Collection of data to monitor quality and effectiveness of nursing care.
   - Analysis of quality data to identify opportunities for improving care.
   - Formulation of recommendations to improve nursing practice and client outcomes.
   - Implementation of activities to enhance the quality of nursing practice.
   - Participation on interdisciplinary teams that evaluate clinical practice or health services.
   - Development of policies and procedures to improve quality of care.

2. The nurse uses the results of quality care activities to initiate changes in practice.

3. The nurse uses the results of quality care activities to initiate changes throughout the health care delivery system, as appropriate.

FIGURE 9-4   ANA Standard I: Quality of Care.

(Reprinted with permission from *Standards of Clinical Nursing Practice*, American Nurses' Association, Washington, DC, 1991.)

provement efforts may focus on the system of stocking intravenous fluids and equipment on the nursing unit to make sure that equipment is readily available when you need it. In summary, quality assurance focuses on your performance whereas quality improvement focuses on the system's performance.

In the following section, each of the measurement criteria in Figure 9-4 are described as they relate to quality assurance or improvement. These steps lead to the systematic evaluation and improvement of the quality of care.

9-2 TEST YOURSELF

Critical Thinking and Evaluation

One of Ted Alexander's postoperative nursing diagnoses was impaired physical mobility related to pain, effects of medication, and prolonged bedrest. On the third day after surgery, you helped Ted get out of bed. You noted that his upper-body strength was decreasing. Even though he had been doing his exercises as instructed, he had difficulty in helping to move himself in bed and assisting to get out of bed. He expressed a desire to become more independent in this process. When asked about his level of comfort, he confirmed that the pain medication was working. On a scale of 1 to 10 he reported the pain level to be a 2.

Use the Critical Thinking format presented below to evaluate Ted's progress in resolving the diagnosis of impaired physical mobility.

1. What is the issue?

2. What information do I need and how can I obtain it?

3. What do the data mean?

4. Based on the facts, what should I do?

5. Are there other questions I should ask?

6. Is this the best way to deal with the issue?

9-2 TEST YOURSELF

Critical Thinking and Evaluation: Answers

1. **What is the issue?**
   The issue is whether or not Ted is making progress toward resolving the nursing diagnosis of impaired physical mobility. If he is not making progress I must determine why not and adjust the plan of care.

2. **What information do I need?**
   I need to evaluate Ted's muscle strength and range of motion (ROM). Does Ted perceive his muscle strength has decreased? Can Ted support and turn himself independently? Does he have full ROM of his arms?

3. **What do the data mean?**
   I have noted that Ted seems to be losing instead of maintaining upper body strength. When getting him out of bed (OOB), he could not assist us in pulling himself up in an upright position. It took three people to get him OOB.

   It seems that the strengthening exercises are not maintaining his upper body strength and he is discouraged that he is not capable of helping the staff in repositioning himself.

4. **Based on the facts, what should I do?**
   The plan of care must be revised. After reviewing his interventions and discussing the situation with some co-workers, it was decided to add a trapeze over his bed. This would allow him to assist the nurses in position changes and can also be used in exercise to strengthen his upper body.

   The findings were also discussed with the physician, who consented to a physical therapy consult.

5. **Are there other questions I should ask?**
   A. How will the use of the trapeze affect the integrity of his incision? (Take special care to assist him with splinting and protecting his incision.)
   B. When will Ted be able to resume eating? He is still NPO. If he does not start consuming calories soon he may need some other kind of nutritional support in order to regain his strength.
   C. Are there physiological reasons why he is weak? What is his hemoglobin? What is his nutritional status? Is he actively bleeding?

6. **Is this the best way to deal with this issue?**
   This is one approach. You have re-evaluated the client and changed the plan of care and the situation needs continued monitoring.

STANDARD II. PERFORMANCE APPRAISAL
The Nurse Evaluates His/Her Own Nursing Practice in Relation to Professional Practice Standards and Relevant Statutes and Regulations

Measurement Criteria

1. The nurse engages in performance appraisal on a regular basis, identifying areas of strength as well as areas for professional/practice development.
2. The nurse seeks constructive feedback regarding his/her own practice.
3. The nurse takes action to achieve goals identified during performance appraisal.
4. The nurse participates in peer review as appropriate.

FIGURE 9-5   ANA Standard II: Performance Appraisal.

(Reprinted with permission from *Standards of Clinical Nursing Practice*, American Nurses' Association, Washington, DC, 1991.)

STANDARD IV. COLLEGIALITY
The Nurse Contributes to the Professional Development of Peers, Colleagues, and Others

Measurement Criteria

1. The nurse shares knowledge and skills with colleagues and others.
2. The nurse provides peers with constructive feedback regarding their practice.
3. The nurse contributes to an environment that is conducive to clinical education of nursing students, as appropriate.

FIGURE 9-6   ANA Standard IV: Collegiality.

(Reprinted with permission from *Standards of Clinical Nursing Practice*, American Nurses' Association, Washington, DC, 1991.)

Examples of High Volume, High Risk, and
Problem Prone Aspects of Care

TYPE OF ASPECT OF CARE	SERVICE	ASPECT OF CARE
High volume	Critical care	Cardiac monitoring
High volume	Postpartum	Providing comfort measures
High volume	Nursing home	Maintaining skin integrity
High risk	Postanesthesia care unit	Maintaining an open airway
High risk	Pediatrics	Administering medications
High risk	Home care	Detecting complications
Problem prone	Surgical unit	Managing the confused elderly postop client
Problem prone	Outpatient clinic	Follow-up on clients who miss appointments
Problem prone	Emergency department	Communicating with a client with a language barrier

FIGURE 9-7　Examples of high risk, high volume, and problem prone aspects of care.

ANA Measurement
Criteria Standard
I-1 (Standard of
Professional
Performance): Qual-
ity of care activi-
ties may include
identification of as-
pects of care im-
portant for quality
monitoring.

Identify Important Aspects of Care

Evaluation activities are based on the most important activities of the nursing department. Highest priority is given to those aspects of care that are high volume, high risk, or problem prone.

High-volume aspects of care occur frequently or affect large numbers of clients.

High-risk aspects of care include those that place clients at risk for serious consequences or deprive them of substantial benefit if the care is not provided correctly.

Problem-prone aspects of care are those that have tended in the past to produce problems for staff or patients.

Figure 9-7 provides examples of high-volume, high-risk, and problem-prone aspects of care for various types of nursing settings.

ANA Measurement
Criteria Standard
I-1 (Standard of
Professional
Performance): Qual-

Identify Indicators

Indicators are the measurable components of the aspects of care. They are identified by the nurses who work within a particular setting and are based on nursing research and documentation of research in the literature. Indicators may evaluate the structure, process, or outcome of care. The *structure* of nursing care includes resources such as the number of nurses, the mix of registered nurses and other support personnel, and the type of equipment that is available.

Examples of Structural Indicators

☐ Number of registered nurses on the day shift

☐ Availability of emergency equipment on each nursing unit

Processes of care focus on the delivery of care. Nursing interventions that are considered processes of care include performing procedures, managing complications, and documentation.

Examples of Process Indicators

☐ Delivery of medications to the unit

☐ Accurate assessment of clients

☐ Management of the client during a seizure

☐ Proper completion of documentation forms

Outcomes of care are the positive results and complications of nursing interventions. Outcome indicators are the prime focus of monitoring.

Examples of Outcome Indicators

☐ Client satisfaction with nursing care

☐ Client understanding of teaching provided

☐ Wound infections

☐ Medication reactions

☐ Falls

Collect and Organize Data

Data are collected from a variety of sources, including reports, medical records, committee minutes, and questionnaires. Interviews, observation, or review of written materials are methods of data collection.

Example. You are part of a multidisciplinary team consisting of dietitians, admitting clerks, and nurses who are evaluating the problem of hospitalized clients who do not receive a meal tray when it is ordered. As a step in solving

ity of care activities may include identification of indicators used to monitor quality and effectiveness of nursing care.

ANA Measurement Criteria Standard I-1 (Standard of Professional Performance): Quality of care activities may include collection of data to monitor quality and effectiveness of care.

ANA Measurement Criteria Standard II-4 (Standard of

Professional Performance): The nurse participates in peer review as appropriate.

ANA Measurement Criteria Standard I-1 (Standard of Professional Performance): The nurse analyzes quality data to identify opportunities for improving care.

ANA Measurement Criteria Standard IV-2 (Standard of Professional Performance): The nurse provides peers with constructive feedback regarding their practice.

ANA Measurement Criteria Standard I-1 (Standard of Professional Performance): Quality of care activities may include formulation of recommendations to improve nursing practice or client outcomes.

this problem the team decides to develop a simple data collection form. Each time a client does not receive a tray that is ordered, the form is completed. The team hopes that the data will show a pattern or trend.

Analyze Data

Once data are collected they are analyzed to determine if there are apparent patterns or trends. Are certain times of the day, types of clients, care-providers, or medical problems consistently appearing in the data?

Example.   A busy emergency department nursing staff discovers that a large number of clients leave the waiting area before they are called into the examining area. Concerned that these individuals are leaving the hospital without being seen, the nurse manager studies the data. He discovers that the largest number of clients leave during the time the nurses are eating dinner.

Once patterns or trends are identified, this information is shared with the appropriate people so that recommendations for changes can be made.

Make Recommendations to Improve Care

There are multiple ways in which care can be improved. These may include changing staffing or supplies, educating nurses or clients, altering policies and procedures, renovating buildings, finding new suppliers—the list is endless.

Example.   The emergency department nurse manager in the previous example recognized that the flow of clients into the examining rooms slowed down at dinner time. He presented the data to the 3-11 shift staff nurses and asked for their suggestions for addressing the problem. The nurses recommended changing the scheduling of the dinner meal times for the nurses. Instead of dividing the nurses into two groups for meals, they were divided into three groups. This solution maintained the flow of clients into the examining rooms and resulted in fewer people leaving without being seen by the physician.

Take Action to Solve Problems

Once recommendations for changes are made, action is taken to solve the problem. The actions that are likely to be most effective are those that are simple, cost effective, and acceptable to those who will be implementing them.

Example.   A large urban hospital is concerned about visitor security. A number of people from outside the hospital are wandering around in areas of the hospital in which they do not belong. A multidisciplinary team decides to eliminate the traditional cardboard pass that is issued to visitors. Instead, they

ANA Measurement Criteria Standard I-1 (Standard of Professional Performance): Quality of care activities may include implementation of activities to enhance the quality of nursing practice.

develop plastic laminated color-coded cards that are worn on a chain around the neck. The hospital employees are now able to quickly spot someone who has slipped through the security system or is in an area of the building that does not correspond to the card.

EVALUATION OF QUALITY OF CARE AND THE NURSING PROCESS

The quality assurance and improvement process uses the same steps as does the nursing process.

Assessment. What is the process that needs to be improved? What information should be collected to understand this process? Who should collect it and when?

Diagnosis. Based on the assessment data, what is the problem that is preventing high-quality care? What is leading to high costs, unhappy people, delays, or waste?

Planning. What changes do the team suggest to improve the process? How will these changes be made? Who needs to be involved in the change process? How will we know the changes have been successfully made?

Implementation. In this phase, the changes are implemented after thorough preparation, planning, and communication.

Evaluation. This phase, like the nursing process, involves measuring the effectiveness of the change. More data are collected and compared with the assessment data to determine if improvement has occurred.

The following example shows the quality improvement process in action.

Example. Clients who were waiting to be admitted to a large hospital are complaining that they have to wait a long time in the admitting office. A multidisciplinary team consisting of nurses, personnel from the admitting office, and housekeeping is assembled. Data are collected to determine:

- ☐ how long clients are kept waiting for a bed.
- ☐ how long it takes from the time a bed is vacated before it is filled by the new client.
- ☐ how many discharged clients leave the hospital each hour of the day.
- ☐ the reason why clients leave the hospital after the official discharge time of 11 AM.

During the analysis of the data, it was discovered that the key to the problem was a lack of communication about the availability of beds on the medical surgical units. Clients were being held in the emergency department, critical care units, and postanesthesia care unit waiting for a medical surgical

---

EVALUATION IS SYSTEMATIC AND ONGOING

EVALUATION AND THE NURSING PROCESS

CRITICAL THINKING AND EVALUATION

EVALUATION OF THE QUALITY OF CARE

EVALUATION OF THE QUALITY OF CARE AND THE NURSING PROCESS

ANA Measurement Criteria Standard I-1 (Standard of Professional Performance): Quality of care activities may include participation on interdisciplinary teams that evaluate clinical practice or health services.

ANA Measurement Criteria Standard I-3 (Standard of Professional Performance): The nurse uses results of quality of care activities to initiate changes throughout the health care delivery system as appropriate.

bed. Clients were delayed in leaving the facility waiting for a ride from a family member or for the rescue squad to take them home. However the primary problem at the heart of the issue was lack of communication between the nurses, housekeepers, and the admitting department. The nurses did not always tell the housekeepers that a bed needed to be washed after the client left. The housekeepers did not always tell the nurses when the bed was ready for the next person. And the admitting department wasn't always told that the bed was ready for the new client.

When planning how to address this problem, the team identified the need to request that physicians discharge clients as early as possible in the day and tell clients the day before the intended discharge so family members could make arrangements to pick up the client before the 11 AM discharge time the next day. It was determined that little could be done about the evening transportation by the rescue squads because they were made up of volunteers who worked during the day.

ANA Measurement Criteria Standard I-3 (Standard of Professional Performance): Quality of care activities may include development of policies and procedures to improve quality of care.

To address the communication problem relating to the availability of beds, the housekeepers were asked to contact the admitting department when the bed was ready. Because the admitting department had only one phone line, a second line was installed with an answering machine to receive the calls that the bed was ready. In addition, the vice president of nursing personally visited clients who had to wait more than one half hour in the admitting area for a bed. Within a month the number of clients waiting more than half an hour for a bed fell from 30 a week to two. The project was evaluated as a success.

SUMMARY

Evaluation is an ongoing and systematic process used to judge each component of the nursing process and to evaluate the quality of care. The term is used most commonly to describe decisions made about the client's achievement of outcomes. If the outcomes are not achieved the nurse evaluates each part of the plan of care and makes revisions as needed. Evaluation of the quality of care given to groups of clients uses a systematic process that parallels the nursing process. Changes are then made to improve the quality of care.

REFERENCE

Roc C. The muddy waters of clinical teaching. Am J Nurs 1992 July; 20.

BIBLIOGRAPHY

Erst D: Total quality management in the hospital setting. J Nurs Care Qual 1994; 8(2):1.
Jones K: Outcomes analysis: methods and issues. Nursing Economics 1993; 11(3):145.

Matz L and Gary G: Patient outcomes measure home health care accomplishments. Nurs Manage 1992; 24(5):96Y.

Oie M and Recker D: Empowerment through collaboration: Implementing a team quality assurance model. J Nurs Care Qual 1992; 6(2):32.

Palmer M and others: Continence outcomes: Documentation on medical records in the nursing home environment. J Nurs Care Qual 1992; 6(3):36.

Patton S and Stanley J: Bridging quality assurance and continuous quality improvement. J Nurs Care Qual 1993; 7(2):15.

Pobojewski B and others: Documenting nursing process in the perioperative setting: continuity of care, patient evaluation. AORN J 1992 July; 98–104.

Zager LR and others: Merging concepts: nursing process, workload management, and quality improvement. J Nurs Staff Develop 1992 Nov/Dec; 254–258.

TEN

LEGAL AND ETHICAL ISSUES AND THE NURSING PROCESS

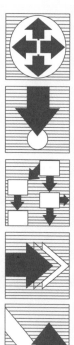

OBJECTIVES

After reading this chapter, you will be able to:

1. Describe four principles of law.
2. Identify two essential rights and responsibilities of nurses and clients.
3. Differentiate between negligence and malpractice.
4. Utilize the steps of the nursing process to resolve an ethical dilemma.

INTRODUCTION

Legal and ethical issues pervade the nursing process. Our nursing activities are guided by legal and ethical principles as we carry out the steps of the nursing process. Legal principles define our responsibilities when providing care, whereas ethical principles affect how we fulfill these responsibilities. Often

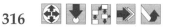

STANDARD V. ETHICS

The Nurse's Decisions and Actions on Behalf of Clients Are Determined in an Ethical Manner

---

Measurement Criteria

1. The nurse's practice is guided by the Code for Nurses
2. The nurse maintains client confidentiality
3. The nurse acts as a client advocate
4. The nurse delivers care in a nonjudgmental and nondiscriminatory manner that is sensitive to client diversity
5. The nurse delivers care in manner that preserves/protects client autonomy, dignity, and rights
6. The nurse seeks available resources to help formulate ethical decisions.

FIGURE 10-1   ANA Standard V: Ethics.

(Reprinted with permission from *Clinical Nursing Practice*. Washington, DC: American Nurses Association, 1991.)

these concepts are intertwined. Figure 10-1 illustrates the nurse's responsibilities to provide care in a legal and ethical manner, as defined by the American Nurses' Association (ANA). The information presented in this chapter addresses four basic principles of law. Ethical content will include definitions of morals and ethics, sources of ethics, ethical theories, examples of ethical dilemmas, and the steps in ethical decision-making.

PRINCIPLES OF LAW

Four basic concepts that guide the legal system are described in this section.

FOUR PRINCIPLES OF LAW

The legal system is constantly evolving

Client's and nurses rights and responsibilities

Law based on fairness and justice

The Legal System Is Constantly Evolving

Changes occur in the legal system in response to societal issues. As new technologies and health care issues raise legal questions, the courts attempt to come up with solutions. For example, as AIDS continues to spread, questions are raised about mandatory testing for AIDS and confidentiality of test results. As issues such as this one appear to be resolved, others arise to take their place. The legal issues being raised in the first half of the 1990s will be different from the ones affecting health care in the second half of the decade. As cases are

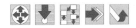

resolved in court, the decisions being made subsequently influence the resolution of future cases and impact on nursing practice.

Each Individual Has Rights and Responsibilities

This principle dictates that each person in the health care environment has rights to be protected and obligations to fulfill. The client's rights are considered when planning and delivering nursing care. Additionally, you have rights and responsibilities as an employee and a professional.

Client Rights

In the mid 1990s the concept of client rights has come under increased scrutiny. Clients as health care consumers have become more aware of their rights as a result of increasing consumer education. The media has effectively taught large segments of the population about wellness practices, treatment options, and how to select a health care practitioner. Nurses are providing primary care as nurse midwives and nurse practitioners. Studies have shown that clients who receive care from nurse practitioners as compared to physicians have equal or greater satisfaction with their care, receive equal or greater education, and have equal or greater compliance with treatment (New study, 1993). Consumers are demanding such meaningful data in order to select a health care facility or provider. Consumers are being given data about the kind of outcomes of care that each hospital can provide.

Consumer and health care groups have fought to protect the consumer by mandating certain rights. There are two well-known bills of rights for clients. The Bill of Rights for Mental Health Patients is a federal law that guarantees client rights in nursing homes and home health agencies. Various state laws describe the rights of mentally or developmentally disabled persons, residents of health facilities, and clients in general (Rosenfield, 1988).

The American Hospital Association has published a voluntary bill of rights for all hospitalized clients in both private and public facilities (Fig. 10-2). This bill of rights describes the type of care the client can expect to receive while hospitalized. A few of these rights will be discussed below.

Right to Considerate and Respectful Care.   As part of the therapeutic relationship you should determine how the client wishes to be addressed. Refrain from using such disparaging forms of address as "Gramps," "Pops," or "Grandma." Research has shown that hospitalized clients equate quality of care with how often they are called by name (Satisfaction Data, 1989).

Right to Agree to or Refuse Treatment to the Extent Permitted by Law and to Be Informed of the Consequences.   Health care practitioners are expected to provide sufficient information about treatments and alternative options so that the client can make an informed decision. A client who is

---

Nurse judged on similarly educated person's actions in similar situation

FOUR PRINCIPLES OF LAW
The legal system is constantly evolving
Client's and nurses rights and responsibilities

ANA Measurement Criteria Standard V-5 (Standard of Professional Performance): The nurse delivers care in a manner that preserves/protects client autonomy, dignity and rights.

Client rights
Considerate and respectful care
Informed consent and informed refusal

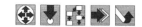

Management Advisory
A PATIENT'S BILL OF RIGHTS
Patient and Community Relations

Introduction

Effective health care requires collaboration between patients and physicians and other health care professionals. Open and honest communication, respect for personal and professional values, and sensitivity to differences are integral to optimal patient care. As the setting for the provision of health services, hospitals must provide a foundation for understanding and respecting the rights and responsibilities of patients, their families, physicians, and other caregivers. Hospitals must ensure a health care ethic that respects the role of patients in decision making about treatment choices and other aspects of their care. Hospitals must be sensitive to cultural, racial, linguistic, religious, age, gender, and other differences as well as the needs of persons with disabilities.

The American Hospital Association presents *A Patient's Bill of Rights* with the expectation that it will contribute to more effective patient care and be supported by the hospital on behalf of the institution, its medical staff, employees, and patients. The American Hospital Association encourages health care institutions to tailor this bill of rights to their patient community by translating and/or simplifying the language of this bill of rights as may be necessary to ensure that patients and their families understand their rights and responsibilities.

Bill of Rights*

1. The patient has the right to considerate and respectful care.
2. The patient has the right to and is encouraged to obtain from physicians and other direct caregivers relevant, current, and understandable information concerning diagnosis, treatment, and prognosis.

    Except in emergencies when the patient lacks decision-making capacity and the need for treatment is urgent, the patient is entitled to the opportunity to discuss and request information related to the specific procedures and/or treatments, the risks involved, the possible length of recuperation, and the medically reasonable alternatives and their accompanying risks and benefits.

(continued)

These rights can be exercised on the patient's behalf by a designated surrogate or proxy decision maker if the patient lacks decision-making capacity, is legally incompetent, or is a minor.

FIGURE 10-2   A Patient's Bill of Rights.

(Reprinted with permission of the American Hospital Association, Copyright 1992.)

Management Advisory
A PATIENT'S BILL OF RIGHTS
Patient and Community Relations–cont'd.

Patients have the right to know the identity of physicians, nurses, and others involved in their care, as well as when those involved are students, residents, or other trainees. The patient also has the right to know the immediate and long-term financial implications of treatment choices, insofar as they are known.

3. The patient has the right to make decisions about the plan of care prior to and during the course of treatment and to refuse a recommended treatment or plan of care to the extent permitted by law and hospital policy and to be informed of the medical consequences of his action. In case of such refusal, the patient is entitled to other appropriate care and services that the hospital provides or transfer to another hospital. The hospital should notify patients of any policy that might affect patient choice within the institution.

4. The patient has the right to have an advance directive (such as a living will, health care proxy, or durable power of attorney for health care) concerning treatment or designating a surrogate decision maker with the expectation that the hospital will honor the intent of that directive to the extent permitted by law and hospital policy.

   Health care institutions must advise patients of their rights under state law and hospital policy to make informed medical choices, ask if the patient has an advance directive, and include that information in patient records. The patient has the right to timely information about hospital policy that may limit its ability to implement fully a legally valid advance directive.

5. The patient has the right to every consideration of privacy. Case discussion, consultation, examination, and treatment should be conducted so as to protect each patient's privacy.

6. The patient has the right to expect that all communications and records pertaining to his/her care will be treated as confidential by the hospital, except in cases such as suspected abuse and public health hazards when reporting is permitted or required by law. The patient has the right to expect that the hospital will emphasize the confidentiality of this information when it releases it to any other parties entitled to review information in these records.

7. The patient has the right to review the records pertaining to his/her medical care and to have the information explained or interpreted as necessary, except when restricted by law.

(continued)

Management Advisory

A PATIENT'S BILL OF RIGHTS
Patient and Community Relations—cont'd.

8. The patient has the right to expect that, within its capacity and policies, a hospital will make reasonable response to the request of a patient for appropriate and medically indicated care and services. The hospital must provide evaluation, service, and/or referral as indicated by the urgency of the case. When medically appropriate and legally permissible, or when a patient has so requested, a patient may be transferred to another facility. The institution to which the patient is to be transferred must first have accepted the patient for transfer. The patient must also have the benefit of complete information and explanation concerning the need for, risks, benefits, and alternatives to such a transfer.

9. The patient has the right to ask and be informed of the existence of business relationships among the hospital, educational institutions, other health care providers, or payers that may influence the patient's treatment and care.

10. The patient has the right to consent to or decline to participate in proposed research studies or human experimentation affecting care and treatment or requiring direct patient involvement, and to have those studies fully explained prior to consent. A patient who declines to participate in research or experimentation is entitled to the most effective care that the hospital can otherwise provide.

11. The patient has the right to expect reasonable continuity of care when appropriate and to be informed by physicians and other caregivers of available and realistic patient care options when hospital care is no longer appropriate.

12. The patient has the right to be informed of hospital policies and practices that relate to patient care, treatment, and responsibilities. The patient has the right to be informed of available resources for resolving disputes, grievances, and conflicts, such as ethics committees, patient representatives, or other mechanisms available in the institution. The patient has the right to be informed of the hospital's charges for services and available payment methods.

The collaborative nature of health care requires that patients, or their families/surrogates, participate in their care. The effectiveness of care and patient satisfaction with the course of treatment depend, in part, on the patient fulfilling certain responsibilities. Patients are responsible for

(continued)

Management Advisory
A PATIENT'S BILL OF RIGHTS
Patient and Community Relations–cont'd.

providing information about past illnesses, hospitalizations, medications, and other matters related to health status. To participate effectively in decision making, patients must be encouraged to take responsibility for requesting additional information or clarification about their health status or treatment when they do not fully understand information and instructions. Patients are also responsible for ensuring that the health care institution has a copy of their written advance directive if they have one. Patients are responsible for informing their physicians and other caregivers if they anticipate problems in following prescribed treatment.

Patients should also be aware of the hospital's obligation to be reasonably efficient and equitable in providing care to other patients and the community. The hospital's rules and regulations are designed to help the hospital meet this obligation. Patients and their families are responsible for making reasonable accommodations to the needs of the hospital, other patients, medical staff, and hospital employees. Patients are responsible for providing necessary information for insurance claims and for working with the hospital to make payment arrangements, when necessary. A person's health depends on much more than health care services. Patients are responsible for recognizing the impact of their life-style on their personal health.

Conclusion

Hospitals have many functions to perform, including the enhancement of health status, health promotion, and the prevention and treatment of injury and disease; the immediate and ongoing care and rehabilitation of patients; the education of health professionals, patients, and the community; and research. All these activities must be conducted with an overriding concern for the values and dignity of patients.

mentally competent has the right to refuse treatment, even when the health care personnel do not agree with that decision or think it is in the client's best interests. For example, a client may refuse to have treatment for a newly diagnosed cancer or to have a feeding tube or IV inserted. In either example, an individual who is of sound mind and understands the consequences of this

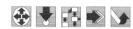

Assault: Suggestion or threat to touch a person without consent

Battery: Intentional touching without another's consent

decision may refuse treatment. If a client refuses treatment and you say you will perform it anyway, you may be held liable for *assault*. If you actually perform the procedure, *battery* has occurred.

Example. A Louisiana nurse inserted a Foley catheter into a quadriplegic man against his wishes. The man objected to the use of the catheter but was told by the nurse to "shut up." The man begged that the catheter not be put in because of past complications. This was verified by the nurse's notes, which stated in part, "Pt became very upset when catheter was inserted and notified his family." In the trial that followed the court ruled that battery was committed (Tammelleo, 1991c).

When a client refuses to consent to a treatment, stop and notify the nursing supervisor. The supervisor and the doctor, depending on the circumstances, may try to convince the client to accept the treatment. In rare instances the doctor may seek a court order to overrule the client's decision. For instance, this is sometimes done when a Jehovah's Witness with minor children refuses to accept a blood transfusion. The courts have held that it is in the state's best interests to protect the children from a parent's decision to risk death.

A mentally competent adult has the right to refuse care even in life-threatening situations.

Example. During an attempt to resuscitate a woman in the intensive care unit the client opened her eyes. She said to the nurse, "Let me go. Leave me alone." The physician, who was standing by her side, verified that the client wanted no further treatment. The resuscitation effort ended and the client was allowed to die.

Client rights

Considerate and respectful care

Informed consent and informed refusal

Confidentiality

ANA Measurement Criteria Standard V-2 (Standard of Professional Performance): The nurse maintains client confidentiality

Right to Expect that All Communications and Records Pertaining to Care Will Be Kept Confidential. The ethical aspects of this issue will be discussed later in this chapter. Nurses are prohibited from sharing information about a client with anyone other than health care professionals directly responsible for the client's care. There are additional stringent rules that protect the privacy of clients who receive treatment for mental health disorders and drug and alcohol addictions. In these cases laws protect their confidentiality to prevent others from knowing that treatment is being received for these problems.

The principle of confidentiality applies to family members who are seeking detailed information. It is best to ask the client's permission before giving information to friends and family. Be sure to determine the procedure to follow if a family member wants to see the client's record. Most facilities require the client to give written permission and expect the nurse to notify the physician of the request.

Do not discuss the client's condition in public areas. The elevator is one such place in which a casual comment could be overheard by a family member or friend. You should be aware that certain information is so sensitive that it should not be discussed at all.

Example. The estate of a New Jersey physician with AIDS won a six million dollar verdict against a hospital because the lab results of HIV positive were widely discussed within the hospital and community, resulting in the destruction of the physician's practice. The physician's family sued the hospital for breach of confidentiality. The verdict was upheld when the hospital appealed the case.

Client Responsibilities

Share Information. Clients have a responsibility to provide you with appropriate information about their health status and medical and nursing problems. You can reasonably expect that a client will share relevant information and should carefully document if you suspect the client is withholding important information.

Example. When you ask Justin Davis if he uses recreational drugs, you observe that he loses eye contact, shrugs his shoulders, acts uncomfortable, and weakly denies using drugs. You notice scars along the course of the veins of his arms and chart: "Denies using drugs, scars noted along course of veins of forearms."

Follow Instructions. Clients are expected to comply with reasonable requests of health care personnel, such as instructions to stay in bed when weak, notify you of significant symptoms, refrain from tampering with medical equipment, and so on. If the client does not follow your instructions and becomes injured as a result, it is unlikely that a jury would be sympathetic if the client sues you. The legal doctrine of *comparative negligence* describes the client's responsibilities for the injuries. The jury may find the client (plaintiff) partially or totally responsible for the injuries. The total amount of money that the plaintiff would otherwise receive would be reduced by the percentage that the plaintiff's negligence contributed to the injuries.

When you encounter a client who does not follow instructions, document carefully. In your charting describe the behavior of the client and indicate that you warned the client of the risk of not following your instructions.

Example. When you enter 13-year-old Brian MacDougall's room, you discover that he has received 800 ml of IV fluid in one hour. In response to your questioning, he admits that he adjusted the flow meter so he "could get the IV finished sooner." You discuss the hazards of fluid overload and document "800 ml of IV fluid infused in one hour. Client admits to tampering with IV flow meter. Advised him of risks of rapid IV infusion. States he understands and will not do it again."

Nurse's Rights

Under this principle of law you have rights and responsibilities as an employee and professional.

Client rights

Considerate and respectful care

Informed consent and informed refusal

Confidentiality

Client responsibilities

Share information

Follow instructions

Comparative negligence: the court assigns partial responsibility for the defendant's alleged negligence to the plaintiff in the case.

FOUR PRINCIPLES OF LAW

The legal system is constantly

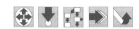
Right to a Safe Environment. You have a right to a safe working environment according to the Occupational Safety and Health Administration (OSHA) laws. The regulations permit you to refuse to work in proven unsafe conditions. Your employer is obligated to provide you with safety equipment and you have a responsibility to use the equipment. For example, you are expected to wear gloves when handling blood and body fluids. If you do not wear gloves when drawing blood and contract hepatitis, you would not be entitled to compensation from the employer.

Right to Be Free from Sexual Harassment. There is no precise definition of what constitutes sexual harassment. The courts have defined three situations that are unlawful:

- Submission to sexual harassment is either explicitly or implicitly a term or condition of an individual's employment.

Example. You are told that tolerating sexual harassment is required in order to keep your job.

- Submission to or rejection of such conduct is used as the basis for employment decisions affecting you.

Example. You are told that if you tolerate sexual harassment you will be promoted.

- Sexual harassment has the effect of substantially interfering with your work performance or creating an intimidating, hostile, or offensive working environment.

Example. Two male employees of an Ohio hospital "groped" a female unit clerk on a deserted elevator. Both lost their jobs following an investigation that they had violated the hospital's rules prohibiting sexual harassment (Tammelleo, 1993).

You have a right to expect your school and your employer to have policies for the reporting of sexual harassment. If you are ever the victim of sexual harassment, you have the responsibility to report it through the appropriate channels.

Nurse's Responsibilities

There are many nursing responsibilities. A few are highlighted below.

Safe Practice. You are expected to practice nursing in such a manner that you do not jeopardize the safety of the clients entrusted to your care. A nursing license is a legal document that permits the nurse to offer certain skills and knowledge to the public of the state, where such practice would otherwise be unlawful without a license (Creighton, 1986). Nurses are required to hold a current license issued by their state in order to practice. You must be in good health to apply for an initial license, to renew your license, or to receive a license in another state (licensure by endorsement). Schools of nursing are expected to screen out those individuals who have physical and mental disabilities that would prevent them from practicing safely. Those with physical or mental disabilities who are applying for a license renewal or obtaining a license by endorsement are required to present evidence that they are able to practice nursing in a safe and competent manner in spite of their disability (Champagne et al, 1987). The Americans with Disabilities Act provides new rights to individuals with handicaps. Physical disabilities that have led to concern about safe practice include legal blindness, severe hearing impairment, and the loss of motor skills and normal speech.

The Board of Nursing is the regulatory agency that is charged with the authority to discipline nurses who do not practice in a safe, professional manner. The Board is expected to take disciplinary action when a nurse has a physical, mental, or substance abuse impairment. Through surveys of state boards of nursing, Champagne et al (1987) and Swenson et al (1987a, 1987b, 1989), found that:

- 99 percent of the boards had dealt with cases of illegal substance abuse.
- 76 percent with alcohol abuse.
- 70 percent with legal substance abuse that impaired practice.
- 20 percent with cases of mental impairment.
- 5 percent with cases of physical impairment.

Murphy and Connell (1987) studied 100 records of Arizona nurses who had violated the state's nurse practice act and discovered that 60 percent of the nurses had been disciplined for substance abuse and 40 percent for incompetence.

Nurses have also been disciplined or lost their licenses for failure to file tax returns and pay taxes, allowing the daughter of a nurse to pose as a nurse (Creighton, 1986a), and failing to comply with regulations for nurse midwives. Advanced nursing practice was the basis of a Missouri case on the role of nurse practitioners. An Idaho nurse named Jolene Tuma provided a client with information on alternative cancer therapies and retained her license after the Idaho board sought to remove it for unprofessional conduct. The Idaho court ruled that the nurse practice act was sufficiently vague on what constituted unprofessional conduct (Cushing, 1986).

You may be disciplined or have your licensed revoked for behavior that occurs within or even outside the scope of your employment. For example, a male nurse anesthetist lost his license after he was found guilty of photographing the male genitalia of three corpses. The court decided that his conduct was such that there was sufficient likelihood that he might invade the privacy and offend the dignity of patients entrusted to his care (Tammelleo, 1992a). Another

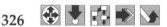

STANDARD III. EDUCATION
The Nurse Acquires and Maintains Current Knowledge in Nursing Practice

---

Measurement Criteria

1. The nurse participates in ongoing educational activities related to clinical knowledge and professional issues
2. The nurse seeks experiences to maintain clinical skills
3. The nurse seeks knowledge and skills appropriate to the practice setting

---

FIGURE 10-3   ANA Standard III: Education.

(Reprinted with permission from *Clinical Nursing Practice*. Washington, DC: American Nurses Association, 1991.)

male nurse lost his license after being convicted of sexual assault of 11- and 12-year-old girls (Tammelleo, 1992b).

As part of maintaining your clinical skills, you are expected to acquire and maintain current knowledge of nursing practice (Fig. 10-3). This is accomplished by:

- attending educational programs presented by your employer or outside seminar companies.
- reading journals and books.
- listening to audiotapes.
- reading self-learning modules.
- watching videotapes.
- using a computer-assisted program.
- utilizing experts in clinical nursing.

Responsibility Not to Abandon Clients.   You have a responsibility to provide care when no other or too few staff are available to provide for the client's safety. No nurse can walk off a unit in these circumstances without being charged with abandoning the clients.

Example.   A New York nurse was advised by her supervisor that due to a shortage of 3-11 nurses, a 7-3 nurse would have to work an additional eight-hour shift. Under the hospital's mandatory overtime the nurse with the least seniority was required to stay. Although the nurse left the unit shortly after

Nurse's Rights

Right to a safe environment

Right to be free from sexual harassment

Nurse's Responsibilities

Safe practice

Not abandon clients

the 3-11 shift began, saying she was going to the supervisor's office, she actually left the hospital for 45 minutes. Her license was suspended for a year after she was found guilty of professional misconduct for abandoning her patients (Tammelleo, 1993b).

Short staffing does not eliminate the principle that each person is accountable for his or her actions. For example, if a person spills water on the floor in a traffic area, that person is responsible for cleaning up the water to prevent injury to others. This individual could not say, "I was too busy to clean it up." The principle of individual accountability must be placed within the perspective of the agency's liability for short staffing. A hospital that fails to provide a safe level of nursing care may be held liable under two separate theories: vicarious liability (or respondeat superior) and corporate liability. *Vicarious liability* refers to the legal principle that a hospital is liable for the acts of its employees because of an employer-employee relationship. *Corporate liability* consists of the hospital's liability for injuries stemming from its own acts and omissions. In one case, a nursing administration yielded to pressure to keep two critical care beds filled with patients instead of closing the beds because of inadequate staffing. The hospital could be held liable for any injuries resulting from short staffing as long as the critical care nurses did what would have been reasonable under the circumstances (Fiesta, 1990).

Vicarious liability: an agency's liability for acts or omissions of its employees.

Corporate liability: an agency's responsibility for its own acts or omissions.

Law Is Based on a Concern for Fairness and Justice

The third principle of law seeks to protect a person's rights from infringement by the actions of another person. It defines appropriate conduct under the law and creates a mechanism to enforce this conduct. The laws are designed to achieve a fair outcome in legal disputes, and to provide structure for managing the complexities of the health care system.

There are guidelines for a nurse's conduct and mechanisms for enforcing those rules. The expectations of professional conduct are defined by the state board of nursing in the nurse practice act, the ANA and other specialty organizations, by standards published by the Joint Commission, and other accrediting bodies. The state board of nursing consists of a group of nurses and, in some states, non-nurses who are appointed by the governor. The board is charged with a number of responsibilities:

FOUR PRINCIPLES OF LAW

The legal system is constantly evolving

Rights and responsibilities

Law based on fairness and justice

1. Approval of the curriculum of schools of nursing located in the state.

2. Inspection of employer records to be sure the nursing employees are credentialed and complying with professional standards (Markowitz, 1982).

3. Rulings on questions that are submitted to it. These questions clarify the scope of nursing practice. For instance, the board may be asked to rule on whether licensed practical nurses may insert intravenous needles.

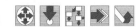

4. Determining who is competent to be licensed as a nurse and the granting of licenses.

5. Disciplining of nurses who are found to be unfit or incompetent to practice nursing.

Four principles of law

The legal system is constantly evolving

Rights and responsibilities

Law based on fairness and justice

Reasonable and prudent person

Reasons for lawsuits

Definitions

A Nurse's Actions Are Judged on the Basis of What a Similarly Educated Reasonable and Prudent Person Would Have Done in a Similar Situation

This fourth principle refers to the concepts that are applied in nursing malpractice cases. In a society that has increasingly turned to the courts for resolution of disputes, standards are needed to judge nursing performance.

Reasons for Lawsuits

The number of lawsuits being filed against nurses is increasing, although physicians are sued with greater frequency. According to the ANA, 6.2 nurses per 10,000 are sued each year. This is in contrast to 1,800 physicians per 10,000 (How likely is a lawsuit, 1990). Despite the relatively small number of nurses who are sued each year, nurses need to continue to be concerned with the legal aspects of nursing practice. Lawsuits against nurses are on the increase for a number of reasons:

1. The consumer has become better educated on what to expect from the health care system and nursing care.

2. Plaintiff attorneys (who represent the client) are becoming more able to identify the case that has merit.

3. Plaintiff attorneys are likely to name as many people as possible when filing a lawsuit. This allows them to potentially tap the pocket of the hospital's and the nurse's insurance companies, as well as the physician's insurance carrier.

4. Plaintiff lawyers are more aware that nurses are professionals and accountable for their own actions.

5. Many nurses are providing increasingly specialized and complex care that exposes the client and the nurse to greater risk (Godkin et al, 1987).

Negligence: deviation from standard of care.

Malpractice: deviation from a professional standard of care.

Definitions

The terms negligence and malpractice are often used to describe the *standard of care*. The standard of care is a concept that defines the expected and appropriate actions should occur. For example, if you take your car to the garage because the brakes are not working, the auto mechanic is expected to follow certain

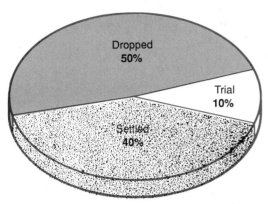

FIGURE 10-4   How malpractice suits are resolved.

procedures to repair or replace the brakes. The mechanic who failed to properly fix the brakes would be considered negligent. *Negligence* is a general term referring to a deviation from the standard of care that a reasonably prudent person would follow in a particular set of circumstances. Any individual could be negligent in carrying out responsibilities. In the wintertime, if you do not clear the ice off your sidewalk and someone slips and breaks a hip, you could be judged to be negligent.

Malpractice is a specific type of negligence that occurs when a professional does not adhere to professional standards of care. If a doctor removes the wrong kidney or a nurse gives blood to the wrong client, they may be judged as having committed malpractice. Lawyers, doctors, dentists, and nurses are some of the professionals who are named in malpractice suits.

Outcomes of Lawsuits

Insurance studies show that of all medical malpractice cases filed, 50 percent are dropped, 40 percent are settled out of court, and 10 percent go to trial (Fig. 10-4). The 40 percent that settle out of court represent those cases that the team defending the nurse or physician believes would result in a verdict in favor of the plaintiff. The client who decides to file a malpractice suit is called the *plaintiff*. This person can be the client, a family member, or some other entity. The cases chosen for trial are either the ones that the defense believes it can win, or those that cannot be settled out of court because the plaintiff will not accept the dollar amount offered by the defense. The defense is successful in winning approximately 60 to 90 percent of the cases that get into court, although this varies from state to state. Daniels (1989) studied 1,886 malpractice cases in various geographical areas and found a 68 percent defense success rate.

A study by Taragin and others (1992) of 8000 cases involving New Jersey physicians found that physician care was considered defensible by the insurance company in 62 percent of the cases and indefensible in 25 percent. The

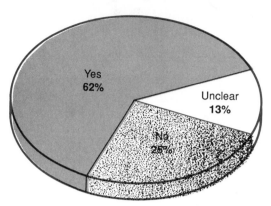

FIGURE 10-5 Can physician's care be defended?

(Based on data from Taragin M and others: The influence of standard of care and severity of injury on the resolution of medical malpractice claims, Ann Intern Med 1992; 117(9),780–784.)

remaining 13 percent of the cases were unclear as to the defensibility (Fig. 10-5). Payment to the plaintiff was made in 43 percent of all cases. Less than $50,000 was given to half of the plaintiffs. Only 15 percent received more than $200,000. It is difficult to find similar studies of nursing malpractice claims.

Student nurses are expected to provide nursing care as would a competent registered nurse. You are obligated to seek help when confronted with a new experience in which you are unclear how to proceed. While lawsuits against students are rare, the plaintiff could sue the student, instructor, facility, physician, and registered nurse staff.

It is now recommended that nurses carry their own malpractice insurance policies in addition to whatever coverage may be provided by their employer. One of the reasons for having personal insurance is the need for coverage for actions outside of the employment setting, such as private duty nursing and giving advice to neighbors. Some nurses believe that if they are covered by an employer's policy and money is paid out on a claim, the employer's insurance company will try to collect this sum from the nurse. This is a misconception and is untrue. Insurance companies work hard to maintain a good relationship with those they insure and are not interested in trying to obtain a nurse's assets.

Anatomy of a Lawsuit

Statute of limitations: laws that specify the length of time within which a person can file specific types of lawsuits.

First the plaintiff must convince an attorney that the case is worth pursuing. The attorney will try to make a determination if (1) malpractice has occurred, (2) if it can be proved, and (3) if there are injuries as a result. The vast majority of people who approach malpractice attorneys are turned away because the attorney judges the case as not being meritorious based on an analysis of these three elements.

When filing a lawsuit against a nurse, the attorney must be aware of the *statute of limitations*. This is a legal time limit that defines how long a suit can be filed after the plaintiff discovers an injury has occurred. For example, a client falls out of bed and breaks a hip in a state with a two-year statute of limitations. The suit must be filed within two years of the accident if the plaintiff intends to try to collect money from the insurance policy covering the nurse believed to be negligent. In another example, a plaintiff finds out four years after an operation that a clamp has been left inside. This person has up to two years after the discovery of the clamp to file a suit. The statute of limitations is often longer when the injured person is an infant or child.

After a plaintiff finds an attorney willing to consider the case the attorney may send the case to an *expert witness*. A nurse expert witness is someone with specialized clinical skill and knowledge who reviews the material and determines if the nurse violated appropriate standards of care. If the expert witness believes that the case has merit, the attorneys exchange *interrogatories*, which are a series of fact-finding questions designed to provide information about the case. The interrogatories, which are filled out by the nurse defendant with the assistance of the attorney, usually include questions about the nurse's education background and additional information about the facts surrounding the incident that led to the client's injuries.

The defense attorney, who is paid by the insurance company to represent the nurse (the defendant), may also have the case reviewed by an expert witness. Depending on the expert's opinion, the defense may settle the case or proceed to the next phase. *Depositions*, which consist of questioning under oath, are taken from the experts and the nurses involved in the case. If the case is not dropped or settled it proceeds to trial, which can occur two or more years after the incident.

In order to win the case the plaintiff must prove four elements:

Duty.   The plaintiff must prove that the nurse had a duty to care for the client as part of the nurse-client relationship. This relationship is established as soon as a client comes under the care of an organization by which the nurse is employed and is not difficult to prove in a lawsuit.

Breach of Duty.   A breach of duty occurs when the nurse does not deliver care according to what a similarly educated reasonably prudent nurse would have done under the same circumstances. Standards such as the state nurse practice act or those written by professional organizations are used to evaluate the nurse's actions. Expert witnesses are used in most cases to establish the standard of care.

At one time a nurse's practice was evaluated against the standard of care of nurses practicing in the same geographical area. With advances in technology, communication, and transportation, the guideline has become obsolete. A nurse's performance is now evaluated on national trends and practices.

Causation.   Causation, also referred to as proximate cause, means that the plaintiff must prove that the nurse's actions actually resulted in the injury.

Expert witness: a person who has special knowledge of a subject about which a court requests testimony.

Interrogatories: a series of written questions submitted to another person having information relevant to a lawsuit. These are usually filled out by the plaintiff and the defendant.

Deposition: a sworn pretrial testimony given by a person in response to questions asked by the attorney for the opposing side.

The plaintiff must prove
Duty
Breach of duty
Causation
Damages

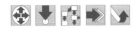
Because there are so many factors involved, this is the most difficult element to prove. In the following case the plaintiff was not able to establish proximate cause:

Example.   The nurse, in violation of the physician's orders that a postoperative abdominal surgery client should not be fed, gave the client solid food. A second operation eight days after the initial one showed the client's condition was worsening. When the client attempted to sue, there was no evidence that the feeding had made the client's condition worsen and the nurse was not held liable (Northrop and Kelly, 1987).

Damages.   The last element that the plaintiff must prove is that there were actual physical or emotional damages that were proximately caused by the nurse's negligent actions. The breach of duty may result in falls, medication errors, burns, equipment-related injuries, complications, deterioration in the client's status, and so on. When the jury decides that more than one health care professional has been negligent the damages will be divided among them. A sum of money is awarded to compensate for pain, suffering, lost income and companionship, medical bills, and so on.

The following three hypothetical cases illustrate reasons why the plaintiff could lose a malpractice suit for failure to prove one of the four elements described above:

Case 1. Rose Lewis developed a wound infection following surgery and believed the nurses were negligent when changing her dressing. However, the nurses used sterile technique and followed the appropriate procedures in cleaning her incision. The plaintiff would lose a malpractice case because she could not prove that there was a **breach** in duty.

Case 2. When Jennifer Watson's baby was born with abnormalities she wanted to sue the labor and delivery nurses. However, she had heavy exposure to toxic chemicals early in her pregnancy. These chemicals are known to cause birth defects. The plaintiff would lose a malpractice case because she cannot prove **causation** or that the labor and delivery nurses caused the genetic defects.

Case 3. Augustus Athena fell out of bed the first night he was in the hospital after receiving a sleeping pill. The standard of care required that the side rails be kept up but they were down at the time of the fall. Augustus did not injure himself when he fell. He would lose a malpractice case because there were no **damages**.

FOUR PRINCIPLES OF LAW

The legal system is constantly evolving

Rights and responsibilities

CRITICAL THINKING AND LEGAL ASPECTS OF THE NURSING PROCESS

Nurses often lose malpractice suits because one or more of the steps of the nursing process are omitted or performed incorrectly as a result of a failure to use critical thinking.

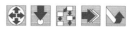

Assessment

The assessment process can result in injury to the client if important information is not obtained or transmitted to the appropriate person.

Example. A New Jersey client was brought to the recovery room by the anesthesiologist, who told the nurse: "The patient got narcotics; please watch his respirations." The nurse assigned to the client stated after the anesthesiologist left the room, she asked another nurse to watch the client. The nurse admitted that she never got a verbal response from the other staff nurse and that when she returned there was no one near the patient. She maintained that upon her return, she checked the client and observed his respiration rate to be 8 breaths/min, a dangerously low rate. When the anesthesiologist returned and inquired about the client's condition, the nurse informed him that the client was fine. However, the anesthesiologist realized the client had stopped breathing. Resuscitation was unsuccessful and the client remained comatose until his death a year later. The plaintiff's expert witnesses testified in the trial that the nurse deviated from the standard of care by

☐ failing to ascertain the drugs administered to the client.

☐ leaving the client without verifying that the client would be monitored.

☐ failing to recognize that the client had stopped breathing.

The jury found the nurse to be 100 percent negligent (Tammelleo, 1991d).

In this case the nurse failed to ensure that the appropriate assessment data would be collected in her absence and failed to act on data that indicated the client was in danger.

Diagnosis

As discussed in Chapter 3, several types of errors can occur in the diagnostic phase of the nursing process. These include:

1. basing the diagnosis on inaccurate or incomplete data collection.
2. inaccurate interpretation of assessment data due to reaching premature conclusions or allowing personal prejudices to affect the interpretation.
3. formulating nursing diagnoses without sufficient clinical knowledge or experience.

Any of these types of diagnostic errors can lead to client injury. In order to avoid making diagnostic errors, use your critical-thinking abilities, and don't be afraid to ask questions.

Example. In *Morreale v. Downing* a critical care nurse was held negligent for failing to discover a hip fracture in a 13-year-old boy. The boy had been in a motor vehicle accident and was hospitalized in the ICU for three weeks. The

Law based on fairness and justice

Reasonable and prudent person

Critical thinking and legal aspects of the nursing process

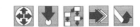
nurses failed to note his impaired physical mobility when he improved to the point that he was able to walk. His mother noted a discrepancy in the length of one leg. The physician ordered an x-ray, which showed a hip fracture. The nurses were held liable because they gave the boy frequent care and had ample opportunity to observe him walking and to notify the physician of unusual findings (Cushing, 1987b).

Planning

In the planning phase of the nursing process, you are expected to use your critical-thinking abilities to come up with a plan that is appropriate for resolving the client's nursing diagnosis. Your plan must address the client's significant problems and include interventions that are likely to be effective. Priority setting is needed to juggle the many demands on your time and to address the issues that are of most concern to your client.

In the following case the nurse failed to develop an effective plan for providing care for a postoperative client, who happened to be a prisoner:

ANA Measurement Criteria Standard V-4 (Standard of Professional Performance): The nurse delivers care in a nonjudgmental and nondiscriminatory manner that is sensitive to client diversity.

Example.   Following David Boretti's surgery for a gunshot wound, he was returned to an infirmary in the jail. The holding cell had no bed and he was forced to sleep on the cement floor. He was not given any dressings for his wound and his crutches, which he needed to walk, were taken away. When he requested something for pain the registered nurse at the facility told him she had no intention of contacting the physician. Motrin, which was ordered for pain, was not given to him until four days later. David informed the nurse that he had to resort to toilet tissue and soap and water to clean the wound area. The nurse responded that she was busy passing out medication and that she did not have the time for him and could not be bothered with his petty problems.

On the next several days David was unable to convince the nurses to contact the physician, who saw him five days after he returned to the jail. Despite the lack of dressings, David's wound healed normally. He brought suit against the nurses. The attorneys representing the nurses filed a motion with the court requesting that the suit be dropped. The judge ruled that a jury should decide if the nurses exhibited deliberate indifference to a serious medical need in violation of the patient's civil and Eighth Amendment rights. The Eighth Amendment prohibits cruel and unusual punishment. The judge stated that the failure of nurses to treat patients with care and compassion, not to mention following a prescribed plan for treatment, is reprehensible (Tammelleo, 1991e).

In this case the nurses' failure to establish a plan of care and attend to even the most basic of the client's needs is hard to justify. Although David did not develop an infection, the treatment that he received could be interpreted as psychological cruelty, and thus he sustained damages from the treatment. It is unreported how the case was resolved.

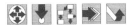

Implementation

The implementation phase of the nursing process is filled with opportunities to provide safe, effective care. It is also the phase in which treatment errors can lead to serious patient injury. The failure to protect the client from injury can lead to a lawsuit. The application of the nursing process requires you to critically think through your questions and assumptions while you are giving care, and to be alert to the signals that warrant further investigation or changing your interventions.

The legal literature is filled with cases involving errors made during the implementation phase of the nursing process. In the following case the plaintiffs were not clients, but the parents of a psychiatric inpatient:

Example. Mr. and Mrs. Thayer were visiting their son, who was in a locked ward of a psychiatric institute. Upon arriving in her son's room, Mrs. Thayer noticed a woman putting her own clothes in Mrs. Thayer's son's dresser. When Mrs. Thayer went to the nursing station to describe what was happening, the staff person on duty said, "Oh, my goodness, is that where she is? We've been looking for her."

Later, as the Thayers were getting ready to leave, the same young woman patient approached Mrs. Thayer and suddenly began to beat and choke her. Severe bruises, chipped teeth, and emotional distress were the result of the attack on Mrs. Thayer. The Thayers brought suit against the hospital. During the course of the trial it was determined that the patient was supposed to have been under constant observation, which meant that the assigned staff member should always be able to see the patient and not be more than six steps away. The constant observation was indicated because the patient had been involved in several recent episodes of assaultive behavior. The nurse assigned to the patient was one of two nurses on the unit. The nurse testified that "Because I was aware of the restrictions which had been placed on the patient were somewhat loose, because I had not noticed any particular problems or concerns with this patient and because there was no one in the living area with the patient at the time, I determined it would be proper to let her out of my sight for the short period of time it would take me to conduct fifteen minute checks." (Tammelleo, 1991a).

The Thayers lost this suit because too much time had elapsed from the time of the incident to the time they filed the suit. The legal battle over the statute of limitations overshadowed the issue of the nurse's responsibility to keep the patient under constant observation as ordered. Another issue that was not resolved was the responsibility of the psychiatric hospital to provide sufficient staff so that constant observation can be maintained.

Evaluation

One of the most difficult phases of the nursing process is the evaluation of information in order to make judgments about progress. As you critically evaluate all of the data that are available about the patient, you are making clinical judgments. Those judgments will direct you to continue or alter the plan of care. Failure to reach the appropriate conclusions about the client's status may lead to injury, as this case illustrates:

Example. Helen Ketchum had been diagnosed as having a subarachnoid hemorrhage (a hemorrhage in her brain) and had surgery that lasted from 11:00 AM to 6:00 PM. Ketchum was placed in the ICU for recovery. There was some question as to the degree to which her condition may have deteriorated during the night shift following her surgery and whether the night nurse appropriately evaluated her condition. There is no indication that the night nurse informed the physician of a series of warning signs, including respiratory distress, elevated pulse, reduced response of her pupils, all signs of Ketchum's deterioration. The end result was that Ketchum sustained severe brain damage, and her family brought suit against the hospital.

The nurse expert witness testified that the client's chart indicated that the night nurse had inadequately assessed and inadequately documented Ketchum's neurological condition. The physician expert witness testified that had Ketchum's physician been informed of the warning signs, he could have prescribed a diuretic to relieve the pressure on the client's brain and the damage causing the client's current condition would probably not have occurred. The initial verdict was in favor of the hospital; however, when Ketchum's family appealed the verdict, the higher court reversed the decision of the lower court and ruled that the case should be retried (Tammelleo, 1991b). The verdict of the second trial has not been reported.

In this case the failure of the night nurse to adequately evaluate Mrs. Ketchum's condition, and to reach a decision about her status that would have included notifying the physician, contributed to the deterioration of Mrs. Ketchum. As you evaluate the information that is relevant to the client's condition, use the resources available to you. When in doubt, act on your concerns, even at the risk of feeling foolish. You may save a client's life by asking questions of the right person or reporting your concerns.

This section of the chapter has presented a brief overview of legal issues that affect the nursing process. Legal principles guide the delivery of nursing care and are used to judge the behavior of health care personnel. You will be able to increase your knowledge of legal aspects of nursing by reading and asking questions. As you develop more knowledge, use your critical-thinking abilities to determine the appropriate actions to carry out the standard of care.

**ETHICAL FOUN-
DATIONS**
Definitions

ETHICAL FOUNDATIONS OF NURSING PRACTICE

The resolution of ethical dilemmas, like the decisions made in providing nursing care, requires critical thinking. Ethical decision making can be complex because it requires careful examination of value systems, and rarely results in

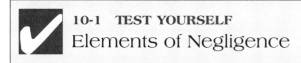

10-1 TEST YOURSELF
Elements of Negligence

Read the following description of an actual legal case and identify the four elements of malpractice: duty, breach of duty, causation, and damages. How much money do you think the plaintiff got when the case was settled out of court?

In April 1988 the plaintiff received a head injury when the driver of a car in which he was a passenger fell asleep at the wheel. His recovery from this accident was steady and uncomplicated. In May 1988 the plaintiff was sent to a head injury rehabilitation hospital for treatment. When he was admitted his diagnoses were "anxiety" and "head injury." On his second day there, the plaintiff struck a nurse, packed his suitcase, and ran up a flight of stairs attempting to leave the facility. Later that evening, while in a confused and agitated state, the plaintiff climbed out an open, unsecured window and fell headfirst seventeen feet to concrete, sustaining a second head injury. A CT scan showed fresh bleeding in his brain. The nurse who was in charge of watching the plaintiff failed to see or transcribe a doctor's order prescribing medication for agitation and restraints as necessary. The plaintiff's expert witnesses testified at a deposition that the standards of care required close supervision of agitated patients and secure windows. They further testified that after the first injury the plaintiff would have returned to employment and his normal roles as husband and father. Since the second injury, his judgment, memory and self control were impaired to the point that he must live in a supervised, structured environment and cannot work.

DUTY
_____

BREACH OF DUTY
_____

CAUSATION
_____

DAMAGES
_____

Source: Head injury rehabilitation hospital had unsecured window from which patient falls. Medical Malpractice Verdicts, Settlements & Experts, January 1993, 1.

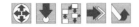

10-1 TEST YOURSELF
Elements of Negligence: Answers

DUTY

The plaintiff was a client being cared for in the rehabilitation facility. The facility had a duty to prevent him from injuring himself.

BREACH OF DUTY

The nurse taking care of the plaintiff had an obligation to implement measures when the client showed signs of agitation, particularly since the client became agitated earlier in the day and tried to escape. The nurse should have given the plaintiff medication to calm him down and applied restraints if needed. The facility had a responsibility to keep locks on the windows to protect the clients.

CAUSATION

The failure of the staff to protect the plaintiff led to a fall which caused new bleeding in the brain.

DAMAGES

Impaired judgment, memory, and self-control resulted from the fall, resulting in confinement to a supervised environment instead of returning home.

OUTCOME

The case was settled out of court for $3.65 million.

Morals: beliefs instilled by society that define right and wrong.

Ethics: broader aspect of morals. Nursing ethics deal with a standard of nursing behavior designed to protect clients.

a clear resolution of a dilemma. In fact, the solution to an ethical dilemma may be the answer that provides more elements of right than wrong, and does the least harm to all concerned.

Definitions

Ethical decision-making is based on an understanding of morals and ethics. *Morals* are the beliefs that are instilled in us by our parents and society as a whole. They include our sense of what is right and wrong. For example, we learn that it is wrong to kill, steal, or tell lies. This set of beliefs forms codes of behavior based on cultural expectations.

The term *ethics* is used to describe a broader aspect of morals. Ethical thinking begins when a person goes beyond the acceptance of the rules of the social group and moves into the realm of thinking and analyzing morals (Fowler and Levine-Ariff, 1987). Nursing ethics concerns itself with a standard of behavior that reflects the profession's desire to protect or ensure the well-being of its clients (Fenner, 1980).

According to Fry (1989) the characteristics of an ethical dilemma include the following:

1. A conflict between human needs or the welfare of others and a need for the nurse to choose between them.
2. A choice to be made guided by moral principles.
3. A choice guided by the process of weighing reasons and assigning priorities to competing values.
4. A choice affected by personal feelings and values and the context of the situation.

Examples of Ethical Dilemmas

Box 10-1 provides examples of ethical dilemmas that may affect nurses. Nurses encounter a variety of ethical dilemmas in health care. Cassells and Redman (1989) reported on a sample of 742 nurses who described the types of ethical dilemmas they had experienced in clinical practice within a year of graduation. The most common ethical issues they had faced included the following:

1. Informed consent by clients prior to surgical procedures and hazardous tests or treatments.
2. Resuscitation when the client experienced sudden unexpected death.
3. Discontinuing life-saving treatment.
4. Moral dilemmas in caring for clients with a poor prognosis or terminal illness.
5. Evaluation of the client's level of competency to make own decisions.
6. Clients refusing treatment.
7. Withholding information from clients.
8. Allocation of scarce resources.

There is a difference between legal and ethical responsibilities. As described earlier in the chapter, nurses have legal responsibilities as professionals. These are defined in the nurse practice act and in other standards set by a variety of agencies. Ethical responsibilities result from the relationship that the nurse forms with the client, the employer, and other health care

**ETHICAL FOUN-
DATIONS**
Definitions
*Examples of ethical
dilemmas*

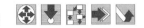

BOX 10-1
Ethical Dilemmas that May Affect Nurses

---

1. Abortion
2. Termination of life sustaining treatment
3. "Blowing the whistle," or exposing illegal and unethical behavior
4. Mistreatment of children, retarded or elderly clients
5. Treatment decisions involving dying clients
6. Equal access to health care for all
7. Allocation of scarce health care resources which requires a decision to deny health care to a needy client (such as a kidney transplant)
8. Protecting confidentiality of client information
9. Providing treatment that conflicts with a nurse's ethical principles.

---

professionals. These ethical duties may be identical to legal responsibilities but may also obligate the nurse to perform actions beyond what the law requires. For example, the ANA states that it is unethical for the nurse to participate in the act of killing a prisoner to fulfill a death sentence, even though the execution is legal. Table 10-1 illustrates how legal and ethical issues can be in conflict.

ETHICAL FOUN-
DATIONS
Definitions
Examples of ethical
dilemmas
Sources of ethics

Sources of Ethics

Ethical duties are often not defined in legal statutes. The ANA Code for Nurses (Fig. 10-6), Standards of Professional Performance, the Social Policy Statement, and the International Code of Nursing Ethics define the responsibilities of nurses to clients, society, and to the nursing profession. In addition, the ANA and other specialty nursing organizations, such as the American Association of Critical Care Nurses, periodically issue statements to guide the ethical behavior of nurses. One such publication is the ANA statement of guidelines for withdrawing or withholding food and fluid (ANA, 1988).

ANA Measurement
Criteria Standard
V-1 (Standard of
Professional
Performance): The
nurse's practice
is guided by the
Code for Nurses.

The Code for Nurses had its beginnings as early as 1897 in the first constitution of the Nurses' Associated Alumnae, which was the forerunner of the ANA. Over the next 88 years, the Code for Nurses was refined to its present format. In 1984 the ANA published explanations of each of the 11 points in the Code (ANA, 1985a). The consequences of failing to follow the Code may include disciplinary action and expulsion from the ANA, as well as legal action taken against the nurse. For example, nurses were being paid by antiabortion groups for the names of women who had abortions. Members of these right-to-life

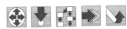

TABLE 10–1   Examples of Ethical and Legal Dilemmas

ETHICAL AND LEGAL

A nurse refuses to follow a physician's order because to obey would clearly violate the nurse's ethical responsibility to the client and the nurse practice act for that state.

ETHICAL AND ILLEGAL

A nurse is asked by a terminally ill client to administer an overdose of narcotic to hasten her inevitable death and end her suffering.

UNETHICAL AND LEGAL

A nurse initiates CPR on a terminally ill client. The physician has not written a "do not resuscitate" order. The nurse believes that the patient would not have wanted to be resuscitated at the time of death.

UNETHICAL AND ILLEGAL

A nurse participates in the unnecessary medication of an elderly nursing home resident to make the resident less troublesome and more compliant.

groups then proceeded to harass the women with abusive phone calls when they returned home from the hospital. The nurses involved in this activity violated the second point in the Code, which states that the nurse safeguards the client's rights to privacy by "judiciously protecting information of a confidential nature" (Benjamin and Curtis, 1986).

Ethical Theories

The nurse is often placed in the role of client advocate in order to protect the rights of clients. An *advocate* is one who protects the rights of another. You act as a client advocate in many ways, including obtaining resources or information for the client, contacting the physician when there is a change in the client's condition, or lobbying for improved health care. While it is important for the nurse to understand the points contained in the Code for Nurses, the nurse needs more substance in order to make ethical decisions. Ethical theories describe approaches for resolving dilemmas commonly faced by nurses. "Philosophers, beginning with Socrates, Plato, and Aristotle, have for centuries attempted to answer two major questions of ethics: What is the meaning of right and of good? What ought I to do?" (Davis, 1983). Ethical theories help answer these questions.

There are two major ethical theories used to help nurses resolve health care dilemmas: deontology and utilitarianism. The *deontologic* approach states that the rightness or wrongness of actions is determined by how the interventions

ETHICAL FOUN-
DATIONS
Definitions
Examples of ethical
dilemmas
Sources of ethics
Ethical theories

Deontology: Right-
ness or wrongness
of actions is de-
termined by how
the interventions
conform to a rule.

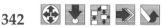

AMERICAN NURSES' ASSOCIATION CODE FOR NURSES

1. The nurse provides services with respect for human dignity and the uniqueness of the client unrestricted by considerations of social or economic status, personal attributes, or the nature of health problems.
2. The nurse safeguards the client's right to privacy by judiciously protecting information of a confidential nature.
3. The nurse acts to safeguard the client and the public when health care and safety are affected by incompetent, unethical, or illegal practice of any person.
4. The nurse assumes responsibility and accountability for individual nursing judgments and actions.
5. The nurse maintains competence in nursing.
6. The nurse exercises informed judgment and uses individual competence and qualifications as criteria in seeking consultation, accepting responsibilities, and delegating nursing activities to others.
7. The nurse participates in activities that contribute to the ongoing development of the profession's body of knowledge.
8. The nurse participates in the profession's efforts to implement and improve standards of nursing.
9. The nurse participates in the profession's efforts to establish and maintain conditions of employment conducive to high quality nursing care.
10. The nurse participates in the profession's effort to protect the public from misinformation and misrepresentation and to maintain the integrity of nursing.
11. The nurse collaborates with members of the health professions and other citizens in promoting community and national efforts to meet the health needs of the public.

FIGURE 10-6   American Nurses' Association Code for Nurses.

(Reprinted with permission of the American Nurses' Association, Washington, DC.)

conform to a rule. For instance, breaking a promise to a client would be considered wrong. Deontologists use rules because they are right, irrespective of the consequences they may produce in a particular situation. When the nurse makes a moral judgment in one given situation, the nurse will make the same judgment in any similar situation regardless of time, place, and persons involved (Davis, 1983).

One of the flaws with this approach is that most situations have extenuating circumstances. For example, in some instances it would be better to break than to keep a promise (Fowler and Levine-Ariff, 1987). You may be asked to keep a promise not reveal that the client has brought a quart of whiskey to the hospital. After thinking it over, you realize that it is better to break the promise so that you can protect the client from the consequences of consuming alcohol while being treated in the hospital.

Utilitarianism: actions are right or wrong based on the consequences of the actions or "the greatest good for the greatest number."

The *utilitarian* approach states that actions are right or wrong on the basis of the consequences of the actions. This philosophy defines "good as happiness or pleasure and right as maximizing the greatest good and least amount of harm for the greatest number of persons. This position assumes that one can weigh and measure harm and benefit and come out with the greatest possible balance of good over evil for most people" (Davis, 1983).

Utilitarians focus on the results of actions rather than on their motivations. According to this approach, the nurse would weigh the consequences of telling the truth. Other factors may take priority, such as the nurse's own survival or the continuation of the system for the benefit of future clients. In this case the nurse may not tell the truth in preference to other interests that promote greater happiness. This view is quite different from the deontologic position, which would maintain that the nurse must tell the truth without exception (ANA, 1985b).

The utilitarian position is often referred to when making decisions in managing scarce health care resources.

Example.   An intensive care unit may have only one empty bed. A young father who is supporting his elderly parents and three young children is in the emergency department with chest pain. Next to him is an elderly man who lives alone and needs treatment for diabetic coma. The utilitarian position would maintain that the bed should go to the young father because it would provide the greatest good for the greatest number of people.

Critics of the utilitarian approach question "whether this position involves the total happiness for a few or the average happiness for all. A crucial question is whether or not what one does in a particular situation contributes to the greatest general good or the least amount of harm for everyone. But how can everyone's welfare really be considered? Others accuse the utilitarian of ignoring the personal nature of good, e.g., truth telling and promise keeping" (Davis, 1983).

Other philosophers have offered alternatives to deontologic and utilitarian positions. These include Franken's Theory of Obligation, Firth's Ideal Observer Theory, and Justice as Fairness by Rawls. The newer positions incorporate components of utilitarian and deontologic thinking.

ETHICAL DECISION-MAKING AND THE NURSING PROCESS

ETHICAL FOUN-DATIONS
Definitions
Examples of ethical dilemmas
Sources of ethics
Ethical theories
Ethical Decision Making and the Nursing Process

In many agencies, an ethics committee is available to assist in resolving dilemmas. It typically consists of representatives from many disciplines, such as nursing, medicine, social service, ministry, administration, and so on. The group usually provides bedside consultations when ethical dilemmas arise. Although the ethics committee may not refer to their guidance as the nursing process, they follow the same elements. The following describes how you as a nurse or how the committee would approach an ethical dilemma.

Assessment

Begin by gathering all relevant information. This includes important information on:

ANA Measurement Criteria Standard V-6: (Standard of Professional

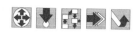
**Performance):
The nurse seeks
available resources
to help formulate
ethical decisions.**

- the circumstances surrounding the dilemma.
- the rights and responsibilities of all involved, including the client, family, and health care team.
- the wishes of the client and family.
- the legal aspects of the situation, including whether any laws govern the resolution of the dilemma.

Diagnosis

Next, define the ethical components of the dilemma. Ask these questions:

- What are the values that are in conflict?
- Who holds each of the values?
- Does the dilemma fall into one of the common types of conflict, such as truth telling versus withholding the truth, treating or letting die, freedom versus authority, or alleviation of pain versus preservation of life?

Planning

Planning should include the individuals who are involved in the dilemma, such as the client, family, and health care team. This phase involves the identification of:

- the goals of treatment.
- the primary decision maker, if not the client.
- all of the possible options.
- the ranking or desirability of the options.
- the application of ethical theories as they relate to the dilemma.
- the selection of the best option.

Implementation

In this phase, the agreed upon solution is implemented. Depending on the nature of the dilemma, this may involve such interventions such as turning off a ventilator, sharing information with others, allowing a client to refuse treatment, or withholding CPR.

Evaluation

In this final phase the decisions that have been made are evaluated. This includes examining the consequences of the actions that were taken, and comparing the results with previous experiences in similar situations.

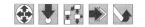

EXAMPLE OF ETHICAL DECISION-MAKING

During the last several years HIV infections have dramatically increased in number and given rise to a host of legal and ethical questions. Many legal concerns have arisen regarding employment practices and discrimination based on having AIDS or a positive HIV blood test. One of the ethical questions centers on the role of the nurse and physician in informing others about a client's diagnosis.

In a situation described in an article (Laufman, 1989), a nurse was assigned to be a case manager for a 32-year-old homosexual man who had developed AIDS. (See Chapter 8 for a discussion of case management.) The client had been sexually active for only the past four years and had few partners. His family was unaware of his homosexuality and his diagnosis until a week before he died.

The client, Jose, told the nurse that he had intended to tell his family the truth about his diagnosis when his illness worsened. He expected his family to react negatively and was concerned that the nurse keep the matter confidential. When his condition deteriorated Jose told his brother about his disease, his lifestyle, and his poor prognosis.

Jose's brother was shocked and demanded to know why the nurse had not told him about Jose's disease. The nurse explained that she could not have done so without the client's consent. Jose's brother said he and his family felt they had a right to know so that they could protect themselves from infection.

Did the client's right to confidentiality supersede the right of the family to prepare for Jose's death and to protect themselves from what they saw as the risk of AIDS?

Assessment

Information About the Circumstances

The client was living at home with his mother, brother, and two cousins. He was his mother's primary source of economic and emotional support since his father's death several years earlier. The nurse provided doses of an experimental drug to treat his eye problem. The *brother was given information about the medications Jose was receiving* but did not display curiosity or ask detailed questions about Jose's illness.

Rights and Responsibilities

Jose.   According to the Patient's Bill of Rights, *Jose had a right to considerate and respectful care.* Additionally, *he had the right to receive complete information about his condition.* The physician had told him he would probably live about two more years. Finally, *he had a right to expect that confidentiality of health information would be maintained.*

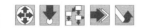
The Nurse. The Code for Nurses specifies that *the nurse had an ethical obligation to safeguard the client's right to privacy* by protecting confidential information. Therefore the nurse must make a diligent effort to obtain the client's consent for release of information.

The Physician. The position of the physician is more complex with respect to confidentiality and the client with AIDS. On one hand the physician is expected to maintain confidentiality of information. *"Disclosure of confidential information by a physician constitutes an invasion of the patient's right to privacy"* (Hirsh, 1989).

On the other hand, the physician is expected to safeguard others who would be affected by the client's actions.

Tarasoff v. The Regents of California: the psychologist had a duty to warn people at risk of injury.

Example. The *Tarasoff v. The Regents of California* case has set a legal precedent that *the physician has a duty to warn people at risk.* In this case a psychologist was treating a client who provided the name of a former girlfriend he was intending to kill. The man carried out his threat and murdered the woman (Ms. Tarasoff). The psychologist, who protected the client's right to privacy by not sharing this information, was held liable for not warning the woman that his client intended to kill her. The court said, "If the exercise of reasonable care to protect the threatened victim requires the therapist to warn the endangered party or those who can reasonably be expected to notify her, we see no sufficient societal interest that would protect and justify concealment. The containment of such risks lies in the public interest" (131 California Reporter, 1976).

The American Medical Association has taken a position that the physician should attempt to persuade the individual with AIDS to stop endangering the sexual or intravenous contacts, to notify authorities if persuasion fails, and if the authorities take no action, to notify and counsel the endangered third parties (Closen and Issacman, 1989). However, with respect to Jose's situation, the legal precedents and advice relate to sexual and needle-sharing contacts, not to family members, who are at very low risk for infection.

Factors that Could Influence the Decision-Making Process

The ethical responsibilities of the nurse and physician have been identified. Legal dictates of the State of California, where Jose lived, need to be considered. The California Health and Safety Code prohibits the willful or negligent disclosure of HIV results to any third party unless a written authorization is signed by the client. However, another statute grants immunity from civil or criminal liability to physicians who wish to warn a spouse that his or her partner has tested positive for HIV (Martello, 1989). The California laws do not require disclosure to family members other than a spouse.

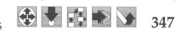

Diagnosis

The ethical dilemma described in Jose's situation involves truth telling versus withholding of the truth. In this case the factors that were being balanced included the client's right to privacy versus the family's right to information.

Planning

In this phase the nurse considered the ethical theories in relation to the dilemma she experienced. The utilitarian position, which emphasizes the greatest good for the greatest number, was rejected. The nurse believed that informing the family of the diagnosis would not be in the client's best interests because they were not at high risk for infection. Rather, the nurse took the deontologic position that the decision to maintain confidentiality was right, irrespective of the consequences. This decision was consistent with the nurse's role as a client advocate. In this situation, the nurse acted as an advocate by maintaining confidentiality. Other alternatives that she rejected included refusing to care for Jose, which was inconsistent with her responsibilities as a nurse. Finally, she could have told the family herself but did not because this disclosure would have been illegal in California and unethical.

> **ANA Measurement Criteria Standard V-3: (Standard of Professional Performance): The nurse acts as a client advocate.**

Implementation

The nurse resolved the dilemma by protecting Jose's rights and his autonomy. She provided the family with the information they needed to avoid exposure to his blood and body fluids and made sure they followed infection control procedures.

Evaluation

The greatest harm Jose could imagine was having his family relationships jeopardized by their reaction to his diagnosis and sexual orientation. When his brother learned the truth of his illness, he refused to let Jose's friends visit him in the hospital. Jose died a week later. The nurse has not had further contact with the family following Jose's death and cannot comment on the aftereffects of the nondisclosure on them.

Commentary

This example illustrates the complex factors that may need to be considered in resolving an ethical dilemma. Jose's case dealt with a nurse who helped a client to keep information from family members. Another difficult aspect of the case involves the sharing of information with Jose's sexual partners. The Center for

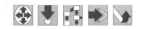

Disease Control recommends that sexual partners of HIV-infected persons and those who share needles should be counseled and tested for HIV antibodies. The American Psychiatric Association recommends that the physician notify the client of the specific limits of the confidentiality of information about HIV status. If the physician has reason to suspect that the HIV-positive client is engaging in behavior that is known to transmit the disease, it is ethically permissible for the physician to notify a person in danger. This assumes that the client does not agree to change the behavior or notify person(s) at risk, or that the physician has good reason to believe that the client will not keep a promise after agreeing to do these things (Haggberg, 1992). The issue of confidentiality and HIV status is a difficult and emotional one. There is no consensus regarding confidentiality. As more of the population becomes HIV positive it is expected that a consensus will emerge.

SUMMARY

Legal aspects of nursing are guided by the four principles defined above. The nurse must maintain awareness of changes in practice to ensure that the client's and the nurse's rights are protected. Critical thinking is essential to safeguard the client's rights and protect the client from harm. Malpractice suits often result in a settlement or jury verdict when a plaintiff is able to prove that the nurse breached a duty, the breach directly led to damages, and that the damages were significant. Ethical issues pervade many aspects of nursing practice. The effective resolution of these dilemmas rests on a foundation of knowledge concerning professional behavior and ethical theories, skill in using the nursing process, and a willingness to take risks.

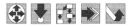

10-2 TEST YOURSELF
Ethical Decision-Making

Consider the following situation and apply the nursing process steps of assessment, diagnosis and planning to this dilemma.

Eighteen-year-old Molly was diagnosed with liver and pancreatic cancer in February and is a patient on your nursing unit. Her doctor and her parents decided to withhold the truth from her and asked the nurses to keep Molly's hopes up. She was told that she would graduate with her class in May. Now, in mid March, Molly is near death and asks you, "What is wrong with me?"

ASSESSMENT

What are the rights and responsibilities of Molly, her parents, and the health care team? What are the wishes of Molly and her family? Do any laws apply to this dilemma?

DIAGNOSIS

What are the values that are in conflict and who holds each of the values?

PLANNING

What are the possible options and how desirable are each? How do deontology and utilitarian approaches apply to this dilemma? What is the best option?

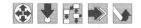

10-2   TEST YOURSELF
Ethical Decision-Making: Answers

Assessment: What are the rights and responsibilities of Molly, her parents and the health care team? What are the wishes of Molly and her family? Do any laws apply to this dilemma?

Molly's rights: According to the Patient's Bill of Rights Point 2 in Figure 10-2, Molly has the right to obtain from physicians and other direct care-givers relevant, current, and understandable information concerning her diagnosis, treatment, and prognosis. Molly has the right to know her diagnosis and prepare for death.

Molly's parents' rights: Molly's parents have a right to express their opinions.

Molly's physician's responsibilities: The doctor is responsible for telling Molly the truth since Molly is 18 and an adult in the eyes of the law.

You have a right to be able to provide support to Molly without having to be deceptive.

Molly wishes to know the truth and her parents and physician wish to withhold the truth.

Diagnosis: What are the values that are in conflict and who holds each of the values?

The values in conflict are truth telling (which Molly is requesting) and withholding the truth (which the parents and physician believe is the best course).

Planning: What are the possible options and how desirable are each? How do deontology and utilitarian approaches apply to this dilemma? What is the best option?

Possible options:

1. You can tell Molly the truth without discussing the issue with Molly's parents or doctor.

2. You can tell Molly that her liver is a bit affected, but she will be ready to graduate with her own class.

3. You can avoid Molly's question and pretend you don't hear her.

4. You can request a conference with Molly's parents and physician to discuss the issue.

5. You can request that the ethics committee become involved in the dilemma.

Continued.

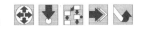

 10-2 TEST YOURSELF
Ethical Decision-Making: Answers–cont'd.

Ethical theories: Deontologists would say that Molly must be told the truth because it is not right to lie to a client. Utilitarians would say that the greatest good for the greatest number means that Molly is outnumbered by those who want to withhold the truth. By not telling her the truth the physician and her parents will be comfortable with the situation.

Best option: Implementing the first option is not the best solution because Molly's parents and physician have clearly indicated that she is not to be told about her diagnosis and prognosis. The second option involves lying to the client, while the third simply postpones the problem and does not resolve the issue. The fourth option is best because it involves all of the crucial parties and is a good beginning step to opening up the issue for discussion. The last option could be a useful resource to Molly's parents, physician, and yourself as you resolve the issue.

This test yourself was based on an ethics poll reported in the Jan/Feb 1983 issue of *Nursing Life* in an article called "Do you tell your patient the truth... do you talk about your patients?" In the real situation, no one told the client the truth and she died without the chance to come to terms with her death.

REFERENCES

American Nurses' Association: Code for Nurses with Interpretive Statements. Kansas City, MO: American Nurses' Association, 1985a.

American Nurses' Association: Ethical Dilemmas Confronting Nurses. Kansas City, MO: American Nurses' Association, 1985b.

American Nurses' Association: Ethics in Nursing. Kansas City, MO: American Nurses' Association, 1988.

Benjamin M and Curtis J: Ethics in Nursing. New York: Oxford University Press, 1986.

131 California Reporter 14, 27-28 (California 1976).

Cassells J and Redman B: Preparing students to be moral agents in clinical nursing practice. Nurs Clin North Am 1989; 24(2):463–73.

Champagne M, Havens B, and Swenson J: State board criteria for licensure and disciplinary procedure regarding impaired nurses. Nurs Outlook 1987; 35(2): 54–57, 101.

Closen M and Issacman S: Notifying private third parties at risk for HIV infection. TRIAL 1989 May; 50–55.

Creighton H: Licensure problems. Nurs Manag 1986; 17(2):16, 18.

Cushing M: How courts look at nurse practice acts. Am J Nurs 1986; 86(2):131–132.

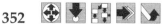
Cushing M: Keeping watch. Am J Nurs 1987; 87(8):1021–1022.

Daniels S: Verdicts in medical malpractice cases. TRIAL 1989 May; 23–30.

Davis S: Ethical Dilemmas and Nursing Practice. East Norwalk, CT: Appleton-Century-Crofts, 1983.

Fenner K: Ethics and the Law in Nursing. New York: Van Nostrand, 1980.

Fiesta J: The nursing shortage: Whose liability problem? Part 1. Nurs Manag 1990 January, 24–25.

Fowler M and Levine-Ariff J: Ethics at the Bedside. Philadelphia: JB Lippincott, 1987.

Fry S: Teaching Ethics in Nursing Curricula. Nurs Clin North Am 1989; 24(2):485–497.

Godkin L, Wooten B, and Godkin J: The jury decides: are registered nurses legally liable for their job-related actions? Nurs Manag 1987; 18(5):73–74, 76, 79.

Haggberg M: AIDS and confidentiality: A legal/ethical dilemma. J Healthcare Qual 1992; 14(2) 32–34.

Hirsh H: Hear all, see all, tell very, very little. Legal Aspects Med Pract, 1989 March; 7–9.

How likely is a lawsuit? Am J Nurs, 1990 January, 42.

Laufman J: AIDS, Ethics and the truth. Am J Nurs 1989; 89(7):924–930.

Markowitz L: How your state board works for you. Nurs Life 1982; 2:25–32.

Martello J: Can you keep a secret? AIDS: Confidentiality versus disclosure. Legal Aspects Med Pract, 1989 February; 7–9.

Murphy J and Connell C: Violations of the state's nurse practice act: How big is the problem? Nurs Manag 1987; 18(9):44–46, 48.

New study shows nurses offer same or better treatment at lower costs. ANA Council Perspect, 1993 Spring; 3.

Rosenfield A: A patient's bill of rights. Legal Aspects Med Pract, 1988 November; 3–5.

Satisfaction Data: Patient perception is reality. Hospitals 1989 July 5; 40.

Swenson J, Havens B, and Champagne M: Interpretations of state board criteria and disciplinary procedures regarding impaired nurses. Nurs Outlook 1987a; 35(3):108–110, 145.

Swenson J, Havens B, and Champagne M: State board members' perceptions of impaired nurses. Nurs Outlook 1987b; 35(4):154–155.

Swenson J, Havens B, and Champagne M: State boards and impaired nurses. Nurs Outlook 1989; 37(2):94–96.

Tammelleo D: "Constant observation" means "constant observation." Regan Report on Nursing Law 1991a March; 4.

Tammelleo, D: Failure to document and communicate: Catastrophic results. Regan Report on Nursing Law 1991b April; 1.

Tammelleo, D: LA: Nurse inserts catheter over patient's objection: Battery. Regan Report on Nursing Law 1991c June; 3.

Tammelleo, D: Recovery room nurse fails to monitor the patient. Regan Report on Nursing Law 1991d July; 2.

Tammelleo, D: Nurse fails to treat prisoner: Civil rights action. Regan Report on Nursing Law 1991e August; 1.

Tammelleo D: OR: Sexually explicit photographs of corpses: License revocation upheld. Regan Report on Nursing Law 1992a, November; 3.

Tammelleo, D: MT: Conviction of sex assault: Revocation of expired license upheld. Regan Report on Nursing Law 1992b December; 3.

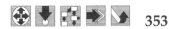

Tammelleo D: OH: Termination for sexual harassment: Hospital policy conflicts with "at will" status. Regan Report on Nursing Law 1993a February; 3.

Tammelleo D: NY: Refused to stay for additional shift: Abandonment charged-suspension results. Regan Report on Nursing Law 1993b March; 3.

Taragin M and others: The influence of standard of care and severity of injury on the resolution of medical practice claims. Ann Intern Med 1992; *117* (9), 780–84.

BIBLIOGRAPHY

American Nurses' Association: Social Policy Statement. Kansas City, MO: American Nurses' Association, 1982.

Bellocq J: Protecting your license. J Profess Nurs 1989; *5*(1):8.

Brooke P: Shopping for liability insurance. Am J Nurs 1989 Feb (2);171–172.

Cleveland H: Labor law issues for health care providers, in Gosfield A (ed): 1989 Health Law Handbook. New York: Clark Boardman Co., 1989.

Ingenito EF and others, Rehabilitation of patients with HIV: Patient confidentiality v treatment team right to know. Am J Phys Med Rehab 1990; *69*(6):330–332.

International Council of Nurses: International Code for Nursing Ethics, in Beauchamp T and Walters L (eds): Contemporary Issues in Bioethics. Encino, CA: Dickenson Publications, 1978.

Ivanic J: Confidentiality of health care information: some notable concerns. Perspect Healthcare Risk Manag 1992 Winter; 13.

Iyer P and Camp N: Nursing documentation: A nursing process approach. 2nd ed. St. Louis: Mosby–Year Book, 1994.

Lund M: The heart of the matter. Am J Nurs 1992 April; 22–24.

Maciorowski LF: The enduring concerns of privacy and confidentiality, Holistic Nurs Pract, 1991 April; *5*(3):51–6.

Miedema F: A practical approach to ethical decisions. Am J Nurs 1991 December; 20–25.

Neumann T: A nurse's guide to fail safe delegating. Nursing 1989; *19*(9):63–64.

Northrop C: Legal content in the nursing curriculum: what students need and how to provide it. Nurs Outlook 1989; *34*(4):200.

Nurses Associated Alumnae of the US and Canada, Constitution, 1897.

Quinley K: Twelve tips for defending yourself in a malpractice suit. Am J Nurs 1990; *90*(1):37–40.

Strother A: Drawing the line between life and death. Am J Nurs 1991 April; 24–25.

Tammelleo D: Nurse refuses to 'float': Sunk. The Regan Report on Nursing Law 1986 December; 1.

Torres CG: Security measures for AIDS and HIV. Am J Public Health 1991 February; *81* (2):210–211.

Viens D: A history of nursing's code of ethics. Nurs Outlook 1989; *37*(1):45–49.

White N and others: Promoting critical thinking skills. Nurse Educ 1990; *15*(5),16–19.

APPROVED NURSING DIAGNOSES

The currently accepted North American Nursing Diagnosis Association (NANDA) diagnoses are organized in a classification known as Taxonomy I. NANDA adopted this grouping to facilitate the organization of nursing diagnoses. Nurses can expect that this ordering may change, since Taxonomy I, as the first step in organizing this information, will be tested, refined, revised, and expanded.

Taxonomy I is organized to reflect the patterns of human responses, which are listed and defined below:

1. *Exchanging:* A human response pattern involving mutual giving and receiving.
2. *Communicating:* A human response pattern involving sending messages.
3. *Relating:* A human response pattern involving established bonds.
4. *Valuing:* A human response pattern involving the assigning of relative worth.
5. *Choosing:* A human response pattern involving the selection of alternatives.
6. *Moving:* A human response pattern involving activity.
7. *Perceiving:* A human response pattern involving the reception of information.
8. *Knowing:* A human response pattern involving meaning associated with information.
9. *Feeling:* A human response pattern involving the subjective awareness of information.

Table A-1 illustrates the groupings of accepted diagnoses, which have been placed under each human response pattern.

This part of the book is organized according to Taxonomy I, including the revisions made at the 1992 NANDA conference. In addition to providing the currently accepted NANDA diagnoses, this section includes the definition, defining characteristics, and related factors for each of the diagnoses. Readers can refer to this section for assistance in formulating correctly stated nursing diagnoses—an important component of nursing care planning.

TABLE A-1   NANDA Taxonomy of Nursing Diagnoses

PATTERN 1:	**EXCHANGING**
1.1.2.1	Altered nutrition: more than body requirements
1.1.2.2	Altered nutrition: less than body requirements
1.1.2.3	Altered nutrition: high risk for more than body requirements[+]
1.2.1.1	High risk for infection[+]
1.2.2.1	High risk for altered body temperature[+]
1.2.2.2	Hypothermia
1.2.2.3	Hyperthermia
1.2.2.4	Ineffective thermoregulation
1.2.3.1	Dysreflexia
1.3.1.1	Constipation
1.3.1.1.1	Perceived constipation
1.3.1.1.2	Colonic constipation
1.3.1.2	Diarrhea
1.3.1.3	Bowel incontinence
1.3.2	Altered patterns of urinary elimination
1.3.2.1.1	Stress incontinence
1.3.2.1.2	Reflex incontinence
1.3.2.1.3	Urge incontinence
1.3.2.1.4	Functional incontinence
1.3.2.1.5	Total incontinence
1.3.2.2	Urinary retention
1.4.1.1	Altered (specify type) tissue perfusion (renal, cerebral, cardiopulmonary, gastrointestinal, peripheral)
1.4.1.2.1	Fluid volume excess
1.4.1.2.2.1	Fluid volume deficit
1.4.1.2.2.2	High risk for fluid volume deficit[+]
1.4.2.1	Decreased cardiac output
1.5.1.1	Impaired gas exchange
1.5.1.2	Ineffective airway clearance
1.5.1.3	Ineffective breathing pattern
1.5.1.3.1	Inability to sustain spontaneous ventilation[*]
1.5.1.3.2	Dysfunctional venilatory weaning response[*]
1.6.1	High risk for injury[+]
1.6.1.1	High risk for suffocation[+]
1.6.1.2	High risk for poisoning[+]
1.6.1.3	High risk for trauma[+]
1.6.1.4	High risk for aspiration[+]
1.6.1.5	High risk for disuse syndrome[+]
1.6.2	Altered protection
1.6.2.1	Impaired tissue integrity
1.6.2.1.1	Altered oral mucous membrane
1.6.2.1.2.1	Impaired skin integrity
1.6.2.1.2.2	High risk for impaired skin integrity[+]

[+]Categories with modified label terminology.
[*]New diagnostic categories, approved 1992.

Continued.

TABLE A-1   NANDA Taxonomy of Nursing Diagnoses–cont'd.

PATTERN 2:	COMMUNICATING
2.1.1.1	Impaired verbal communication

PATTERN 3:	RELATING
3.1.1	Impaired social interaction
3.1.2	Social isolation
3.2.1	Altered role performance

PATTERN 3:	RELATING
3.2.1.1.1	Altered parenting
3.2.1.1.2	High risk for altered parenting+
3.2.1.2.1	Sexual dysfunction
3.2.2	Altered family processes
3.2.2.1	Care-giver role strain*
3.2.2.2	High risk for care-giver role strain*
3.2.3.1	Parental role conflict
3.3	Altered sexuality patterns

PATTERN 4:	VALUING
4.1.1	Spiritual distress (distress of the human spirit)

PATTERN 5:	CHOOSING
5.1.1.1	Ineffective individual coping
5.1.1.1.1	Impaired adjustment
5.1.1.1.2	Defensive coping
5.1.1.1.3	Ineffective denial
5.1.2.1.1	Ineffective family coping: disabling
5.1.2.1.2	Ineffective family coping: compromised
5.1.2.2	Family coping: potential for growth
5.2.1	Ineffective management of therapeutic regimen (individual)*
5.2.1.1	Noncompliance (specify)
5.3.1.1	Decisional conflict (specify)
5.4	Health-seeking behaviors (specify)

PATTERN 6:	MOVING
6.1.1.1	Impaired physical mobility
6.1.1.1.1	High risk for neurovascular dysfunction*
6.1.1.2	Activity intolerance
6.1.1.2.1	Fatigue
6.1.1.3	High risk for activity intolerance+
6.2.1	Sleep pattern disturbance
6.3.1.1	Diversional activity deficit
6.4.1.1	Impaired home maintenance management
6.4.2	Altered health maintenance
6.5.1	Feeding self-care deficit
6.5.1.1	Impaired swallowing

+Categories with modified label terminology.
*New diagnostic categories, approved 1992.

TABLE A-1   NANDA Taxonomy of Nursing Diagnoses–cont'd.

PATTERN 6:	MOVING
6.5.1.2	Ineffective breast-feeding
6.5.1.2.1	Interrupted breast-feeding*
6.5.1.3	Effective breast-feeding
6.5.1.4	Ineffective infant feeding pattern*
6.5.2	Bathing/hygiene self-care deficit
6.5.3	Dressing/grooming self-care deficit
6.5.4	Toileting self-care deficit
6.6	Altered growth and development
6.7	Relocation stress syndrome*
PATTERN 7:	**PERCEIVING**
7.1.1	Body image disturbance
7.1.2	Self-esteem disturbance
7.1.2.1	Chronic low self-esteem
PATTERN 7:	**PERCEIVING**
7.1.2.2	Situational low-self-esteem
7.1.3	Personal identity disturbance
7.2	Sensory/perceptual alterations (specify) (visual, auditory, kinesthetic, gustatory, tactile, olfactory)
7.2.1.1	Unilateral neglect
7.3.1	Hopelessness
7.3.2	Powerlessness
PATTERN 8:	**KNOWING**
8.1.1	Knowledge deficit (specify)
8.3	Altered thought processes
PATTERN 9:	**FEELING**
9.1.1	Pain
9.1.1.1	Chronic pain
9.2.1.1	Dysfunctional grieving
9.2.1.2	Anticipatory grieving
9.2.2	High risk for violence: self-directed or directed at others+
9.2.2.1	High risk for self-mutilation*
9.2.3	Post-trauma response
9.2.3.1	Rape-trauma syndrome
9.2.3.1.1	Rape-trauma syndrome: compound reaction
9.2.3.1.2	Rape-trauma syndrome: silent reaction
9.3.1	Anxiety
9.3.2	Fear

+Categories with modified label terminology.
*New diagnostic categories, approved 1992.

ALPHABETICAL INDEX OF NANDA-APPROVED DIAGNOSES

Activity intolerance
Activity intolerance, high risk for†
Adjustment, impaired
Airway clearance, ineffective
Anxiety
Aspiration, high risk for†
Body image disturbance
Body temperature, high risk for altered†
Breast-feeding, effective
Breast-feeding, ineffective
Breast-feeding, interrupted*
Breathing pattern, ineffective
Cardiac output, decreased
Care-giver role strain*
Care-giver role strain, high risk for*
Communication, impaired verbal
Conflict, decisional (specify)
Conflict, parental role
Constipation
Constipation, colonic
Constipation, perceived
Coping, defensive
Coping, family: ineffective, compromised
Coping, family: ineffective, disabling
Coping, family: potential for growth
Coping, individual: ineffective
Denial, ineffective
Diarrhea
Disuse syndrome, high risk for†
Diversional activity deficit
Dysreflexia
Family processes, altered
Fatigue
Fear
Fluid volume deficit
Fluid volume deficit, high risk for†
Fluid volume excess
Gas exchange, impaired
Grieving, anticipatory
Grieving, dysfunctional
Growth and development, altered
Health maintenance, altered

Health-seeking behaviors (specify)
Home maintenance management, impaired
Hopelessness
Hyperthermia
Hypothermia
Incontinence, bowel
Incontinence, functional
Incontinence, reflex
Incontinence, stress
Incontinence, total
Incontinence, urge
Infant feeding pattern, ineffective*
Infection, high risk for†
Injury, high risk for†
Knowledge deficit (specify)
Mobility, impaired physical
Neurovascular dysfunction, high risk for peripheral*
Noncompliance (specify)
Nutrition, altered: high risk for more than body requirements†
Nutrition, altered: less than body requirements
Nutrition, altered: more than body requirements
Oral mucous membrane, altered
Pain
Pain, chronic
Parenting, altered
Parenting, altered: high risk for†
Personal identity disturbance
Poisoning, high risk for†
Post-trauma response
Powerlessness
Protection, altered
Rape-trauma syndrome
Rape-trauma syndrome: compound reaction
Rape-trauma syndrome: silent reaction
Relocation stress syndrome*
Role performance, altered
Self-care deficit (bathing/hygiene, dressing/grooming, feeding, toileting)
Self-esteem, chronic low
Self-esteem disturbance
Self-esteem, situational low
Self-mutilation, high risk for*
Sensory/perceptual alterations (specify) (visual, auditory, kinesthetic, gustatory, tactile, olfactory)

†Modified label terminology, 1992.
*New diagnoses, 1992.

Sexual dysfunction

Sexuality patterns, altered

Skin integrity, high risk for impaired†

Skin integrity, impaired

Sleep pattern disturbance

Social interaction, impaired

Social isolation

Spiritual distress

Suffocation, high risk for†

Swallowing, impaired

Therapeutic regimen (individual), ineffective management of*

Thermoregulation, ineffective

Thought processes, altered

Tissue integrity, impaired

Tissue perfusion, altered (specify type) (cardiopulmonary, cerebral, gastrointestinal, peripheral, renal)

Trauma, high risk for†

Unilateral neglect

Urinary elimination, altered patterns of

Urinary retention

Ventilation, inability to sustain spontaneous*

Ventilatory weaning response, dysfunctional

Violence, high risk for: self-directed or directed at others

† Modified label terminology, 1992.
* New diagnoses, 1992.

Alcohol Drinking Patterns, Dysfunctional

Community Coping, Ineffective

Community Coping, Potential for Enhanced

Confusion, Acute

Disorganized Behavior, Infant

Disorganized Infant Behavior, High Risk For

Environmental Interpretation Syndrome, Impaired

Family Processes, Altered: Addictive Behavior (Individual and Family)

Idiopathic Fecal Incontinence

Impaired Skin Integrity, High Risk For: Pressure Ulcer

Labor Pain

Loneliness, High Risk For

Organized Infant Behavior, Potential for Enhanced

Parent/Infant Attachment, Altered

Preservation/Quality of Life, Alteration in

Self Care Deficit, Medication Administration

Spasticity

Spiritual Well Being, Opportunity for Enhanced

Therapeutic Regimen, Ineffective Management of (Families)

Terminal Illness Response

Urinary Filtration Syndrome, Impaired

North American Nursing Diagnosis Association
1994 Diagnoses in Progress

EXCHANGING

A Human Response Pattern Involving Mutual Giving and Receiving

Diagnosis
Altered Nutrition: More than Body Requirements

Definition

The state in which the individual consumes more than adequate nutritional intake in relation to metabolic demands

Defining Characteristics

Weight 10%–20% over ideal for height and frame □ Triceps skin fold greater than 15 mm in men, 25 mm in women □ Measured food consumption exceeds American Diabetic Association recommendations for activity level, age, sex □ Reported or observed dysfunctional eating patterns: pairing food with other activities; concentrating food intake at end of day; eating in response to external cues, such as time of day or social situation; eating in response to internal cues other than hunger, such as anxiety or stress □ Sedentary activity level

Related Factors

Lack of: physical exercise; social support for weight loss; knowledge regarding nutritional needs □ Decreased activity pattern □ Imbalance between activity level and caloric intake □ Eating in response to stress or emotional trauma □ Eating as a comfort measure/substitute gratification □ Learned eating behaviors □ Decreased metabolic need □ Weight gain during pregnancy over current recommendations □ Effects of drug therapy (appetite-stimulating) □ Ethnic and cultural values □ Negative body image □ Perceived lack of control □ Decreased self-esteem □ Feelings of anxiety, depression, guilt, boredom, frustration

Diagnosis
Altered Nutrition: Less than Body Requirements

Definition

The state in which the individual consumes insufficient nutritional intake in relation to metabolic demands

Defining Characteristics

Loss of weight with adequate food intake □ Body weight 20% or more less than ideal for height and frame □ Reported altered taste sensation □ Satiety immediately after ingesting food □ Abdominal pain with or without pathology □ Sore, inflamed buccal cavity □ Capillary fragility □ Abdominal cramping □ Diarrhea and/or steatorrhea □ Hyperactive bowel sounds □ Pale conjunctival and mucous membranes □ Poor muscle tone or skin turgor □ Excessive hair loss □ Decreased serum albumin or total protein □ Decreased serum transferrin or iron-binding capacity □ Metabolic demands in excess of intake □ Anemia □ Lack of interest in food □ Perceived inability to ingest food □ Reported or evidence of lack of food □ Aversion to eating □ Reported inadequate food intake less than recommended daily allowance (RDA) □ Weakness of muscles required for swallowing or mastication □ Lack of information, misinformation □ Misconceptions

Related Factors

Inability to ingest or digest food or absorb nutrients owing to biological, psychological, or economic factors; for example: impaired absorption; alteration in taste or smell; dysphagia; dyspnea; stomatitis; nausea and vomiting; fatigue; inability to chew; decreased appetite; decreased salivation; effects of hyperanabolic or catabolic states: cancer, burns, infections; decreased level of consciousness; stress; effects of aging—decreased sense of taste; knowledge deficit; inadequate finances

High-Risk Diagnosis
Altered Nutrition: High Risk for More than Body Requirements

Definition

The condition in which the individual is at risk of experiencing excessive nutritional intake in relation to metabolic demands

Risk Factors

Reported or observed obesity in one or both parents □ Rapid transition across growth percentiles in infants or children □ Reported use of solid food as major food source before 5 months of age □ Observed use of food as reward or comfort measure □ Reported or observed higher baseline weight at beginning of each pregnancy □ Dysfunctional eating patterns: pairing food with other activities; concentrating food intake at end of day; eating in response to external cues such as time of day, social situation; eating in response to internal cues other than hunger, such as anxiety, stress

High-Risk Diagnosis
High Risk for Infection

Definition

The state in which an individual is at increased risk for being invaded by pathogenic organisms

Risk Factors

Inadequate primary defenses: broken skin; traumatized tissue; decreased ciliary action; stasis of body fluids; change in pH of secretions; altered peristalsis; □ Inadequate secondary defenses; decreased hemoglobin; leukopenia; suppressed inflammatory response □ Tissue destruction and increased environmental exposure □ Effects of: chronic disease; immunosuppression; inadequate acquired immunity; invasive treatments/procedures; malnutrition; pharmaceutical agents; trauma □ Rupture of amniotic membranes □ Insufficient knowledge to avoid exposure to pathogens

High-Risk Diagnosis
High Risk for Altered Body Temperature

Definition

The state in which the individual is at risk for failure to maintain body temperature within normal range

Risk Factors

Dehydration □ Inactivity or vigorous activity □ Altered metabolic rate □ Medications causing vasoconstriction/vasodilation □ Sedation □ Illness or trauma affecting temperature regulation □ Extremes of age □ Extremes of weight □ Exposure to cold/cool or warm/hot environments □ Inappropriate clothing for environmental temperature

Diagnosis
Hypothermia

Definition

The state in which an individual's body temperature is reduced to below the normal range

Defining Characteristics

Major: reduction in body temperature below the normal range; shivering (mild); cool skin; pallor (moderate); □ Minor: slow capillary refill; tachycardia; cyanotic nail beds; hypertension; piloerection; verbalization of feeling cold

Related Factors

Effects of: aging; exposure to cool or cold environment; illness or trauma; damage to hypothalamus; inability or decreased ability to shiver; medications causing vasodilation □ Malnutrition □ Inadequate clothing □ Consumption of alcohol □ Evaporation from skin in cool environment □ Decreased metabolic rate □ Inactivity

Diagnosis
Hyperthermia

Definition

The state in which the individual is at risk because the body temperature is elevated above the individual's normal range

Defining Characteristics

Major: increase in body temperature above normal range ☐ Minor: skin flushed or warm to the touch; increased respiratory rate; tachycardia; seizures/convulsions; shivering; weakness, faintness; perspiration; verbal reports of feeling hot;

Related Factors

Exposure to hot environment ☐ Increased metabolic rate ☐ Effects of: medications/anesthesia; illness or trauma involving temperature regulation; aging; obesity ☐ Dehydration ☐ Inability or decreased ability to perspire ☐ Vigorous activity ☐ Inappropriate clothing ☐ Inability to regulate environmental temperature: no air conditioning; isolette temperature for infants

Diagnosis
Ineffective Thermoregulation

Definition

The state in which the individual's temperature fluctuates between hypothermia and hyperthermia

Defining characteristics

Fluctuation in body temperature above and below the normal range ☐ See also major and minor characteristics present in hypothermia and hyperthermia

Related Factors

Effects of: trauma or illness; immaturity; confusion; aging; fluctuating environmental temperature; sedation; medications causing vasoconstriction or vasodilation; extremes of age; extremes of weight; ☐ Inappropriate clothing for environmental temperature

Diagnosis
Dysreflexia

Definition

The state in which an individual with a spinal cord injury at T7 or above experiences a life-threatening uninhibited sympathetic response of the nervous system to a noxious stimulus

Defining Characteristics

Major: Individual with spinal cord injury (T7 or above) with: paroxysmal hypertension (sudden periodic elevated blood pressure where systolic pressure is > 140mmHg and diastolic pressure is > 90 mmHg); bradycardia or tachycardia (pulse rate < 60 or > 100 beats/min); diaphoresis (above the injury); red splotches on skin (above the injury); pallor (below the injury); headache (a diffuse pain in different portions of the head and not confined to any nerve distribution on the head) ☐ Minor: chilling; conjunctival congestion; horner's syndrome (constriction of the pupil, partial ptosis of the eyelid, enophthalmos, and sometimes loss of sweating over the affected side of the face); paresthesia; pilomotor reflex (gooseflesh formation when skin is cooled); blurred vision; chest pain; metallic taste in mouth; nasal congestion

Related Factors

Bladder distention ☐ Bowel distention ☐ Constipation ☐ Skin irritation ☐ Lack of client/care-giver knowledge

Diagnosis
Constipation

Definition

The state in which the individual experiences a change in normal bowel habits characterized by a decrease in frequency and/or passage of hard, dry stools

Defining Characteristics

Decreased activity level ☐ Frequency less than usual pattern ☐ Hard, formed stools ☐ Palpable mass ☐ Straining at stool ☐ Palpable hard stool on rectal examination ☐ Less than usual amount of stool ☐ Decreased bowel sounds ☐ Gas pain and flatulence ☐ Abdominal or back pain ☐ Reported feeling of abdominal or rectal fullness/pressure ☐ Reported use of laxatives ☐ Impaired appetite ☐ Headache ☐ Nausea ☐ Irritability ☐ Interference with daily living

Related Factors

Less than adequate: dietary intake; fiber intake; fluid intake; ☐ Gastrointestinal lesions ☐ Pain/discomfort on defecation ☐ Effects of: aging; diagnostic procedures; medication; neuromuscular/musculoskeletal impairment; pregnancy; presence of anatomical obstruction; stress or anxiety; ☐ Weak abdominal musculature ☐ Immobility or less than adequate physical activity ☐ Chronic use of laxatives and enemas ☐ Personal habits ☐ Ignoring urge to defecate ☐ Fear of rectal or cardiac pain

Diagnosis
Perceived Constipation

Definition

The state in which an individual makes a self-diagnosis of constipation and ensures a daily bowel movement through abuse of laxatives, enemas, and suppositories

Defining Characteristics

Major: expectation of a daily bowel movement with the resulting overuse of laxatives, enemas, or suppositories; expected passage of stool at the same time every day

Related Factors

Cultural/family health beliefs ☐ Faulty appraisal ☐ Impaired thought processes

Diagnosis
Colonic Constipation

Definition

The state in which an individual's pattern of elimination is characterized by hard, dry stool that results from a delay in passage of food residue

Defining Characteristics

Major: decreased frequency; hard, dry stool; straining at stool; painful defecation; abdominal distention; palpable mass; ☐ Minor; rectal pressure; headache; appetite impairment; abdominal pain

Related Factors

Less than adequate: fluid intake; dietary intake; fiber intake; physical activity ☐ Immobility ☐ Lack of privacy ☐ Emotional disturbances ☐ Chronic use of medication and enemas ☐ Stress ☐ Change in daily routine ☐ Metabolic problems: hypothyroidism; hypocalcemia; hypokalemia

Diagnosis
Diarrhea

Definition

The state in which the individual experiences a change in normal bowel habits characterized by the frequent passage of fluid, loose or unformed stools

Defining Characteristics

Abdominal pain ☐ Anorexia ☐ Change in color or odor of stool ☐ Chills ☐ Cramping ☐ Fatigue ☐ Fever ☐ Increased frequency of bowel sounds ☐ Increased frequency of stool ☐ Irritated anal area ☐ Loose, liquid stools ☐ Malaise ☐ Mucoid stool ☐ Muscle weakness ☐ Thirst ☐ Urgency ☐ Weight loss

Related Factors

Allergies ☐ Effects of: medications; radiation; surgical intervention ☐ Infectious process ☐ Inflammatory process ☐ Malabsorption syndrome ☐ Nutritional disorders ☐ Stress and anxiety ☐ Dietary alterations: food intolerances; high-cellulose foods; increased caffeine consumption; hyperosmolar tube feeding ☐ Excessive use of laxatives ☐ Ingestion of contaminated water or food

Diagnosis
Bowel Incontinence

Definition

The state in which an individual experiences a change in normal bowel habits characterized by involuntary passage of stool

Defining Characteristics

Involuntary passage of stool ☐ Lack of awareness of need to defecate ☐ Lack of awareness of passage of stool ☐ Rectal oozing of stool ☐ Urgency

Related Factors

Diarrhea ☐ Impaction ☐ Effects of: cognitive impairment; medications; neuromuscular impairment; perceptual impairment ☐ Large stool volume ☐ Depression ☐ Severe anxiety ☐ Physical or psychological barriers that prevent access to an acceptable toileting area ☐ Excessive use of laxatives

Diagnosis
Altered Patterns of Urinary Elimination

Definition

The state in which an individual experiences a disturbance in urine elimination

Defining Characteristics

Distended bladder ☐ Dysuria ☐ Frequency ☐ Hesitancy ☐ Incontinence ☐ Increase or decrease in total urine voided in 24 hours, in proportion to intake ☐ Nocturia ☐ Retention ☐ Urgency

Related Factors

Anatomical obstruction ☐ Constipation/fecal impaction ☐ Dehydration ☐ Fatigue ☐ Obesity ☐ Mechanical trauma ☐ Pain/spasm in bladder or abdomen ☐ Urinary tract infection ☐ Decreased attention to bladder cues: depression; sedation; confusion ☐ Fear ☐ Inability to express needs ☐ Stress ☐ Change in environment ☐ Effects of: aging; immobility; indwelling catheter; medications; pregnancy; sensorimotor impairment; surgery ☐ Lack of privacy ☐ Prolonged bedrest

Diagnosis
Stress Incontinence

Definition

The state in which an individual experiences a loss of urine of less than 50 ml occurring with increased abdominal pressure

Defining Characteristics

Major: dribbling associated with increased abdominal pressure/exercise ☐ Minor: frequency (more often than every 2 hours); loss of urine in standing position; urgency

Related Factors

Degenerative changes in pelvic muscles and structural supports associated with increased age ☐ Effects of: pregnancy; high abdominal pressure; obesity ☐ Incompetent bladder outlet ☐ Overdistention between voidings ☐ Weak pelvic muscles and structural supports

Diagnosis
Reflex Incontinence

Definition

The state in which an individual experiences an involuntary passage of urine occurring at predictable intervals when a specific bladder volume is reached

Defining Characteristics

Lack of; awareness of being incontinent; awareness of bladder filling; urge to void or feelings of fullness □ Somewhat predictable voiding pattern □ Uninhibited bladder contractions/spasm at regular intervals □ Voiding in large amounts

Related Factors

Effects of neurological impairment: cerebral loss; interruption of spinal nerve impulse above the level of S3

Diagnosis
Urge Incontinence

Definition

The state in which an individual experiences involuntary passage of urine occurring soon after a strong sense of urgency to void

Defining Characteristics

Major: bladder contracture/spasm; frequency (voiding more often than every 2 hours); urinary urgency □ Minor: nocturia (more than twice per night); voiding in large amounts (> 500 ml); voiding in small amounts (< 100 ml); inability to reach toilet in time

Related Factors

Bladder infection/irritation □ Changes in urine concentration □ Decreased bladder capacity associated with abdominal surgeries; history of pelvic inflammatory disease; indwelling catheter □ Overdistention of bladder □ Diuretic therapy □ Ingestion of: alcohol; caffeine; increased fluids

Diagnosis
Functional Incontinence

Definition

The state in which an individual experiences involuntary and unpredictable passage of urine

Defining Characteristics

Urge to void or bladder contractions sufficiently strong to result in loss of urine before reaching an appropriate site or receptacle □ Unpredictable voiding pattern □ Unrecognized signals of bladder fullness

Related Factors

Effects of: cognitive deficits; motor deficits; sensory deficits □ Altered environment

Diagnosis
Total Incontinence

Definition

The state in which an individual experiences a continuous and unpredictable passage of urine

Defining Characteristics

Constant flow of urine occurs at unpredictable times without distention □ Incontinence refractory to therapy □ Lack of awareness of: perineal or bladder filling; incontinence □ Nocturia □ Uninhibited bladder contractions/spasms □ Unsuccessful incontinence refractor treatments

Related Factors

Effects of: fistulas secondary to trauma; independent contraction of detrusor reflex due to surgery; neurological dysfunction causing triggering of micturition at unpredictable times; neuromuscular trauma related to surgical procedures; neuropathy preventing transmission of reflex indicating bladder fullness; trauma or disease affecting spinal cord/nerves

Diagnosis
Urinary Retention

Definition

The state in which an individual experiences incomplete emptying of the bladder

Defining Characteristics

Bladder distention □ Diminished force of urinary stream □ Dribbling □ Dysuria □ Hesitancy □ High residual urine (> 150 ml, or 20% of voided urine) □ Nocturia □ Overflow incontinence □ Sensation of bladder fullness □ Small, frequent voiding or absence of urine output

Related Factors

Effects of: anxiety (fear of postoperative pain) diminished or absent sensory and/or motor impulses inhibition of reflex arc medications: anesthetics, opiates, psychotropics; high urethral pressure caused by weak detrusor; strong sphincter; urethral blockage associated with: fecal impaction, postpartum edema, prostate hypertrophy, surgical swelling

Diagnosis
Altered (Specify Type) Tissue Perfusion: Renal, Cardiopulmonary, Cerebral, Gastrointestinal, Peripheral

Definition

The state in which an individual experiences a decrease in nutrition and oxygenation at the cellular level due to a deficit in capillary blood supply

Defining Characteristics

Renal: diminished urine output; edema □ Cardiopulmonary: chest pain (relieved by rest); increased heart rate; increased respiratory rate; shortness of breath □ Cerebral: alteration in thought processes; blurred vision; changes in level of consciousness; confusion; restlessness; syncope/vertigo □ Gastrointestinal: constipation; nausea and vomiting; pain □ Peripheral: altered sensory or motor function; burning; changes in hair pattern; claudication; coolness of skin; diminished pulse quality; edema; erythema; extremity pain; flushing; inflammation; pallor; positive Homans' sign; shining skin; slow growth, brittle nails; tissue necrosis (gangrene); trophic skin changes; ulcerated skin/poorly healing areas

Related Factors

Exchange problems □ Hypervolemia □ Hypovolemia □ Interruption of flow: arterial; venous

Diagnosis
Fluid Volume Excess

Definition

The state in which an individual experiences increased fluid retention and edema

Defining Characteristics

Abnormal breath sounds; rales (crackles) □ Anasarca □ Azotemia □ Changes in: blood pressure; central venous pressure; electrolytes; hemoglobin and hematocrit; mental status; pulmonary artery pressure; respiratory pattern; specific gravity □ Edema □ Effusion □ Intake greater than output □ Jugular vein distention □ Muscular twitching/weakness □ Nausea and/or vomiting □ Oliguria □ Positive hepatojugular reflex □ Pulmonary congestion on chest x-ray □ Shortness of breath, orthopnea □ S3 heart sound □ Weight gain □ Restlessness and anxiety

Related Factors

Compromised regulatory mechanisms: aldosterone; antidiuretic hormone; reninangiotensin □ Effects of: age extremes; medications; pregnancy □ Excessive fluid or sodium intake □ Low protein intake

Diagnosis
Fluid Volume Deficit

Definition

The state in which an individual experiences vascular, cellular, or intracellular dehydration

Defining Characteristics

Changes in: urine output; urine concentration; serum sodium □ Sudden weight loss or gain □ Decreased venous filling □ Hemoconcentration □ Hypotension □ Thirst □ Increased: pulse rate; body temperature □ Decreased: skin turgor; pulse volume/pressure □ Change in mental state □ Dry skin □ Dry mucous membranes □ Weakness

Related Factors

Active fluid volume loss □ Failure of regulatory mechanisms

High-Risk Diagnosis
High Risk for Fluid Volume Deficit

Definition

The state in which an individual is at risk of experiencing vascular, cellular, or intracellular dehydration

Risk Factors

Extremes of age □ Extremes of weight □ Excessive losses through normal routes, e.g., diarrhea □ Losses through abnormal routes, e.g., indwelling tubes □ Deviations affecting access to or intake or absorption of fluids, e.g., physical immobility □ Factors influencing fluid needs, e.g., hypermetabolic state □ Knowledge deficit related to fluid volume □ Effects of medications, e.g., diuretics

Diagnosis
Decreased Cardiac Output

Definition

A state in which the blood pumped by an individual's heart is sufficiently reduced that it is inadequate to meet the needs of the body's tissues

Defining Characteristics

Abnormal heart sounds □ Altered blood gases □ Anorexia □ Changes in: blood pressure; color of skin or mucous membranes; mental status □ Cold, clammy skin □ Cough □ Decreased peripheral pulses □ Dyspnea □ Dysrhythmias, electrocardiographic changes □ Edema of trunk, sacrum, or extremities □ Fatigue □ Frothy sputum □ Gallop rhythm □ Jugular vein distention □ Oliguria □ Orthopnea □ Rales □ Restlessness □ Shortness of breath □ Sudden weight gain □ Syncope □ Tachycardia □ Variations in hemodynamic readings □ Vertigo □ Weakness

Related Factors

Reduction in stroke volume as a result of: electrical malfunction; alteration in conduction; alteration in rate; alteration in rhythm; mechanical malfunction □ Alteration in afterload □ Alteration in inotropic changes in heart □ Alteration in preload: structural problems secondary to congenital abnormalities, trauma

Diagnosis
Impaired Gas Exchange

Definition

The state in which an individual experiences a decreased passage of oxygen and/or carbon dioxide between the alveoli and the vascular system

Defining Characteristics

Clubbing of fingers □ Confusion □ Cyanosis □ Fatigue and lethargy □ Hypercapnea □ Hypoxia □ Inability to move secretions □ Irritability □ Restlessness □ Somnolence □ Tachycardia □ Use of accessory muscles

Related Factors

Ventilation-perfusion imbalance □ Altered: blood flow; oxygen-carrying capacity of blood; oxygen supply □ Alveolar-capillary membrane changes □ Aspiration of foreign matter □ Decreased surfactant production □ Effects of: anesthesia; medications (narcotics, sedatives, tranquilizers) □ Hypo-/hyperventilation □ Inhalation of toxic fumes or substances

Diagnosis
Ineffective Airway Clearance

Definition

The state in which an individual is unable to clear secretions or obstructions from the respiratory tract to maintain airway patency

Defining Characteristics

Absent or adventitious breath sounds □ Air hunger □ Change in respiratory rate or depth □ Cough, effective or ineffective, with or without sputum □ Cyanosis □ Diaphoresis □ Dyspnea □ Fever □ Restlessness □ Stridor □ Substernal, intercostal retraction □ Tachycardia □ Tachypnea □ Anxiety

Related Factors

Decreased energy, fatigue □ Effects of: anesthesia; infection; medication (narcotics, sedatives, tranquilizers); perceptual/cognitive impairment; presence of artificial airway; trauma □ Inability to cough effectively □ Tracheobronchial secretions or obstruction □ Aspiration of foreign matter □ Environmental pollutants □ Inhalation of toxic fumes or substances

Diagnosis
Ineffective Breathing Pattern

Definition

The state in which an individual's inhalation and/or exhalation pattern does not enable adequate pulmonary inflation or emptying

Defining Characteristics

Abnormal blood gases □ Altered chest excursion □ Assumption of three-point position □ Cough □ Cyanosis □ Dyspnea □ Fremitus □ Increased anteroposterior diameter □ Nasal flaring □ Pursed-lip breathing and prolonged expiratory phase □ Respiratory rate, depth changes □ Shortness of breath □ Tachypnea □ Use of accessory muscles

Related Factors

Decreased: energy; lung expansion □ Effects of: anesthesia; cognitive/perceptual impairment; medication (narcotics, sedatives, tranquilizers); neuromuscular/musculoskeletal impairment; obesity □ Fatigue □ Immobility, inactivity □ Inflammatory process □ Pain, discomfort □ Tracheobronchial obstruction □ Anxiety

Diagnosis
Inability to Sustain Spontaneous Ventilation

Definition

A state in which the response pattern of decreased energy reserves results in an individual's ability to maintain breathing adequate to support life

Defining Characteristics

Major: dyspnea; increased metabolic rate □ Minor: increased restlessness; apprehension; increased use of accessory muscles; decreased tidal volume; increased heart rate; decreased pO_2; increased pCO_2; decreased cooperation; decreased SaO_2

Related Factors

Metabolic factors □ Respiratory muscle fatigue

Diagnosis
Dysfunctional Ventilatory Weaning Response (DVWR)

Definition

A state in which a patient cannot adjust to lowered levels of mechanical ventilator support, which interrupts and prolongs the weaning process

Defining Characteristics

Mild DVWR ☐ Major: responds to lowered levels of mechanical ventilator support with: restlessness; slightly increased respiratory response ☐ Minor: responds to lowered levels of mechanical ventilator support with: expressed feelings of increased need for oxygen; breathing discomfort, fatigue, warmth; queries about possible machine malfunction; increased concentration on breathing ☐ Moderate DVWR ☐ Major: responds to lowered levels of mechanical ventilator support with: slight increase from baseline blood pressure < 20 mmHg; slight increase from baseline heart rate < 20 beats/min; baseline increase in respiratory rate < 5 breaths/min ☐ Minor: hypervigilence to activities; inability to respond to coaching; inability to cooperate; apprehension; diaphoresis; eye widening, "wide-eyed look"; decreased air entry on auscultation; color changes; pale, slight cyanosis; slight respiratory accessory muscle use ☐ Severe DVWR ☐ Major: responds to lowered levels of mechanical ventilator support with: agitation; deterioration in arterial blood gases from current baseline; increase from baseline blood pressure > 20 mmHg; increase from baseline heart rate > 20 beats/min; respiratory rate increases significantly from baseline ☐ Minor: profuse diaphoresis; full respiratory accessory muscle use; shallow, gasping breaths; paradoxical abdominal breathing; discoordinated breathing with the ventilator; decreased level of consciousness; adventitious breath sounds, audible airway secretions; cyanosis

Related Factors

Physical: ineffective airway clearance; sleep pattern disturbance; inadequate nutrition; uncontrolled pain or discomfort ☐ Psychosocial: knowledge deficit of the weaning process, patient role; patient-perceived inefficiency about the ability to wean; decreased motivation; decreased self-esteem; anxiety: moderate, severe; fear; hopelessness; powerlessness; insufficient trust in the nurse ☐ Situational: uncontrolled episodic energy demands or problems; inappropriate pacing of diminished ventilator support; inadequate social support; adverse environment (noisy, active environment, negative events in the room, low nurse-to-patient ratio, extended nurse absence from the bedside); history of ventilator dependence > 1 week; history of multiple unsuccessful weaning attempts

High-Risk Diagnosis
High Risk for Injury

Definition

The state in which an individual is at risk of injury as a result of environmental conditions interacting with the individual's adaptive and defensive resources

Risk Factors

Internal: biochemical; regulatory dysfunction (sensory, integrative, effector dysfunction; tissue hypoxia); malnutrition; immune/autoimmune; abnormal blood profile (leukocytosis/leukopenia, altered clotting factors, thrombocytopenia, sickle cell, thalassemia, decreased hemoglobin); physical (broken skin, altered mobility); developmental age (physiological, psychosocial); psychological (affective, orientation) ☐ External: biological (immunization level of community, microorganism); chemical (pollutants, poisons, drugs, pharmaceutical agents, alcohol, caffeine, nicotine, preservatives, cosmetics and dyes); nutrients (vitamins, food types); physical (design, structure and arrangement of community, building, and/or equipment); mode of transport/transportation; people/provider (nosocomial agents, staffing patterns; cognitive, affective, and psychomotor factors)

High-Risk Diagnosis
High Risk for Suffocation

Definition

The state in which an individual has accentuated risk of accidental suffocation (inadequate air available for inhalation)

Risk Factors

Internal (Individual): disease or injury process; lack of: safety education, safety precautions; reduced: motor abilities, olfactory sensation; cognitive or emotional difficulties □ External (Environmental): children: inserting small objects into mouth or nose, left unattended in tubs or pools, playing with plastic bags, balloons; discarded or unused refrigerators, freezers with doors not removed; household gas leaks; immobile client incorrectly positioned on abdomen; low-strung clothesline; pacifier hung around infant's neck; person who eats large mouthfuls of food; pillows placed: in an infant's crib, incorrectly under the head of client with a compromised airway; propped bottle placed in an infant's crib; smoking in bed; use of fuel-burning heaters not vented to outside; vehicle engine running in closed garage; ventilator connectors improperly monitored

High-Risk Diagnosis
High Risk for Poisoning

Definition

The state in which an individual has accentuated risk for accidental exposure to or ingestion of drugs or dangerous products in doses sufficient to cause poisoning

Risk Factors

Internal (Individual): reduced vision; cognitive or emotional difficulties; inadequate drug education; combination of drugs/alcohol, consumption of outdated drugs, use of drugs prescribed for others; insufficient finances; lack of safety, proper precautions; □ External (Environmental): availability of illicit drugs contaminated by poisonous additives; chemical contamination of food, water; dangerous products, medicines placed or stored within the reach of children or confused persons; flaking, peeling paint or plaster in presence of young children; large supplies of drugs in home; paint, lacquer in poorly ventilated areas or without effective protection; poisons stored in food containers; presence of: atmospheric pollutants, poisonous vegetation; unprotected contact with heavy metals or chemicals; unsafe work environment

High-Risk Diagnosis
High Risk for Trauma

Definition

The state in which an individual has accentuated risk of accidental tissue injury associated with internal or external factors

Risk Factors

Internal (Individual): balancing difficulties; confusion; fatigue; hypotension: orthostatic, postural; pain; poor vision; reduced; hand-eye coordination, large, small muscle coordination, mobility of arms, legs, temperature, tactile sensation; side effects of medications; visual, hearing impairment; weakness; history of: previous trauma, substance abuse; insufficient finances to purchase safety equipment or make repairs; lack of: safety education, safety precautions; language barrier □ External (Environmental): bathing: in very hot water, without hand grips, without anti-slip equipment; children: carried on adult bicycles, playing near vehicle pathways, playing with candles, cigarettes, matches, sharp-edged toys, playing without safety gates near stairs, unsupervised, riding bicycles without headgear, riding in front seat of car or without seat restraints; contact with: acids or alkalis, dangerous machinery, intense cold, rapidly moving machinery, industrial belts, or pulleys; driving: after partaking of alcohol, drugs, at excessive speeds, cycles without headgear, mechanically unsafe vehicle, without necessary visual aids, without seat restraints; electrical hazards: faulty electrical plugs, frayed wires, or defective appliances, overloaded electrical outlets, fuse boxes, unanchored electrical wires; fire hazards: experimenting with chemicals, gasoline, gas leaks, delayed lighting of burner or oven, grease waste collected on stoves, highly flammable toys, clothing, incorrectly stored combustibles or corrosives, playing with fireworks, gunpowder, pot handles facing front of stove, smoking in bed or near oxygen, unscreened fires or heaters, use of thin, worn potholders or mitts, wearing plastic flammable clothing; safety hazards: entering unlighted rooms, guns or ammunition stored unlocked, high beds, high-crime neighborhood and vulnerable client, knives stored uncovered, large icicles hanging from roof, litter or liquids on floor, stairway, obstructed passageways, slippery floors, snow or ice on stairs, walkways, unanchored rugs, unsafe road or crossing, unsafe window protection, unsturdy or absent stair rails, unsteady ladders, chairs, use of cracked dishware, glasses; miscellaneous: inappropriate call-for-aid mechanism for client on bedrest, sliding on coarse bed linen, struggling within bed restraints, overexposure to sun, sunlamps, radiotherapy

High-Risk Diagnosis
High Risk for Aspiration

Definition
The state in which an individual is at risk for entry of gastrointestinal secretions, oropharyngeal secretions, solids, or fluids into tracheobronchial passages

Risk Factors
Reduced level of consciousness □ Depressed cough and gag reflexes □ Presence of tracheostomy or endotracheal tube □ Incomplete lower esophageal sphincter □ Gastrointestinal tubes □ Tube feedings □ Medication administration □ Situations hindering elevation of upper body □ Increased intragastric pressure □ Increased gastric residual □ Decreased gastrointestinal motility □ Delayed gastric emptying □ Impaired swallowing □ Facial, oral, or neck surgery or trauma □ Wired jaw

High-Risk Diagnosis
High Risk for Disuse Syndrome

Definition
The state in which an individual is at risk for deterioration of body systems as the result of prescribed or unavoidable musculoskeletal inactivity

Risk Factors
Paralysis □ Mechanical immobilization □ Prescribed immobilization □ Severe pain □ Altered level of consciousness

Diagnosis
Altered Protection

Definition
The state in which an individual experiences a decrease in the ability to guard the self from internal or external threats such as illness or injury

Defining Characteristics
Major: deficient immunity; impaired healing; altered clotting; maladaptive stress response; neurosensory alterations □ Minor: chilling; perspiring; dyspnea; cough; itching; restlessness; insomnia; fatigue; anorexia; weakness; immobility; disorientation; pressure sores

Related Factors

Effects of extremes of age ☐ Inadequate nutrition ☐ Alcohol abuse ☐ Abnormal blood profiles (leukopenia, thrombocytopenia, anemia, coagulation) ☐ Drug therapies (antineoplastic, corticosteroid, immune, anti-coagulant, thrombolytic) ☐ Treatments (surgery, radiation) ☐ Diseases (cancer, immune disorders)

Diagnosis
Impaired Tissue Integrity

Definition

The state in which an individual experiences damage to mucous membrane or corneal, integumentary, or subcutaneous tissue

Defining Characteristics

Damaged or destroyed tissue: cornea; mucous membrane; integumentary; subcutaneous

Related Factors

Altered circulation ☐ Effects of therapeutic radiation ☐ Fluid deficit/excess ☐ Impaired mobility ☐ Irritants: chemical: body excretions, body secretions, medications; mechanical: friction, pressure, shear; thermal: temperature extremes; ☐ Nutritional deficit/excess ☐ Knowledge deficit

Diagnosis
Altered Oral Mucous Membrane

Definition

The state in which an individual experiences disruption in the tissue layers of the oral cavity

Defining Characteristics

Atrophy of gums ☐ Coated tongue ☐ Dry mouth (xerostomia) ☐ Edema of mucosa ☐ Halitosis ☐ Hemorrhagic gingivitis ☐ Hyperemia ☐ Lack of or decreased salivation ☐ Oral: carious teeth; desquamation; lesions; pain or discomfort; plaque; redness; ulcers; vesicles ☐ Stomatitis

Related Factors

Dehydration ☐ Effects of: chemotherapy; medication; radiation to head/neck; surgery ☐ Immunosuppression ☐ Inadequate oral hygiene ☐ Infection ☐ Lack of or decreased salivation ☐ Mouth breathing ☐ Malnutrition/vitamin deficiency ☐ NPO for more than 24 hours ☐ Trauma: chemical associated with: acidic foods, alcohol, drugs, noxious agents, tobacco; mechanical associated with: braces, broken teeth, endotracheal tube, ill-fitting dentures, nasogastric tube placement ☐ Vomiting

Diagnosis
Impaired Skin Integrity

Definition

The state in which an individual experiences an alteration or disruption of the skin

Defining Characteristics

Disruption of: skin surface ☐ Invasion of body structures

Related Factors

External: chemical substance; humidity; hyperthermia; hypothermia; mechanical factors: shearing forces, pressure, restraints; physical immobilization; radiation ☐ Internal (somatic): altered: circulation, metabolic state, nutritional state, emaciation, obesity, pigmentation, sensation, turgor (change in elasticity); developmental factors; effects of medication; immunological deficit; skeletal prominence

High-Risk Diagnosis
High Risk for Impaired Skin Integrity

Definition

The state in which an individual is at risk of experiencing an alteration or disruption of the skin

Risk Factors

External: chemical substance; excretions or secretions; humidity; hyperthermia; hypothermia; mechanical factors: shearing forces, pressure, restraints; physical immobilization, radiation □ Internal (somatic): altered: circulation, metabolic state, nutritional state, emaciation, obesity, pigmentation, sensation, turgor (change in elasticity); developmental factors; effects of medication; immunological deficit; psychogenic; skeletal prominence

COMMUNICATING

A Human Response Pattern Involving Sending Messages

Diagnosis
Impaired Verbal Communication

Definition

The state in which an individual experiences a decreased or absent ability to use or understand language in human interaction

Defining Characteristics

Difficulty with phonation □ Disorientation □ Dyspnea □ Flight of ideas □ Impaired articulation □ Inability to: find words; identify objects; modulate speech; name words □ Lack of desire to speak, speak dominant language, speak in sentences □ Incessant verbalization □ Loose association of ideas □ Stuttering/slurring

Related Factors

Altered thought processes □ Auditory impairment □ Decreased circulation to the brain □ Effects of: surgery; trauma □ Inflammation □ Mental retardation □ Oral deformities □ Physical barrier: intubation; Tracheostomy □ Respiratory embarrassment □ Speech pattern dysfunction □ Inability to read or write □ Ineffective listening skills □ Language barrier □ Psychological barriers: anxiety; fear

RELATING

A Human Response Pattern Involving Established Bonds

Diagnosis
Impaired Social Interaction

Definition

The state in which an individual participates in an insufficient or excessive quantity or ineffective quality of social exchange

Defining Characteristics

Major: verbalized or observed discomfort: in social situations; in receiving or communicating a satisfying sense of belonging, caring, interest, or shared history; observed use of unsuccessful socialization behaviors; dysfunctional interaction with peers, family, and/or others □ Minor: family report of change of style or pattern of interaction

Related Factors

Knowledge/skills deficit about ways to enhance mutuality □ Communication barriers □ Self-concept disturbances □ Absence of available significant others or peers □ Limited physical mobility □ Therapeutic isolation □ Sociocultural dissonance □ Environmental barriers

Diagnosis
Social Isolation

Definition

The state in which an individual experiences aloneness that is perceived as imposed by others and as negative or threatening

Defining Characteristics

Objective: absence of supportive significant other(s) (family, friends, group); sad, dull affect; inappropriate or immature interests/activities for developmental age/stage; uncommunicative, withdrawn, no eye contact; preoccupation with own thoughts; repetitive, meaningless actions; projects hostility in voice, behavior;

seeks to be alone or exists in a subculture; evidence of physical/mental handicap or altered state of wellness; shows behavior unaccepted by dominant cultural group ☐ Subjective: expresses feelings of: aloneness imposed by others, rejection; experiences feelings of difference from others; inadequacy in or absence of significant purpose in life; inability to meet expectations of others; insecurity in public; expresses: values acceptable to the subculture but unacceptable to the dominant cultural group, interests inappropriate to the developmental age/state

Related Factors

Factors contributing to the absence of satisfying personal relationships such as: delay in accomplishing developmental tasks; immature interests; alterations in: mental status, physical appearance, state of wellness; unacceptable: social behavior, values; inability to engage in satisfying personal relationships; inadequate personal resources; inadequate support systems: living alone, recent retirement, recent/frequent change of residence, loss of a significant other; stress

Diagnosis
Altered Role Performance

Definition

The state in which an individual experiences a change, conflict, or denial of role responsibilities or inability to perform role responsibilities

Defining Characteristics

Changes in: self-perception of role; others' perception of role; physical capacity to resume role; usual patterns of responsibility ☐ Conflicts in roles ☐ Disparity between self and others in defining roles ☐ Denial of role ☐ Lack of knowledge of role ☐ Observed difficulty performing role function ☐ States inability to perform role expectations

Related Factors

Change in: employment; family structure; financial status; health status ☐ Combination of role loss and acquisition ☐ Cultural transition ☐ Developmental crisis ☐ Ineffective coping mechanisms ☐ Loss of support group ☐ Role acquisition ☐ Role loss

Diagnosis
Altered Parenting

Definition

The state in which a nurturing figure(s) experiences inability to create an environment which promotes optimal growth and development of another human being

Defining Characteristics

Abandonment ☐ Runaway ☐ Verbalizes: inability to control child; disappointment in gender or physical characteristics of an infant/child (constant); resentment toward infant/child; role inadequacy; frustration; disgust at body functions of infant/child; desire to have child call him/her by first name versus traditional cultural tendencies ☐ Lack of parental attachment behaviors ☐ Inappropriate visual, tactile, auditory stimulation ☐ Negative: identification of infant's/child's characteristics; attachment of meanings to infant's/child's characteristics ☐ Inattention to infant's/child's needs ☐ Inappropriate caretaking behaviors: toilet training; sleep and rest; feeding ☐ Noncompliance with health appointments for infant/child ☐ Inappropriate or inconsistent discipline practices ☐ Frequent: accidents; illnesses ☐ Growth and development lag in child ☐ History of child abuse or abandonment by primary care-taker ☐ Child receives care from multiple care-takers without consideration of the needs of the infant/child ☐ Compulsively seeks role approval from others

Related Factors

Ineffective role model □ Effects of: physical and psychosocial abuse of nurturing figure; unmet social/emotional maturational needs of parenting figures; interruption in bonding process, i.e., maternal, paternal, other; unrealistic expectations for self, infant, partner; intensive or special care requirements; multiple pregnancies; physical or mental handicaps; acute/chronic mental or physical illnesses; limited cognitive functioning □ Lack of: available role model; support between/from significant other(s); knowledge; role identity; or inappropriate response of child to relationship □ Perceived threat to own survival, physical and emotional □ Presence of stress (financial, legal, recent crisis, cultural move)

High-Risk Diagnosis
High Risk for Altered Parenting

Definition

The state in which a nurturing figure(s) is at risk to experience an inability to create an environment that promotes the optimal growth and development of another human being

Risk Factors

Ineffective role model □ Effects of: physical and psychosocial abuse of nurturing figure; unmet social/emotional maturational needs of parenting figures; interruption in bonding process, i.e., maternal, paternal, other; unrealistic expectations for self, infant, partner; intensive or special care requirements; multiple pregnancies; physical or mental handicaps; acute/chronic mental or physical illnesses; limited cognitive functioning; □ Lack of: available role model; support between/from significant other(s); knowledge; role identity; or inappropriate response of child to relationship □ Perceived threat to own survival, physical and emotional □ Presence of stress (financial, legal, recent crisis, cultural move)

Diagnosis
Sexual Dysfunction

Definition

The state in which an individual experiences a change in sexual function that is viewed as unsatisfying, unrewarding, or inadequate

Defining Characteristics

Verbalization of problem □ Alterations in: achieving perceived sex role; achieving sexual satisfaction; relationship with significant other □ Actual or perceived limitation imposed by disease and/or therapy □ Conflicts involving values □ Inability to achieve desired satisfaction □ Seeking confirmation of desirability □ Change of interest in self and others

Related Factors

Biopsychosocial alteration of sexuality: ineffective or absent role models, physical abuse, psychosocial abuse, e.g., harmful relationships, vulnerability, values conflict lack of: privacy, significant other, knowledge; effects of altered body structure/function: pregnancy, recent childbirth, drugs, surgery, anomalies, disease process, trauma, radiation; misinformation

Diagnosis
Altered Family Processes

Definition

The state in which a family that normally functions effectively experiences a dysfunction

Defining Characteristics

Family system unable or unwilling to: meet physical, spiritual, security, emotional needs of all its members; communicate openly and effectively; express or accept a wide range of feelings from other family members; relate to each other for mutual growth and maturation;

demonstrate flexibility in function and roles; demonstrate respect for individuality and autonomy of its members; accomplish current or past developmental tasks; make effective decisions; become involved in community activities; seek or accept help appropriately; adapt to change or deal with traumatic experience constructively ☐ Presence of inappropriate or poorly communicated: direction and level of energy; family rules, rituals, or symbols

Related Factors

Situational or developmental transitions and/or crises ☐ Reduced income ☐ Unemployment ☐ Relocation ☐ Large number of family members ☐ Multigenerational family ☐ Single-parent family ☐ Loss or gain of significant other ☐ Conflict or change in family role ☐ Absent or ineffective family role models ☐ Effects of chronic illness

Diagnosis
Care-giver Role Strain

Definition

A care-giver's felt difficulty in performing the family care-giver role

Defining Characteristics

Care-givers report that they: do not have enough resources to provide the care needed; find it hard to do specific caregiving activities; worry about such issues as the care-receiver's health and emotional state, having to put the care-receiver in an institution, and who will care for the individual if something should happen to the care-giver; feel that care-giving interferes with other important roles in their lives; feel loss because the care-receiver is like a different person, compared with before care-giving began, or in the case of a child, feel that he/she was never the child the care-giver expected; feel family conflict related to issues of providing care; feel stress or nervousness in their relationship with the care-receiver; feel depressed

Related Factors

Pathophysiological/Physiological: illness severity of the care-receiver; addiction or codependency; premature birth/congenital defect; discharge of family member with significant home care needs; care-giver health impairment; care-giver is female ☐ Developmental: care-giver is not developmentally ready for care-giver role, e.g., young adult needed to provide care for a middle-aged parent; developmental delay or retardation of the care-receiver or care-giver ☐ Psychosocial: psychological or cognitive problems in the care-receiver; marginal family adaptation or dysfunction prior to care-giving situation; marginal care-giver's coping patterns; past history of poor relationship between care-giver and care-receiver; care-giver is spouse; care-receiver exhibits deviant, bizarre behavior ☐ Situational: presence of abuse or violence; presence of situational stressors that normally affect families, such as significant loss; disaster or crisis; poverty or economic vulnerability; major life events, e.g., birth, hospitalization, leaving home, returning home, marriage, divorce, employment, retirement, death; duration of care-giving required; inadequate physical environment for providing care, e.g., housing, transportation, community services, equipment; family/care-giver isolation; lack of respite and recreation for care-giver; inexperience with care-giving; care-giver's competing role commitments; complexity/amount of care-giving tasks

High-Risk Diagnosis
High Risk for Care-giver Role Strain

Definition

A care-giver is vulnerable for felt difficulty in performing the family care-giver role

Risk Factors

Pathophysiological: illness severity of the care-receiver; addiction or codependency; premature birth/congenital defect; discharge of family member with significant home care needs; care-giver health impairment; unpredictable illness course or instability in the care-receiver's health; care-giver is female; psychological or cognitive problems in the care-receiver □ Developmental: care-giver is not developmentally ready for care-giver role, e.g., young adult needed to provide care for a middle-aged parent; developmental delay or retardation of the care-receiver or care-giver □ Psychosocial: marginal family adaptation or dysfunction prior to care-giving situation; marginal care-giver's coping patterns; past history of poor relationship between care-giver and care-receiver; care-giver is spouse; care-receiver exhibits deviant, bizarre behavior □ Situational: presence of abuse or violence; presence of situational stressors that normally affect families, such as significant loss; disaster or crisis; poverty or economic vulnerability; major life events, e.g., birth, hospitalization, leaving home, returning home, marriage, divorce, employment, retirement, death; duration of care-giving required; inadequate physical environment for providing care, e.g., housing, transportation, community services, equipment; family/care-giver isolation; lack of respite and recreation for care-giver; inexperience with care-giving; care-giver's competing role commitments; complexity/amount of care-giving tasks

Diagnosis
Parental Role Conflict

Definition
The state in which a parent experiences role confusion and conflict in response to a crisis

Defining Characteristics
Major: parent(s) expresses: concerns/feelings of inadequacy to provide for child's physical and emotional needs during hospitalization or in the home, concerns about changes in parental role, family functioning, family communication, family health; demonstrated disruption in care-taking routines □ Minor: expresses concern about perceived loss of control over decisions relating to child; reluctant to participate in usual care-taking activities, even with encouragement and support; verbalizes/demonstrates feelings of guilt, anger, fear, anxiety, and/or frustration about effect of child's illness on family process

Related Factors
Separation from child because of chronic illness □ Intimidation with invasive or restrictive modalities (isolation, intubation), specialized care centers, policies □ Home care of a child with special needs (apnea monitoring, postural drainage, hyperalimentation) □ Interruptions of family life because of home care regimen (treatments, care-givers, lack of respite) □ Change in marital status

Diagnosis
Altered Sexuality Patterns

Definition
The state in which individuals express concern regarding their sexuality

Defining Characteristics
Major: Reported difficulties, limitations, or changes in sexual behaviors or activities

Related Factors
Effects of illness or medical treatment: drugs; radiation; anomalies □ Extreme fatigue □ Obesity □ Pain □ Performance anxiety □ Knowledge/skill deficit about alternative responses to health-related transitions: pregnancy; surgery; recent childbirth; trauma; menopause □ Impaired relationship with a significant other □ Lack of significant other □ Fear of pregnancy or of acquiring a sexually transmitted disease □ Conflicts with sexual orientation or variant preferences □ Ineffective or absent role models □ Loss of job or ability to work □ Separation from or loss of significant other

VALUING

A Human Response Pattern Involving the
Assigning of Relative Worth

Diagnosis
Spiritual Distress

Definition

The state in which an individual experiences a
disruption in the life principle that pervades a
person's entire being and that integrates and
transcends one's biological and psychosocial
nature

Defining Characteristics

Self-destructive behavior or threats □ Alteration in behavior or mood evidenced by anger,
crying, preoccupation, anxiety, hostility
□ Sleep pattern disturbances □ Feeling separated or alienated from deity □ Feelings of
helplessness or hopelessness □ Depression
□ Expresses concerns about meaning of life and
death and/or belief systems □ Verbalizes inner
conflict about beliefs □ Questions moral and
ethical implications of therapeutic regimen
□ Inability to participate in usual religious practices □ Regards illness as punishment □ Requests spiritual assistance for a disturbance in
belief system □ Displacement of anger toward
clergy □ Does not experience that God is for-
giving □ Engages in self-blame

Related Factors

Loss of significant others □ Challenged belief
and value system, e.g., result of moral or ethical
implications associated with disease process,
therapy, or intense suffering □ Beliefs opposed
by family, peers, or health care providers
□ Disruption in usual religious activity □ Effects of personal and family disasters or major
life changes

CHOOSING

A Human Response Pattern Involving the
Selection of Alternatives

Diagnosis
Ineffective Individual Coping

Definition

The state in which an individual demonstrates
impaired adaptive behaviors and problem-
solving abilities in meeting life's demands and
roles

Defining Characteristics

Insomnia □ Physical inactivity □ Stress related disorders: ulcers; hypertension; irritable
bowel □ Substance abuse □ Inappropriate
use of defense mechanisms: withdrawal; depression; overeating; blaming;
scapegoating; manipulative behavior; self-pity
□ Change in usual communication patterns
□ Inability to meet or take responsibility for basic
needs □ Chronic anxiety □ Exaggerated fear
of pain, death □ General irritability □ Fear of
pain, death □ Inability to problem solve
□ High rate of accidents or illnesses □ Frequent
headaches/neckaches □ Emotional tension
□ Verbalizes inability to cope or inability to ask
for help □ Use of magical thinking □ Inability
to perform expected roles □ Indecisiveness
□ Violence toward others □ Self-destructive
behavior □ Unfamiliar environment

Related Factors

Effects of acute or chronic illness □ Loss of
control over body part or body function □ Lack
of support systems □ Separation from or loss of
significant other □ Low self-esteem □ Major
changes in lifestyle □ Unrealistic perceptions
□ Situational or maturational crises □ Inadequate leisure activities □ Knowledge deficit
regarding: therapeutic regimen; disease process;
prognosis □ Sensory overload

Diagnosis
Impaired Adjustment

Definition
The state in which the individual is unable to modify lifestyle/behavior in a manner consistent with a change in health status

Defining Characteristics
Verbalizes nonacceptance of health status change □ Extended period of shock, disbelief, or anger regarding health status change □ Lack of future-oriented thinking □ Nonexistent or unsuccessful ability to be involved in problem solving or goal setting □ Lack of movement toward independence

Related Factors
Effects of disability requiring change in lifestyle □ Sensory overload □ Impaired cognition □ Incomplete grieving □ Assault to self-esteem □ Altered locus of control □ Inadequate support systems

Diagnosis
Defensive Coping

Definition
The state in which an individual repeatedly projects falsely positive self-evaluation based on a self-protective pattern that defends against underlying perceived threats to positive self-regard

Defining Characteristics
Major: denial of obvious problems/weaknesses; projection of blame/responsibility; rationalization of failures; hypersensitivity to slight criticism; grandiosity □ Minor: superior attitude toward others; difficulty establishing/maintaining relationships; hostile laughter or ridicule of others; difficulty in reality-testing perceptions; lack of follow-through or participation in treatment or therapy

Diagnosis
Ineffective Denial

Definition
The state in which an individual consciously or unconsciously attempts to disavow the knowledge or meaning of an event to reduce anxiety/fear to the detriment of health

Defining Characteristics
Major: delays in seeking or refuses health care attention to the detriment of health; does not perceive personal relevance of symptoms or danger □ Minor: uses home remedies (self-treatment) to relieve symptoms; does not admit fear of death or invalidism; minimizes symptoms; displaces source of symptoms to other organs; unable to admit impact of disease on life pattern; makes dismissive gestures or comments when speaking of distressing events; displaces fear of impact of the condition; displays inappropriate affect

Diagnosis
Ineffective Family Coping: Disabling

Definition
The state in which the behavior of a significant person (family member or other primary person) disables their capacities to address effectively tasks essential to either person's adaptation to a health challenge

Defining Characteristics
Assumption of dependency role □ Excessive vigilance over family member □ Adopting symptoms/signs of ill family member □ Denial of existence or severity of illness of family member □ Exploitation or neglect of family members □ Child, spousal, or elder abuse □ Despair □ Unresolved anger or depression □ Rejection or desertion □ Intolerance □ Impaired decision making □ Substance abuse

Related Factors

Effects of major life events   □ Major changes in social/cultural environment   □ Effects of recent or impending death of family member   □ Marital discord   □ Chronically unexpressed feelings of guilt, despair, anxiety, or hostility   □ Highly ambivalent family relationships   □ Dissonant discrepancy of coping styles   □ Unmet psychosocial needs of child or parent   □ Lack of economic resources or support systems

Diagnosis
Ineffective Family Coping: Compromised

Definition

The state in which a usually supportive primary person (family member or close friend) is providing insufficient, ineffective, or compromised support, comfort, assistance, or encouragement that may be needed by the client to manage or master adaptive tasks related to a health challenge

Defining Characteristics

Ineffective responses to illness, disability, or situational crises withdrawal; overprotection; preoccupation with personal reactions, i.e., blaming or scapegoating; manipulative behaviors   □ Inability to demonstrate supportive behaviors   □ Expressed concern about significant other's response to health problem   □ Impaired intimacy or closeness   □ Attempted assistive behaviors with less than satisfactory results

Related Factors

Isolation of family members from one another □ Lack of support for family members   □ Temporary family disorganization and role changes □ Effects of acute or chronic illness   □ Incompatible or differing values, beliefs, or goals   □ Unrealistic expectations   □ Knowledge deficit □ Temporary preoccupation resulting in inability to perceive or act effectively in regard to health needs

Wellness Diagnosis
Family Coping: Potential

Definition

Effective managing of adaptive tasks by family member involved with the client's health challenge, who now is exhibiting desire and readiness for enhanced health and growth in regard to self and in relation to the client

Defining Characteristics

Family members attempt to describe growth impact of crises on their own values, priorities, goals, or relationships   □ Individual expresses interest in making contact on a one-to-one basis or on a mutual and group basis with another person who has experienced a similar situation □ Family member is moving in direction of health-promoting and enriching lifestyle that supports and monitors maturational processes, audits and negotiates treatment programs, and generally chooses experiences that optimize wellness

Related Factors

The family's basic needs are sufficiently gratified and adaptive tasks effectively addressed to enable goals of self-actualization to surface

Diagnosis
Ineffective Management of Therapeutic Regimen (Individual)

Definition

A pattern of regulating and integrating into daily living a program for treatment of illness and the sequelae of illness that is unsatisfactory for meeting specific health goals

Defining Characteristics

Major: choices of daily living ineffective for meeting the goals of a treatment or prevention program □ Minor: acceleration (expected or unexpected) of illness symptoms; verbalized desire to manage the treatment of illness and prevention of sequelae; verbalized difficulty with regulation/integration of one or more prescribed regimens for treatment of illness and its effects or prevention of complications; verbalized that did not take action to include treatment regimens in daily routines; verbalized that did not take action to reduce risk factors for progression of illness and sequelae

Related Factors

Complexity of health care system □ Complexity of therapeutic regimen □ Decisional conflicts □ Economic difficulties □ Excessive demands made on individual or family □ Family conflict □ Family patterns of health care □ Inadequate number and types of cues to action □ Knowledge deficits □ Mistrust of regimen and/or health care personnel □ Perceived seriousness □ Perceived susceptibility □ Perceived barriers □ Perceived benefits □ Powerlessness □ Social support deficits

Diagnosis
Noncompliance (Specify)

Definition

The state in which an individual makes an informed decision not to adhere to a therapeutic recommendation

Defining Characteristics

Observed or reported: evidence of development of complications; evidence of exacerbation of symptoms; failure to progress; clinical data (blood/urine levels); failure to resolve health problems; nonadherence to therapeutic regimen; nonadherence after education; failure to keep appointments; inability to set or attain mutual goals; failure to seek care when disease status warrants

Related Factors

Side effects of medications □ Impaired ability to perform tasks □ Concurrent illness of family member □ Increasing amount of disease-related symptoms despite adherence to advised regimen □ Denial □ Depression □ Forgetfulness □ Feeling of lack of control □ Knowledge deficit □ Lack of perceived benefits of treatment □ Cultural or spiritual values □ Complexity of therapeutic regimen □ Client and provider relationships □ Previous unsuccessful experience with advised regimen □ Lack of support system □ Lack of economic resources (money, transportation)

Diagnosis
Decisional Conflict (Specify)

Definition

The state in which an individual experiences uncertainty about the course of action to be taken when choice among competing actions involves risk, loss, or challenge to personal life values

Defining Characteristics

Major: verbalized uncertainty about choices; verbalized undesired consequences of alternative actions being considered; vacillation among alternative choices; delayed decision-making □ Minor: verbalized feelings of distress while attempting a decision; self-focusing; physical signs of distress or tension (increased heart rate, increased muscle tension, restlessness); questioning personal values and beliefs while attempting a decision

Related Factors

Unclear personal values/beliefs □ Perceived threat to value system □ Lack of experience or interference with decision-making □ Lack of relevant information □ Multiple or divergent sources of information □ Support system deficit

Wellness Diagnosis
Health-Seeking Behaviors (Specify)

Definition

The state in which an individual in stable health is actively seeking ways to alter personal health habits and/or the environment in order to move toward a higher level of health (stable health status is defined as follows: age-appropriate illness prevention measures are achieved, client reports good or excellent health, and signs and symptoms of disease, if present, are controlled)

Defining Characteristics

Major: expressed or observed desire to seek a higher level of wellness □ Minor: expressed or observed desire for increased control of health practice; expressed concern about current environmental conditions on health status; stated or observed unfamiliarity with wellness community resources; demonstrated or observed lack of knowledge in health promotion behaviors

MOVING

A Human Response Pattern Involving Activity

Diagnosis
Impaired Physical Mobility

Definition

The state in which an individual experiences limitation of ability needed for independent physical movement

Defining Characteristics

Reluctance to attempt movement □ Imposed restrictions on movement □ Limited range of motion □ Decreased muscle strength, control, and/or mass □ Inability to move purposefully within the physical environment, including bed mobility, transfer, and ambulation □ Impaired coordination □ Falling or stumbling

Related Factors

Neuromuscular impairment □ Sensory-perceptual impairment □ Fatigue, decreased strength and endurance □ Intolerance to activity □ Effects of: neuromuscular impairment; sensory-perceptual impairment; trauma or surgery □ Inflammation □ Pain □ Obesity □ Side effects of sedatives, narcotics, or tranquilizers □ Depression □ Severe anxiety □ Fear of movement □ Architectural barriers □ Lack of assistive devices

High-Risk Diagnosis
High Risk for Peripheral Neurovascular Dysfunction

Definition

A state in which an individual is at risk of experiencing a disruption in circulation, sensation, or motion of an extremity

Risk Factors

Fractures □ Mechanical compression, e.g., tourniquet, cast, brace, dressing, or restraint □ Orthopedic surgery □ Trauma □ Immobilization □ Burns □ Vascular obstruction

Diagnosis
Activity Intolerance

Definition

The state in which an individual has insufficient physiological or psychological energy to endure or complete required or desired daily activities

Defining Characteristics

Increased or decreased heart rate, blood pressure, respirations □ Electrocardiographic changes reflecting dysrhythmias or ischemia □ Exertional discomfort or dyspnea □ Redness, cyanosis, or pallor of skin during activity □ Dizziness during activity □ Impaired ability to change position or stand or walk without support □ Weakness □ Requiring frequent rest periods □ Worried or uneasy facial expression □ Verbal report of fatigue or weakness □ Confusion

Related Factors

Electrolyte imbalance □ Hypovolemia □ Malnourishment □ Interrupted sleep □ Impaired sensory or motor function □ Deconditioned status □ Imbalance between oxygen supply and demand □ Effects of: aging; impaired sensory or motor function; medications (sedatives, tranquilizers, narcotics) □ Generalized weakness □ Pain □ Fatigue □ Bedrest □ Immobility □ Depression □ Lack of motivation □ Sedentary lifestyle

Diagnosis
Fatigue

Definition

The state in which an individual experiences an overwhelming sense of exhaustion and decreased capacity for physical and mental work

Defining Characteristics

Major: verbalization of an unremitting and overwhelming lack of energy: inability to maintain usual routines □ Minor: perceived need for additional energy to accomplish routine tasks; increase in physical complaints; impaired ability to concentrate; decreased performance; lethargy or listlessness; disinterest in surroundings/introspection; decreased libido; accident-prone; emotionally labile or irritable

Related Factors

Decreased/increased metabolic energy production □ Increased energy requirements to perform activities of daily living □ Overwhelming psychological or emotional demands □ Excessive social and/or role demands □ States of discomfort □ Altered body chemistry: medications; drug withdrawal; chemotherapy

High-Risk Diagnosis
High Risk for Activity Intolerance

Definition

The state in which an individual is at risk of experiencing insufficient physiological or psychological energy to endure or complete required or desired daily activities

Risk Factors

History of previous intolerance □ Deconditioned status □ Presence of circulatory/respiratory problems □ Inexperience with the activity

Diagnosis
Sleep Pattern Disturbance

Definition

The state in which disruption of sleep time causes discomfort or interferes with desired lifestyle

Defining Characteristics

Verbal complaints of: difficulty falling asleep; awakening earlier or later than desired; interrupted sleep; not feeling well-rested □ Changes in behavior or performance; increasing: irritability; restlessness; disorientation; lethargy; listlessness □ Physical signs: mild fleeting nystagmus; slight hand tremor; ptosis of eyelid; expressionless face; headache; dark circles under eyes, reddened eyes; frequent yawning; changes in posture □ Thick speech with mispronunciation and incorrect words □ Napping during day □ Mood alterations □ Difficulty in concentration

Related Factors

Effects of: pregnancy; medications; sensory alterations: internal (illness, psychological stress), external (environmental changes, social cues) □ Pain □ Inactivity □ Diarrhea □ Urinary frequency □ Incontinence □ Nausea □ Lifestyle disruptions □ Demands of caring for others □ Stress □ Fear or anxiety □ Depression □ Nightmares □ Sensory overload □ Unfamiliar environment □ Circadian rhythm disturbances (shift work)

Diagnosis
Diversional Activity Deficit

Definition

The state in which an individual experiences a decreased stimulation from or interest or engagement in recreational or leisure activities

Defining Characteristics

Weight loss or gain □ Yawning □ Crying □ Restlessness □ Preoccupation with self □ Napping during day □ Apathy or hostility □ Complaints of boredom □ Verbalizations of desire for activity □ Depression □ Inability to participate in usual hobbies because of physical limitations or hospitalization

Related Factors

Effects of chronic illness □ Frequent, lengthy treatments □ Unwillingness to learn new skills or acquire new interests □ Social isolation □ Confined to bedrest □ Preoccupation with job □ Decreased economic resources

Diagnosis
Impaired Home Maintenance Management

Definition

The state in which an individual experiences the inability to maintain independently a safe, growth-producing immediate environment

Defining Characteristics

Subjective household members: express difficulty in maintaining home in a comfortable fashion; request assistance with home maintenance; describe outstanding debt or financial crisis □ Objective: disorderly surroundings: unwashed or unavailable: cooking equipment, clothes, linen; offensive odors; presence of rodents or vermin; inappropriate household temperature; accumulation of: dirt, food wastes, hygienic wastes; overtaxed family members (exhausted, anxious); lack of necessary equipment or aids; repeated: hygienic disorders, infestations, infections

Related Factors

Individual/family member disease or injury □ Impaired mental status □ Substance abuse □ Effects of chronic debilitating disease □ Depression □ Lack of: knowledge; motivation; role modeling □ Decreased financial resources □ Insufficient: family organization or planning; finances □ Inadequate support systems □ Unfamiliarity with neighborhood resources

Diagnosis
Altered Health Maintenance

Definition

The state in which an individual experiences inability to identify, manage, and/or seek out help to maintain health status

Defining Characteristics

Demonstrated lack of: knowledge regarding basic health practices; adaptive behaviors to internal or external environmental changes; □ Reported or observed: inability to take responsibility for meeting basic health practices in any or all functional pattern areas; lack of equipment, financial, and/or other resources; impairment of personal support systems; history of lack of health-seeking behavior; expressed interest in improving health behaviors; failure to schedule routine examinations or immunizations; failure to adjust lifestyle to demands of chronic or acute illness

Related Factors

Learning disability □ Knowledge deficit □ Stress □ Substance abuse □ Unachieved developmental tasks □ Dysfunctional grieving □ Ineffective individual or family coping □ Lack of or significant alteration in: communication skills (written, verbal, and/or gestural); ability to make deliberate and thoughtful judgments; motivation; support systems □ Effects of perceptual/cognitive impairment (complete/partial lack of gross and/or fine motor skills) □ Ineffective individual/family coping □ Dysfunctional grieving □ Unachieved developmental tasks □ Disabling spiritual distress □ Lack of material resources □ Feelings of helplessness □ Fear of the unknown □ Religious or cultural values □ Loss of independence □ Inaccessibility of adequate health care services

Diagnosis
Feeding Self-Care Deficit

Definition

The state in which an individual experiences impaired ability to perform or complete feeding activities for self

Defining Characteristics

Inability to bring food from a receptacle to the mouth   □ Inability to cut food   □ Spilled food   □ Untouched food   □ Weight loss

Related Factors

Effects of: aging; chronic illness; cognitive/perceptual/neurovascular impairment; loss of limbs; medications; trauma; surgery; visual impairment   □ Lack of: coordination; motivation; self-confidence   □ Muscular weakness   □ Fatigue   □ Pain, discomfort   □ Contractures   □ Stiffness   □ Presence of external devices—IV lines, casts, slings, traction, splints, restraints Immobility Psychotic states   □ Depression   □ Knowledge deficit   □ Confusion   □ Anxiety   □ Grieving   □ Dependency

Diagnosis
Impaired Swallowing

Definition

The state in which an individual has decreased ability to pass fluids and/or solids voluntarily from the mouth to the stomach

Defining Characteristics

Major: observed evidence of difficulty in swallowing: stasis of food in oral cavity, regurgitation of fluids and/or solids through mouth or nose, choking/coughing   □ Minor: evidence of aspiration; reported pain on swallowing; dehydration; weight loss

Related Factors

Effects of: neuromuscular impairment: decreased or absent gag reflex, decreased strength or excursion of muscles of mastication; perceptual impairment: facial paralysis; mechanical obstruction: edema, tracheostomy tube, tumor   □ Excessive/inadequate salivation   □ Fatigue   □ Reddened, irritated oropharyngeal cavity   □ Limited awareness

Diagnosis
Ineffective Breast-Feeding

Definition

The state in which a mother, infant, or child experiences dissatisfaction or difficulty with the breast-feeding process

Defining Characteristics

Major: unsatisfactory breastfeeding process   □ Minor: actual or perceived inadequate milk supply; infant inability to attach correctly onto maternal breast; no observable signs of oxytocin release; observable signs of inadequate infant intake; nonsustained suckling at the breast; insufficient emptying of each breast per feeding; persistence of sore nipples beyond first week of breast-feeding; insufficient opportunity for suckling at the breast; infant exhibiting fussiness and crying within first hour after breast-feeding, unresponsive to other comfort measures; infant arching and crying at the breast, resisting latching on

Related Factors

Infant anomaly   □ Prematurity   □ Maternal breast anomaly   □ Previous breast surgery   □ Previous history of breast-feeding failure   □ Infant receiving supplemental feedings with artificial nipple   □ Poor infant sucking reflex   □ Nonsupportive partner/family   □ Knowledge deficit   □ Interruption to breast-feeding   □ Maternal anxiety or ambivalence

Diagnosis
Interrupted Breast-Feeding

Definition

A break in the continuity of the breast-feeding process as a result of inability or inadvisability of putting baby to breast for feeding

Defining Characteristics

Major: infant does not receive nourishment at the breast for some or all of feedings   □ Minor: maternal desire to maintain lactation and provide (or eventually provide) her breast milk for her infant's nutritional needs; separation of mother and infant; lack of knowledge regarding expression and storage of breast milk

Related Factors

Maternal or infant illness   □ Prematurity   □ Maternal employment   □ Contraindications to breastfeeding (e.g., drugs, true breast milk jaundice)   □ Need to wean infant abruptly

Wellness Diagnosis
Effective Breast-Feeding

Definition

The state in which a mother-infant dyad/family exhibits adequate proficiency and satisfaction with the breast-feeding process

Defining Characteristics

Major: mother able to position infant at breast to promote a successful latch-on response; infant is content after feedings; regular and sustained suckling/swallowing at the breast; adequate infant weight gain   □ Minor: signs and/or symptoms of oxytocin release (let down or milk ejection reflex); soft stools; over six wet diapers per day of unconcentrated urine; eagerness of infant to nurse; maternal/family verbalization of satisfaction with the breast-feeding process

Related Factors

Basic breast-feeding knowledge   □ Normal breast structure   □ Normal infant oral structure   □ Infant gestational age greater than 34 weeks   □ Support sources   □ Maternal confidence

Diagnosis
Ineffective Infant Feeding Pattern

Definition

A state in which an infant demonstrates an impaired ability to suck or coordinate the suck-swallow response

Defining Characteristics

Major: inability to initiate or sustain an effective suck; inability to coordinate sucking, swallowing, and breathing   □ Minor: none

Related Factors

Prematurity   □ Neurological impairment/delay   □ Oral hypersensitivity   □ Prolonged NPO status   □ Anatomical abnormality   □ Maternal confidence

Diagnosis
Bathing/Hygiene Self-Care Deficit

Definition

The state in which an individual experiences impaired ability to perform or complete bathing/hygiene activities for self

Defining Characteristics

Dirt or stains on body   □ Requests help in bathing   □ Body odor   □ Halitosis   □ Inability to: obtain or get to water source; regulate water temperature or flow; wash body or body parts

Related Factors

Effects of: aging; chronic illness; cognitive/perceptual impairment; loss of limbs; medications; musculoskeletal/neuromuscular impairment; surgery; trauma; visual impairment   □ Lack of: coordination; motivation; self-confidence   □ Muscular weakness   □ Fatigue   □ Pain, discomfort   □ Contractures   □ Stiffness   □ Presence of external devices—IV lines, casts, slings, traction, splints, restraints   □ Immobility   □ Psychotic states   □ Depression   □ Knowledge deficit   □ Confusion   □ Anxiety   □ Dependency   □ Intolerance to activity   □ Decreased strength, endurance

Diagnosis
Dressing/Grooming Self-Care Deficit

Definition

The state in which an individual experiences impaired ability to perform or complete dressing and grooming activities for self

Defining Characteristics

Unshaven face ☐ Uncombed hair ☐ Unfastened clothes ☐ Untied shoes ☐ Overgrown fingernails and toenails ☐ Wearing pajamas during day or daytime clothes to sleep in ☐ Inability to: maintain appearance at satisfactory level; obtain, replace, or wash clothes; put on or take off necessary items of clothing; fasten clothing

Related Factors

Effects of: aging; chronic illness; cognitive/perceptual impairment; loss of limbs; medications; neuromuscular/musculoskeletal impairment; surgery; trauma; visual impairment ☐ Lack of: coordination; motivation; self-confidence ☐ Muscular weakness ☐ Fatigue ☐ Pain, discomfort ☐ Contractures ☐ Stiffness ☐ Presence of external devices—IV lines, casts, slings, traction, splints, restraints ☐ Immobility ☐ Psychotic states ☐ Depression ☐ Knowledge deficit ☐ Confusion ☐ Anxiety ☐ Grieving ☐ Dependency ☐ Intolerance to activity ☐ Decreased strength and endurance

Diagnosis
Toileting Self-Care Deficit

Definition

The state in which an individual experiences impaired ability to perform or complete toileting activities for self

Defining Characteristics

Unable to: get to commode or toilet; sit on or rise from toilet/commode; carry out proper toilet hygiene; manipulate clothing for toileting; flush toilet or empty commode

Related Factors

Effects of: aging; chronic illness; cognitive/perceptual impairment; loss of limbs; medications; neuromuscular/musculoskeletal impairment; surgery; trauma; visual impairment ☐ Lack of: coordination; motivation; self-confidence ☐ Muscular weakness ☐ Fatigue ☐ Pain, discomfort ☐ Contractures ☐ Stiffness ☐ Presence of external devices—IV lines, casts, slings, traction, splints, restraints ☐ Immobility ☐ Psychotic states ☐ Depression ☐ Knowledge deficit ☐ Confusion ☐ Anxiety ☐ Grieving ☐ Dependency ☐ Impaired transfer ability, mobility ☐ Intolerance to activity ☐ Decreased strength and endurance

Diagnosis
Altered Growth and Development

Definition

The state in which an individual deviates from the norms characteristic of age group

Defining Characteristics

Major: altered physical growth; delay or difficulty in performing skills that are typical of age group: motor, social, expressive; inability to perform self-care or self-control activities appropriate for age ☐ Minor: flat affect; decreased responses; listlessness; anxiety; feelings of loneliness, rejection, fear

Related Factors

Effects of physical disability ☐ Environmental and stimulation deficiencies ☐ Inadequate caretaking: indifference; inconsistent responsiveness; multiple caretakers ☐ Prescribed dependence ☐ Separation from significant others

Diagnosis
Relocation Stress Syndrome

Definition
Physiological and/or psychological disturbances as a result of transfer from one environment to another

Defining Characteristics
Major: change in environment/location; anxiety; apprehension; increased confusion (elderly population); depression; loneliness □ Minor: verbalization of unwillingness to relocate; sleep disturbance; change in eating habits; dependency; gastrointestinal disturbances; increased verbalization of needs; insecurity; lack of trust; restlessness; sad affect; unfavorable comparison of post-/pre-transfer staff; verbalization of being concerned/upset about transfer; vigilance; weight change; withdrawal

Related Factors
Past, concurrent, and recent losses □ Losses involved with decision to move □ Feeling of powerlessness □ Lack of adequate support system □ Little or no preparation for impending move □ Moderate to high degree of environmental change □ History and types of previous transfers □ Impaired psychosocial health status □ Decreased physical health status

PERCEIVING

A Human Response Pattern Involving the Reception of Information

Diagnosis
Body Image Disturbance

Definition
The state in which an individual experiences a negative or distorted perception of the body

Defining Characteristics
Either of the following must be present to justify the diagnosis of disturbance in body image: verbal response to actual or perceived change in structure and/or function; nonverbal response to actual or perceived change in structure and/or function □ Subjective: verbalization of: change in lifestyle, fear of rejection or of reaction by others, focus on past strength, function, or appearance, negative feelings about body, feelings of helplessness or powerlessness, preoccupation with change or loss; emphasis on remaining strengths, heightened achievement; extension of body boundary to incorporate environmental objects; refusal to verify actual change or loss; depersonalization of part or loss by use of impersonal pronouns; personalization of part or loss by name □ Objective: missing body part; actual change in structure and/or function; not looking at or touching body part; change in ability to estimate spatial relationship of body to environment; hiding or overexposing body part (intentional or unintentional); trauma to nonfunctioning part; change in social involvement

Related Factors
Effects of loss of body part(s) □ Effects of loss of body function □ Biophysical □ Cognitive/perceptual □ Cultural or spiritual □ Psychosocial

Diagnosis
Self-Esteem Disturbance

Definition
The state in which an individual has negative self-evaluation/feelings about self or self-capabilities, which may be directly or indirectly expressed

Defining Characteristics
Self-negating verbalization □ Expressions of shame/guilt □ Evaluates self as unable to deal with events □ Rationalizes away/rejects positive feedback and exaggerates negative feedback about self □ Hesitant to try new things/situations □ Denial of problems obvious to others □ Projection of blame/responsibility for problems □ Rationalizes personal failures □ Hypersensitive to a slight or criticism □ Grandiosity

Related Factors
To be developed

Diagnosis
Chronic Low Self-Esteem

Definition
The state in which an individual has long-standing negative self-evaluation/feelings about self or self-capabilities

Defining Characteristics
Major: long-standing or chronic: self-negating verbalization, expressions of shame/guilt, evaluates self as unable to deal with events, rationalizes away/rejects positive feedback and exaggerates negative feedback about self, hesitant to try new things/situations □ Minor: frequent lack of success in work or other life events; overly conforming or dependent on others' opinions; lack of eye contact; nonassertive/passive behavior; indecisive; excessively seeks reassurance

Related Factors
To be developed

Diagnosis
Situational Low Self-Esteem

Definition
The state in which an individual has negative self-evaluation/feelings about self that develop in response to a loss or change in an individual who previously had a positive self-evaluation

Defining Characteristics
Major: episodic occurrence of negative self-appraisal in response to life events in a person with a previously positive self-evaluation; verbalization of negative feelings about the self (helplessness, uselessness) □ Minor: self-negating verbalizations; expressions of shame/guilt; evaluates self as unable to handle situations/events; difficulty making decisions

Related Factors
To be developed

Diagnosis
Personal Identity Disturbance

Definition
The state in which an individual experiences an inability to distinguish between self and non-self

Defining Characteristics
To be developed

Related Factors
Developmental crises □ Role changes □ To be developed

Diagnosis
Sensory-Perceptual Alterations (Specify): Visual, Auditory, Kinesthetic, Gustatory, Tactile, Olfactory

Definition
A state in which an individual experiences a change in the amount or pattern of in-coming stimuli accompanied by a diminished, exaggerated, distorted, or impaired response to such stimuli

Defining Characteristics
Change in muscle tension □ Fatigue □ Visual and auditory distortions □ Motor incoordination □ Alteration in posture □ Exaggerated emotional responses □ Rapid mood swings □ Anxiety □ Change in behavior pattern □ Apathy □ Restlessness □ Irritability □ Fear □ Anger □ Depression □ Inappropriate responses □ Hallucinations □ Disor-

dered thought sequence □ Bizarre thinking □ Daydreaming □ Noncompliance □ Lack of concentration □ Altered conceptualization □ Altered communication patterns □ Indication of body image alteration □ Change in usual response to stimuli □ Reported or necessitated change in sensory acuity □ Change in problem-solving abilities □ Altered abstraction □ Disoriented as to time, place, or person

Related Factors

Sleep deprivation □ Pain □ Chemical alteration: endogenous (electrolyte imbalance, elevated blood-urea nitrogen, elevated ammonia, hypoxia); exogenous (central nervous system stimulants or depressants, mind-altering drugs); □ Altered status of sense organs □ Effects of neurological disease, trauma, or deficit □ Inability to communicate, understand, speak, or respond □ Psychological stress or narrowed perceptual fields caused by anxiety □ Altered sensory reception, transmission, and/or integration □ Socially restricted environment (institutionalization, homebound, aging, chronic illness, dying, infant deprivation, bereaved, stigmatized, mentally ill, mentally retarded, or mentally handicapped) □ Environmental factors: therapeutically restricted environment (isolation, intensive care, bedrest, traction, incubator)

Visual

Defining Characteristics

Headache □ Blurring □ Spots □ Double vision □ Excessive tearing □ Inflammation □ Lack of blink or corneal reflex □ Squinting □ Holding objects too close or at a distance for viewing □ Bumping into objects □ Abnormal results of vision testing

Related Factors

Restriction of head/neck motion □ Effects of: aging; stress; neurological impairment □ Failure to use protective eye devices □ Improper use of contact lens □ Difficulty in adjustment to corrective lens □ Persistent visual stimulation

Auditory

Defining Characteristics

Tinnitus □ Abnormal hearing test □ Lack of startle reflex: failure to respond to verbal stimuli □ Cupping of ears □ Inattentiveness □ Withdrawal □ Daydreaming □ Auditory hallucinations □ Inappropriate responses □ Delayed speech or language development

Related Factors

Effects of aging □ Neurological impairment □ Effects of certain antibiotics □ Excessive ear wax, fluid, or foreign body in ear □ Social isolation □ Stress □ Failure to use protective ear devices □ Continuous exposure to excessive noise □ Psychoses

Kinesthetic

Defining Characteristics

Falling □ Vertigo □ Stumbling □ Nausea □ Motion sickness □ Motor incoordination □ Alteration in posture □ Inability to sit or stand

Related Factors

Effects of inner ear inflammation □ Neurological impairment □ Side effects of tranquilizers, sedatives, muscle relaxants, or antihistamines □ Sleep deprivation

Gustatory

Defining Characteristics

Decreased sensitivity to tastes □ Decreased appetite □ Increased use of seasoning

Related Factors

Inflammation of nasal mucosa □ Side effects of certain medications □ Aging □ Effects of trauma to tongue □ Neurological impairment

Tactile

Defining Characteristics
Paresthesias ☐ Hyperesthesias ☐ Anesthesias

Related Factors
Circulatory impairment ☐ Inflammation ☐ Effects of anesthesia ☐ Nutritional deficiencies ☐ Effects of aging ☐ Effects of burns ☐ Neurological impairment ☐ Pain ☐ Persistent tactile stimulation

Olfactory

Defining Characteristics
Decreased sensitivity to smells ☐ Decreased appetite

Related Factors
Inflammation of nasal mucosa ☐ Foreign body in nasal passage ☐ Effects of aging ☐ Neurological impairment

Diagnosis
Unilateral Neglect

Definition
The state in which an individual is perceptually unaware of and inattentive to one side of the body

Defining Characteristics
Major: consistent inattention to stimuli on affected side ☐ Minor: does not look toward affected side; leaves food on plate on the affected side; inadequate self-care, positioning, and/or safety precautions in regard to affected side

Related Factors
Effects of disturbed perceptual abilities, e.g., hemianopsia; one-sided blindness ☐ Effects of neurological illness or trauma

Diagnosis
Hopelessness

Definition
The subjective state in which an individual sees limited or no alternatives or personal choices available and is unable to mobilize energy on own behalf

Defining Characteristics
Major: passivity; decreased verbalization; verbal cues (despondent content, "I can't," sighing) ☐ Minor: increased or decreased sleep; decreased appetite; closing eyes; turning away from speaker; lack of involvement in care or passively allowing care; shrugging in response to speaker; decreased response to stimuli; lack of initiative; flat affect

Related Factors
Chronic pain ☐ Effects of: deteriorating physiological condition; long-term stress; abandonment; role disruption; loss of significant other ☐ Grieving ☐ Depression ☐ Prolonged activity restriction creating isolation ☐ Lost belief in religious values

Diagnosis
Powerlessness

Definition
The state in which an individual experiences the perception that one's own actions will not significantly affect an outcome or a perceived lack of control over a current situation or immediate happening

Defining Characteristics

Severe: Verbal expressions of: having no control or influence over situation, having no control or influence over outcome, having no control over self-care, depression over physical deterioration that occurs despite patient's compliance with regimen; apathy; expressions of uncertainty about fluctuating energy levels; passivity □ Moderate: nonparticipation in care or decision making when opportunities are provided; expressions of dissatisfaction and frustration over inability to perform tasks and/or activities; no attempt to monitor progress; expressions of doubt about self-worth or role performance; reluctance to express true feelings; fearing alienation from caregivers; passivity; inability to seek information regarding care; dependence on others that may result in: irritability, resentment, anger, guilt; does not defend self-care practices when challenged

Related Factors

Immobility □ Difficulty in performing self-care □ Illness-related regimen □ Social isolation □ Low self-esteem □ Cultural role □ Communication barriers □ □ Loss of financial independence □ Lifestyle of helplessness □ Interpersonal interactions □ Lack of knowledge or skills □ Health care environment

KNOWING

A Human Response Pattern Involving Meaning Associated with Information

Diagnosis
Knowledge Deficit (Specify)

Definition

The state in which an individual lacks specific knowledge or skills that affect ability to maintain health

Defining Characteristics

Verbalizes the problem □ Inaccurate: follow-through of instruction; use of health-related vocabulary; performance of test □ Expresses inaccurate perception of problem □ Inability to explain therapeutic regimen or describe personal health status □ Repeatedly requests information □ Failure to seek help or follow therapeutic regimen □ Inappropriate or exaggerated behaviors, e.g., hysteria, hostility, apathy, agitation, depression □ Failure to take medication

Related Factors

Effects of: aging; sensory deficits; language barrier; cognitive limitations □ Information misinterpretation □ Unfamiliarity with information resources □ Lack of: interest in learning; exposure; recall □ Denial □ Substance abuse □ Self-destructive patterns □ Inadequate economic resources

Diagnosis
Altered Thought Processes

Definition

The state in which the individual experiences a disruption in cognitive operations and activities

Defining Characteristics

Agitation or depressed behavior □ Altered sleep patterns □ Inappropriate affect or social behavior □ Non-reality-based thinking □ Fabrication □ Confabulations □ Egocentricity □ Obsessions □ Cognitive dissonance □ Hyper-/hypovigilance □ Nonsensical speech □ Inability to perceive and/or repeat message clearly □ Inaccurate interpretation of environment □ Memory deficits □ Distractibility □ Disorientation as to time, place, person □ Impaired ability to make decisions, problem solve, reason, abstract, conceptualize, calculate □ Delusions or hallucinations □ Ideas of reference □ Decreased response to simple requests

Related Factors

Effects of: aging; medications: sedatives, narcotics, anesthetics, sleep deprivation; psychological conflicts; loss of memory; depression; stress; anxiety; social isolation; emotional trauma; fear of the unknown   □ Negative reactions from others   □ Actual loss of: control; familiar objects; routine surroundings; income; significant other   □ Limited attention span   □ Impaired judgment   □ Sensory overload or deprivation   □ Exposure to unfamiliar environment

FEELING

A Human Response Pattern Involving the Subjective Awareness of Information

Diagnosis
Pain

Definition

The state in which an individual experiences and reports the presence of severe discomfort or an uncomfortable sensation

Defining Characteristics

Subjective: communication (verbal or coded) of pain descriptors   □ Objective: guarding behavior, protective; self-focusing; narrowed focus; altered time perception, withdrawal from social contact, impaired thought process   □ Distraction behavior: moaning; crying; pacing; seeking out other people and/or activities; restlessness   □ Clutching of painful area   □ Trembling   □ Facial mask of pain: eyes lack luster; "beaten" look; fixed or scattered movement; grimace   □ Changes in posture or gait   □ Positive response to palpation   □ Withdrawal reflex   □ Changes in muscle tone (may range from list-

less to rigid)   □ Autonomic responses (not seen in chronic stable pain): increased blood pressure, pulse, respirations; diaphoresis; dilated pupils;   □ Reports of pain

Related Factors

Inflammation   □ Muscle spasm   □ Effects of surgery or trauma   □ Immobility   □ Obstructive processes   □ Pressure points   □ Infectious process   □ Experiences during diagnostic tests   □ Overactivity   □ Injury agents: biological; chemical; physical; psychological

Diagnosis
Chronic Pain

Definition

The state in which an individual experiences pain that continues for more than six months

Defining Characteristics

Major: verbal report or observed evidence of pain experienced for more than six months   □ Minor: facial masks of pain; anorexia; weight changes; changes in sleep patterns; insomnia; guarded movement; depression; personality changes; irritability; fear of reinjury; altered ability to continue previous activities; physical and social withdrawal

Related Factors

Effects of chronic or terminal illness   □ Muscle spasm   □ Inflammation   □ Chronic psychosocial disability

Diagnosis
Dysfunctional Grieving

Definition

The state in which an individual experiences an exaggerated response to an actual or potential loss of person, relationship, object, or functional abilities

Defining Characteristics

Verbal expression of distress at loss □ Expression of unresolved issues □ Crying □ Weight loss □ Amenorrhea □ Changes in: sleep patterns; activity; eating patterns; dream patterns; libido □ Feelings of: anger; guilt; worthlessness; denial; sadness; sorrow □ Decreased interest in personal appearance □ Interference with life functioning □ Reliving of past experiences □ Difficulty in expressing loss □ Alterations in concentration and/or pursuit of tasks □ Developmental regression □ Hyperactivity □ Fear of future □ Absence of emotion □ Suicidal thoughts □ Social withdrawal □ Labile affect

Related Factors

Effects of actual or perceived loss of significant other, health or social status, or valued object: people; possessions; job status; home; ideals; parts and processes of the body □ Absence of anticipatory grieving □ Thwarted grieving in response to a loss □ Effects of multiple losses or crises □ Lack of resolution of previous grieving response □ Ambivalent feelings toward loss □ Changes in lifestyle □ Decreased support system

Diagnosis
Anticipatory Grieving

Definition

The state in which an individual experiences responses to an actual or perceived loss of a person, relationship, object, or functional abilities before the loss occurs

Defining Characteristics

Altered affect □ Anger □ Guilt □ Sorrow □ Choked feelings □ Expressed distress at potential loss □ Altered libido □ Denial of potential loss □ Changes in activity levels, sleeping, or eating habits □ Crying □ Altered communication patterns

Related Factors

Effects of actual or potential loss of significant other, health status, social status, or valued object

High-Risk Diagnosis
High Risk for Violence: Self-Directed or Directed at Others

Definition

The state in which an individual experiences behaviors that can be physically harmful to self or others

Risk Factors

Substance abuse or withdrawal □ Toxic reaction to medication □ Explosive, impulsive, immature personality □ Paranoia □ Panic states □ Rage reactions □ Manic excitement □ Loneliness □ Perceived threat to self-esteem □ Response to catastrophic event □ Suicidal behavior □ Antisocial characteristics □ Dysfunctional communication patterns □ Change in mental or physical health status □ Feelings of alienation □ Catatonic excitement □ Physical, sexual, or psychological abuse (battered women, children, or elderly) □ Manipulative behavior □ Developmental crisis □ Lack of support systems □ Actual or potential loss of significant other □ Social isolation □ Significant change in lifestyle □ Effects of: organic brain syndrome; temporal lobe epilepsy

High-Risk Diagnosis
High Risk for Self-Mutilation

Definition

A state in which an individual is at high risk for performing an act on the self to injure, not kill, which produces tissue damage and tension relief

Risk Factors

Groups at risk: clients with borderline personality disorder, especially females 16–25 years of age; clients in psychotic state—frequently males in young adulthood; emotionally disturbed and/or battered children; mentally retarded and autistic children; clients with a history of self-injury; history of physical, emotional, or sexual abuse □ Inability to cope with increased psychological/physiological tension in a healthy manner □ Feelings of depression, rejection, self-hatred, separation anxiety, guilt, and depersonalization □ Fluctuating emotions □ Command hallucinations □ Need for sensory stimuli □ Parental emotional deprivation □ Dysfunctional family

Diagnosis
Post-Trauma Response

Definition
The state in which an individual experiences a sustained painful response to an overwhelming traumatic event

Defining Characteristics
Major: re-experiencing traumatic event through: flashbacks, intrusive thoughts, repetitive dreams or nightmares, excessive verbalization of traumatic event, verbalization of survival guilt or guilt about behavior required for survival □ Minor: psychic/emotional numbness: impaired interpretation of reality, confusion, dissociation or amnesia, vagueness about traumatic event, constricted affect; altered lifestyle: substance abuse, suicide attempt or other acting-out behavior, difficulty with interpersonal relationships, development of phobia regarding trauma, decreased impulse control/irritability and explosiveness

Related Factors
Effects of: disasters; wars; epidemics; rape; assault; torture; catastrophic illness or accident

Diagnosis
Rape-Trauma Syndrome

Definition
Forced, violent sexual penetration against the victim's will and consent. The trauma syndrome that results from this attack or attempted attack includes an acute phase of disorganization of the victim's lifestyle and a long-term reorganization of lifestyle.

Defining Characteristics
Acute phase: emotional reactions: anger, crying, overcontrol, panic, denial, revenge, self-blame, emotional shock, embarrassment, fear of being alone, humiliation, fear of physical violence and death, desire for revenge, change in sexual behavior, mistrust of opposite sex; multiple physical symptoms: muscle tension, pain, sleep pattern disturbance, gastrointestinal irritability, genitourinary discomfort □ Long-term phase: mentally reliving rape; ambivalence about own sexuality; seeking family or social network support; changes in lifestyle: changes in residence, dealing with repetitive nightmares and phobias; depression; anxiety; loss of self-confidence

Diagnosis
Rape-Trauma Syndrome: Compound Reaction

Definition
Forced, violent sexual penetration against the victim's will and consent. The trauma syndrome that results from this attack or attempted attack includes an acute phase of disorganization of the victim's lifestyle and a long-term reorganization of lifestyle.

Defining Characteristics
Acute phase: emotional reactions: anger, embarrassment, fear of physical violence and death, humiliation, revenge, self-blame; multiple physical symptoms: gastrointestinal irritability, genitourinary discomfort, muscle tension, sleep pattern disturbance: reactivated symptoms of previous conditions: physical illness, psychiatric illness; reliance on alcohol or drugs □ Long-term phase: change in lifestyle: change in residence, dealing with repetitive nightmares and phobias, seeking family support, seeking social network support

Diagnosis
Rape-Trauma Syndrome: Silent Reaction

Definition
Forced, violent sexual penetration against the victim's will and consent. The trauma syndrome that results from this attack or attempted attack includes an acute phase of disorganization of the victim's lifestyle and a long-term reorganization of lifestyle.

Defining Characteristics

Abrupt changes in relationships with opposite sex □ Increase in nightmares □ Increasing anxiety during interviews, e.g., blocking of associations, long periods of silence, minor stuttering, physical distress □ Marked changes in sexual behavior □ No verbalization of the occurrence of rape □ Sudden onset of phobic reactions

Diagnosis
Anxiety

Definition

The state in which an individual experiences a vague uneasy feeling, the source of which is often nonspecific or unknown

Defining Characteristics

Subjective: increased tension; apprehension; painful and persistent increased helplessness; uncertainty; fearfulness; scared; regretful; overexcited; rattled; distressed; jittery; feelings of inadequacy; shakiness; fear of unspecified consequences; expressed concerns regarding change in life events; worried; anxious □ Objective: sympathetic stimulation: cardiovascular excitation, superficial vasoconstriction, pupil dilation, increased perspiration; restlessness; insomnia; glancing about; lack of eye contact; trembling/hand tremors; extraneous movement: foot shuffling, hand/arm movements; facial tension; voice quivering; focus on self; increased wariness

Related Factors

Loss of possessions □ Effects of actual or perceived loss of significant others □ Threat to or change in health status, socioeconomic status, relationships, role functioning, support systems, environment, self-concept, or interaction patterns □ Situational and maturational crises □ Unmet needs □ Threat of death □ Unconscious conflict about essential values and goals of life □ Lack of knowledge □ Loss of control □ Feelings of failure □ Disruptive family life □ Interpersonal transmission and contagion □ Threat to self-concept

Diagnosis
Fear

Definition

The state in which the individual experiences feelings of dread related to an identifiable source perceived as dangerous

Defining Characteristics

Ability to identify object of fear □ Sympathetic stimulation: cardiovascular excitation; superficial vasoconstriction; increased blood pressure, pulse, and respirations □ Wide-eyed appearance □ Crying □ Voice tremors □ Diaphoresis □ Urinary frequency □ Regressive behavior, pacing □ Withdrawing □ Insomnia □ Terror □ Panic □ Apprehension □ Aggression □ Increased alertness □ Decreased self-assurance □ Increased questioning/verbalization □ Feelings of loss of control

Related Factors

Sensory impairment, deprivation, or overload □ Pain □ Effects of loss of body part or function □ Effects of chronic disabling illness □ Language barrier □ Threat of death, actual or perceived □ Anticipation of events posing a threat to self-esteem □ Phobias □ Feelings of failure □ Knowledge deficit □ Learned response, conditioning □ Loss of significant other □ Separation from support system

NORTH AMERICA NURSING DIAGNOSIS ASSOCIATION 1994 DIAGNOSES IN PROGRESS

Alcohol Drinking Patterns, Dysfunctional:
Continuous or intermittent abuse of the beverage alcohol resulting in breakdown of social, emotional, spiritual or physical levels of health for the individual.

Community Coping, Ineffective:
A pattern of community activities for adaptation and problem solving that is unsatisfactory for meeting the demands or needs of the community.

Community Coping, Potential for Enhanced:
A pattern of community activities for adaptation and problem solving that is satisfactory for meeting the demands or needs of the community but can be improved for management of current and future problems/stressors.

Confusion, Acute:
The abrupt onset of a cluster of global, transient changes and disturbances in attention cognition, psychomotor activity, level of consciousness, and/or sleep-wake cycle.

Disorganized Behavior, Infant:
Alteration in integration and modulation of the physiological and behavioral systems of functioning (i.e., autonomic, motor, state, organizational, self regulatory, and attentional-interactional systems).

Disorganized Infant Behavior, Risk for:
Risk for alteration in integration and modulation of the physiological and behavioral sub-systems of functioning (i.e., autonomic, motor, state, organizational, self regulatory, and attentional-interactional systems) which impacts homeostasis and adaption.

Environmental Interpretation Syndrome, Impaired:
Consistent lack of orientation to person, place, time or circumstances over more than three to six months necessitating a protective environment.

Family Processes, Altered: Addictive Behavior (Individual & Family):
The state in which the psychosocial, spiritual, and physiological functions of a family unit are chronically disorganized, leading to conflict, denial of problems, resistance to change, ineffective problem-solving, and a series of self-perpetuating crises.

Idiopathic Fecal Incontinence:
A change in an individual's pattern of elimination characterized by a loss of ability to voluntarily control the passage of feces/gas and occasional/frequent loss of normal stool.

Impaired Skin Integrity, High Risk for: Pressure Ulcer:
A state in which the individual's skin is at risk of being adversely affected.

Labor Pain:
A subjective measure of an unpleasant sensation which lasts the duration of a contraction, and may linger between contractions. The feeling subsides with delivery of a fetus.

Loneliness, High Risk for:
A subjective state in which an individual is at risk of experiencing vague dysphoria.

Organized Infant Behavior, Potential for Enhanced:
Integration and modulation of the physiological and neurobehavioral systems of functioning (i.e., physiologic/autonomic, motor, state, organizational, self regulatory and attentional-interactional systems).

Parent/Infant Attachment, Altered:
Disruption of the interactive process between parent/significant other and infant that fosters the development of a protective and nurturing reciprocal relationship.

Preservation/Quality of Life, Alteration in:
Quality of life is that continuum for measuring how well one meets and takes care of one's own needs. Preservation of life is the ability to prolong life naturally or on a life support system.

Self-Care Deficit, Medication Administration:
The state in which the individual experiences an impaired motor function or cognitive function, causing a decreased ability to feed, bathe, dress, toilet and/or administer his/her own medications.

Spasticity:
The state in which an individual with an upper motor neuron injury experiences increased muscle tone and abnormal reflexes in response to internal or external stimuli which interfere with functional abilities such as mobility, hygiene, eating, dressing, and toileting.

Spiritual Well-Being, Opportunity for Enhanced:
The process of an individual's developing/unfolding of mystery through harmonious interconnectedness that springs from inner strengths.

Therapeutic Regimen, Ineffective Management of (Families):
A pattern of regulating and integrating into family processes a program for treatment of illness and the sequelae of illness that is unsatisfactory for meeting health goals.

Terminal Illness Response:

The state in which an individual with a terminal affliction attempts to deal with end of life decisions, the pending existential loss of loved ones, possessions, and his/her own body image, as well as the debilitating physical symptoms of dying. The family or caregiver are reciprocally affected, and sometimes if the patient is unconscious, they experience the phenomena alone.

Urinary Filtration Syndrome, Impaired:

A state in which the individual is experiencing urinary filtration dysfunction. The urinary filtration system is characterized by changes in glomerular permeability which allow the passage of particles into the urine resulting in compromised urinary function/filtration.

B

EXERCISES

Review the following case study on Ted Alexander. Take the underlined data and classify it according to the Functional Health Pattern Framework. Note that some data may fall into more than one category.

Mr. Ted Alexander, a 50-year-old white divorced salesman from Las Vegas, was on a business trip to Atlantic City when he developed pain in the left upper abdominal quadrant. He took Alka-Seltzer with little relief, and the pain persisted for the next two days. He was busy with appointments during the day and evening and was able to ignore the pain. He ate very little and took two sleeping pills at night. On the afternoon of the third day, the pain became much more intense, and when it continued for several hours and he began to vomit bloody fluid, he went to the emergency department.

Physical examination and laboratory data at this time revealed an alert, well-groomed man with generalized abdominal tenderness, rigidity of the abdominal wall, absent bowel sounds, and a Hgb of 11.6 (normal = 16 +/− 2) with a Hct of 38 (normal 47 +/− 5). The diagnosis of bleeding gastric ulcer was made. He was admitted to the hospital for initial medical management, with surgery anticipated at a later date.

Your examination of the patient reveals the following: B/P 104/60, P 120, R 26, T 98.2°. The patient indicates that he is 6 ft, 2 in tall and weighs 196 lb. He is alert and oriented and states, "I've never had this bleeding before—it's serious, isn't it?" His skin is cool to the touch and slightly diaphoretic. The patient states that he had been a heavy drinker for 15 years and was admitted to the hospital with cirrhosis two years ago by his family doctor, Dr. Martland, but has never had surgery. He denies drinking for the past two years but smokes two packs of cigarettes daily.

Mr. Alexander is tense throughout your conversation but shares a number of concerns with you, including his separation from his two teenage children who live with him. He is also anxious about being cared for by an unfamiliar physician. The emergency department nurse indicates that he wears contact lenses and is concerned because he has left his case and supplies as well as his glasses in his hotel. He gives you $750.00 in cash and traveler's checks to deposit in the hospital safe. He has a partial lower plate of dentures and caps on his four front teeth. Further inquiry reveals that the patient prefers a low-fat diet, occasionally uses laxatives, and has had several occurrences of urinary urgency and nocturia in the last six months.

The physician states that his treatment plan includes gastric suction, anti-ulcer medications, and replacement therapy with IV fluid, blood, electrolytes, and vitamins until the patient is stabilized enough for exploratory surgery. Mr. Alexander agrees to this plan but is concerned about

Continued.

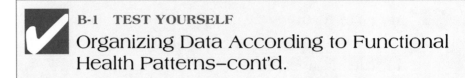
his job demands and wonders how he will deal with "getting back home when all of this is over."

FUNCTIONAL HEALTH PATTERN

Health Perception–Health Management:

Nutritional–Metabolic:

Elimination:

Activity–Exercise:

Sleep–Rest:

Cognitive–Perceptual:

Self-Perception:

Role–Relationship:

Sexuality–Reproductive:

Coping–Stress Tolerance:

Value–Belief:

Physical Assessment:

B-1 TEST YOURSELF

Organizing Data According to Functional Health Patterns: Answers

Health Perception–Health Management:
 Pain in left upper abdominal quadrant, vomiting bloody fluid. Bleeding gastric ulcer. Diagnosis of cirrhosis two years ago. No drinking alcohol for two years. Smokes two packs cigarettes daily. Agrees to plan of care.

Nutritional–Metabolic:
 Low-fat diet

Elimination:
 Occasional laxatives
 Urinary urgency and nocturia

Activity–Exercise:
 Salesman

Sleep–Rest:
 Sleeping pills

Cognitive–Perceptual:
 Wears contacts lenses/glasses

Self-Perception:
 "I've never had this bleeding before—it's serious, isn't it?"

Role–Relationship:
 Lives with two teenage children
 Divorced

Sexuality–Reproductive:

Coping–Stress Tolerance:
 Agrees to plan of care
 Tense, anxious about being cared for by an unfamiliar physician
 Concerned about job demands
 Smokes two packs of cigarettes daily

Value–Belief:

Physical Assessment:
 Pain in left upper abdominal quadrant. Vomiting bloody fluid, alert and oriented, well-groomed, generalized abdominal tenderness, absent bowel sounds, Hgb 11.6, Hct 38, BP 104/60, P 120, R 26, T 98.2. 6 ft, 2 in tall, 196 lb. Cool to touch, diaphoretic. Partial lower plate and caps.

B-2 TEST YOURSELF
Identification of Inferences

Read the cues/clusters in column I and identify possible inferences in column II.

CUE/CLUSTER (DEFINING CHARACTERISTICS)	INFERENCE
1. B/P 90/50 (normally 120/70)	
2. Female, age 25 with bright red vaginal bleeding (one pad in six hours)	
3. Urine glucose 2% (normal = 0)	
4. Dilated pupils in an alert, oriented client without injury and taking medication	
5. Height 5 ft, 1 in; weight 220 lb; pendulous abdomen	
6. B/P 190/104; states, "I wasn't supposed to eat salt."	
7. Whimpering 1-year-old child; restlessness; pulling left ear	
8. Insomnia; P 110; irritability; states, "I feel nervous."	
9. History of accidents; unsteady gait; impaired vision	
10. Newly diagnosed diabetic; states, "I've never tested my blood for sugar before."	

Identification of Inferences: Answers

CUE/CLUSTER (DEFINING CHARACTERISTICS)	INFERENCE
1. B/P 90/50 (normally 120/70)	Abnormally low for client
2. Female, age 25 with bright red vaginal bleeding (one pad in six hours)	Menstruation
3. Urine glucose 2% (normal = 0)	Abnormal glucose level
4. Dilated pupils in an alert, oriented client without injury and taking medication	Effects of medication
5. Height 5 ft, 1 in; weight 220 lb; pendulous abdomen	Obesity
6. B/P 190/104; states, "I wasn't supposed to eat salt."	Abnormally elevated blood pressure
7. Whimpering 1-year-old child; restlessness; pulling left ear	Pain in left ear
8. Insomnia; P 110; irritability; states "I feel nervous."	Anxiety
9. History of accidents; unsteady gait; impaired vision	At risk for injury
10. Newly diagnosed diabetic; states, "I've never tested my blood for sugar before."	Lack of knowledge about blood sugar testing

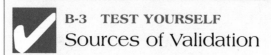

Sources of Validation

Identify methods of validation that might be used by the nurse in the situations described below.

VALIDATION

- **A.** Directly with the client or significant others
- **B.** Collaboration with health care professionals
- **C.** Reference sources

SITUATION

1. Jeremy Pressman is seen in the outpatient clinic for a well baby visit. He is 18 months old and weighs 18 lb. His mother asks, "Is he underweight?" How can this be validated?

2. A 17-year-old teenager is brought into the emergency department complaining of abdominal pain. Shortly after he is placed on a stretcher, he vomits brown liquid. You realize that the vomitus could be old blood but know that certain liquids, such as coffee or hot chocolate, can resemble old blood. What should you do to pursue this?

3. Pat Derby, a 19-year-old college sophomore, is seen at the university student health center because he claims that voices are telling him to kill his accounting professor. The nurse practitioner interviews Pat to obtain more information about his thought processes. During the discussion, Pat indicates that Dr. Johnson saw him three weeks ago when he had these same feelings. What would be an appropriate next step?

4. Ann Bahrami is brought to the hospital by her son. You suspect that she is profoundly depressed and she does not respond to your questions regarding her health history. What should you do next?

5. Carl Pucay is admitted for anorexia nervosa. You recognize that she was on your unit about two months ago with the same problem. When questioned about her attendance at counseling sessions, Carol says she has gone but she avoids eye contact. You suspect that she has not attended regularly. How might you pursue this?

B-3   TEST YOURSELF

Sources of Validation: Answers

1. C—Consult a growth chart (reference source).
2. A—Ask the client or family about intake of coffee or hot chocolate.
3. B—Contact Dr. Johnson.
4. A—Ask the client's son about symptoms and possible causes of depression.
5. B—Call the group facilitator or social worker to verify the client's attendance at counseling sessions.

Identification of Correctly and Incorrectly Written Nursing Diagnoses

The following is a list of nursing diagnostic statements. Decide whether each statement is correctly or incorrectly written. If incorrectly stated, identify the rule(s) violated, by number, from the list below.

GUIDELINES FOR WRITING A NURSING DIAGNOSIS

1. Write the diagnosis in terms of the client's response rather than nursing needs.
2. Use "related to" rather than "due to" or "caused by" to connect the two parts of the diagnosis.
3. Write the diagnosis in legally advisable terms.
4. Write the diagnosis without value judgments.
5. Avoid reversing the two parts of the diagnosis.
6. Avoid using signs and symptoms in the first part of the diagnosis.
7. Be sure that the two parts of the diagnosis do not mean the same thing.
8. Express the related factors in terms that can be changed.
9. Do not include medical diagnoses in the nursing diagnosis.
10. State the diagnosis clearly and concisely.

	CORRECT	INCORRECT	RULE(S)
1. Spiritual distress related to challenged belief about God			
2. Insomnia related to sleep pattern disturbance			
3. Hypothermia caused by lack of appropriate clothing			
4. Altered patterns of urinary elimination related to benign prostatic hypertrophy			

Continued.

Identification of Correctly and Incorrectly Written Nursing Diagnoses–cont'd.

	CORRECT	INCORRECT	RULE(S)
5. Dysfunctional ventilatory weaning response related to uncooperative client			
6. Altered growth and development related to the infant being taken care of by a different caregiver each day			
7. Body image disturbance related to loss of breast			
8. Hyperthermia related to elevated temperature			
9. High risk for trauma related to failure of nurses to put up side rails			
10. Ineffective airway clearance related to pneumonia			
11. Sleep deprivation related to visual sensory perceptual alteration			
12. Needs neurovascular checks every four hours			

B-4   TEST YOURSELF

Identification of Correctly and Incorrectly Written Nursing Diagnoses: Answers

	CORRECT	INCORRECT	RULE(S)
1. Spiritual distress related to challenged belief about God	✔		
2. Insomnia related to sleep pattern disturbance		✔	#5, 6, 7
3. Hypothermia caused by lack of appropriate clothing		✔	#2
4. Altered patterns of urinary elimination related to benign prostatic hypertrophy		✔	#9
5. Dysfunctional ventilatory weaning response related to uncooperative client		✔	#4
6. Altered growth and development related to the infant being taken care of by a different caregiver each day		✔	#10

Continued.

B-4   TEST YOURSELF

Identification of Correctly and Incorrectly Written Nursing Diagnoses: Answers–cont'd.

	CORRECT	INCORRECT	RULE(S)
7. Body image disturbance related to loss of breast		✔	#8
8. Hyperthermia related to elevated temperature		✔	#7
9. High risk for trauma related to failure of nurses to put up side rails		✔	#3
10. Ineffective airway clearance related to pneumonia		✔	#9
11. Sleep deprivation related to visual sensory perceptual alteration		✔	#5
12. Needs neurovascular checks every four hours		✔	#1

B-5   TEST YOURSELF

Revision of Incorrectly Written Diagnoses

The nursing diagnoses that were incorrectly written in the previous exercise are listed below. Revise each nursing diagnosis to make it correct.

NURSING DIAGNOSIS	REVISION
1. Insomnia related to sleep pattern disturbance	
2. Hypothermia caused by lack of appropriate clothing	
3. Altered patterns of urinary elimination related to benign prostatic hypertrophy	
4. Dysfunctional ventilatory weaning response related to uncooperative client	
5. Altered growth and development related to the infant being taken care of by a different caregiver each day	

B-5 TEST YOURSELF

Revision of Incorrectly Written Diagnoses—cont'd.

NURSING DIAGNOSIS	REVISION
6. Body image disturbance related to loss of breast	
7. Hyperthermia related to elevated temperature	
8. High risk for trauma related to failure of nurses to put up side rails	
9. Ineffective airway clearance related to pneumonia	
10. Sleep deprivation related to visual sensory perceptual alteration	
11. Needs neurovascular checks every four hours	

B-5   TEST YOURSELF
Revision of Incorrectly Written Diagnoses: Answers

NURSING DIAGNOSIS	REVISION
1. Insomnia related to sleep pattern disturbances	Sleep pattern disturbance related to excessive noise
2. Hypothermia caused by lack of appropriate clothing	Hypothermia related to lack of appropriate clothing
3. Altered patterns of urinary elimination related to benign prostatic hypertrophy	Altered patterns of urinary elimination related to catheter obstruction
4. Dysfunctional ventilatory weaning response related to uncooperative client	Dysfunctional ventilatory weaning response related to client perceived inefficacy regarding the ability to wean
5. Altered growth and development related to the infant being taken care of by a different caregiver each day	Altered growth and development related to inconsistency in caregiving
6. Body image disturbance related to loss of breast	Body image disturbance related to effects of loss of breast
7. Hyperthermia related to elevated temperature	Hyperthermia related to prolonged exposure to hot environment
8. High risk for trauma related to failure of nurses to put up side rails	Potential for trauma related to decreased level of consciousness
9. Ineffective airway clearance related to pneumonia	Ineffective airway clearance related to retained secretions
10. Sleep deprivation related to visual sensory perceptual alteration	Sensory perceptual alteration (visual) related to sleep deprivation
11. Needs neurovascular checks every four hours	High risk for peripheral neurovascular dysfunction related to mechanical compression secondary to cast

B-6 TEST YOURSELF

Identification of Correctly and Incorrectly Written Client Outcomes

The following is a set of nursing diagnostic statements and outcomes. Decide whether each outcome is correctly or incorrectly written. If incorrectly stated, identify, by number, the rule(s) violated from the list below.

RULES

Outcomes should:
1. Be derived from the diagnoses.
2. Be documented as measurable goals.
3. Be formulated with client and healthcare providers.
4. Be realistic in relation to client's capabilities.
5. Be attainable in relation to available resources.
6. Include a time estimate for attainment.
7. Provide direction for continuity of care.

NURSING DIAGNOSIS	OUTCOME	CORRECT	INCORRECT	RULE(S)
1. Feeding self-care deficit related to impaired physical mobility	Client will receive help to eat			
2. Ineffective breast-feeding related to decreased infant sucking	Demonstrates adequate breast-feeding as manifested by infant weight gain of 3 oz in four days			

Continued.

B-6 TEST YOURSELF

Identification of Correctly and Incorrectly Written Client Outcomes–cont'd.

NURSING DIAGNOSIS	OUTCOME	CORRECT	INCORRECT	RULE(S)
3. Anticipatory grieving related to impending death of child	By time of child's death, family verbalizes complete acceptance			
4. Pain related to muscle spasm	Verbalizes decreased pain within 45 minutes after pain medication			
5. High risk for infection related to hazards associated with invasive equipment	Absence of redness, edema, purulent drainage, temperature elevation, and increased WBCs			
6. High risk for aspiration related to decreased level of consciousness	Prevent aspiration			
7. Social isolation related to obesity, perceived unattractiveness	Loses 1 lb per week until achieves goal of 150 lb			

B-6   TEST YOURSELF

Identification of Correctly and Incorrectly Written Client Outcomes: Answers

NURSING DIAGNOSIS	OUTCOME	CORRECT	INCORRECT	RULE(S)
1. Feeding self-care deficit related to impaired physical mobility	Client will be fed by staff		✔	This is an intervention; 6
2. Interrupted breast-feeding due to maternal illness	Infant maintains current weight during mother's illness	✔		
3. Anticipatory grieving related to impending death of child	By time of child's death, family verbalizes complete acceptance		✔	4
4. Pain related to muscle spasm	Verbalizes decreased pain within 45 minutes after pain medication	✔		
5. High risk for infection related to hazards associated with invasive equipment	No evidence of infection		✔	6

Continued.

B-6   TEST YOURSELF

Identification of Correctly and Incorrectly Written Client Outcomes: Answers–cont'd.

NURSING DIAGNOSIS	OUTCOME	CORRECT	INCORRECT	RULE(S)
6. High risk for aspiration related to decreased level of consciousness	Prevent aspiration		✔	2, 6
7. Social isolation related to obesity, perceived unattractiveness	Loses 1 lb per week until achieves goal of 150 lb		✔	1

B-7   TEST YOURSELF
Revision of Incorrectly Written Client Outcomes

The outcomes that were incorrectly written are listed below. A nursing diagnosis has been identified for each outcome to assist you in formulating a new outcome. Revise each outcome so that it is correctly stated.

NURSING DIAGNOSIS	OUTCOME	REVISED OUTCOME
1. Feeding self-care deficit related to impaired physical mobility	Client will receive help to eat	
2. Anticipatory grieving related to impending death of child	By time of child's death, family verbalizes complete acceptance	
3. High risk for infection related to hazards associated with invasive equipment	No evidence of infection	
4. High risk for aspiration related to decreased level of consciousness	Prevent aspiration	
5. Social isolation related to obesity, perceived unattractiveness	Loses 1 lb per week until achieves goal of 150 lb	

B-7   TEST YOURSELF

Revision of Incorrectly Written Client Outcomes: Answers

The following are suggested answers for the preceding exercise. Keep in mind that there is more than one way to revise an outcome.

NURSING DIAGNOSIS	OUTCOME	REVISED OUTCOME
1. Feeding self-care deficit related to impaired physical mobility	Client will receive help to eat	Prior to discharge feeds self using adaptive equipment
2. Anticipatory grieving related to impending death of child	By time of child's death, family verbalizes complete acceptance	Prior to child's death family verbalizes feelings regarding impending loss
3. High risk for infection related to hazards associated with invasive equipment	No evidence of infection	While CVP line in place, no evidence of infection
4. High risk for aspiration related to decreased level of consciousness	Prevent aspiration	No evidence of aspiration throughout hospitalization
5. Social isolation related to obesity, perceived unattractiveness	Loses 1 lb per week until achieves goal of 150 lb	Interacts with peers after school at least two times per week

B-8 TEST YOURSELF

Identification of Correctly and Incorrectly Written Nursing Interventions

The following is a list of interventions. Decide whether each intervention is written correctly or incorrectly. Identify the rule violated from the list below:

RULES

Nursing interventions should:

1. Include precise action verbs and modifiers.
2. Specify who, what, where, how, and how much.
3. Be individualized for the client.
4. Be signed and dated.

DATE/INIT	NURSING INTERVENTIONS	CORRECT	INCORRECT	RULE(S)
7/11 P.I.	1. Create a safe environment			
3/4 R.N.	2. Assist to cough and deep breathe q2h			
10/15 B.A.	3. Ambulates in room three times daily			
	4. Weigh daily prior to breakfast using bed scale			
6-11 N. I.	5. Teach colostomy care			

B-8 TEST YOURSELF

Identification of Correctly and Incorrectly Written Nursing Interventions: Answers

DATE/INIT	NURSING INTERVENTIONS	CORRECT	INCORRECT	RULE(S)
7/17 P.I.	1. Create a safe environment		✓	1
3/4 R.W.	2. Assist to cough and deep breathe q2h	✓		
10/15 B.A.	3. Ambulates in room three times daily		✓	This is an outcome
	4. Weigh daily prior to break-fast using bed scale		✓	4
6-11 N.I.	5. Teach colos-tomy care		✓	2, 3

B-9 TEST YOURSELF

Revision of Incorrectly Written Nursing Interventions

DATE/INIT	NURSING INTERVENTIONS	REVISED INTERVENTIONS
7/17 P.J.	1. Create a safe environment	
10/15 B.A.	2. Ambulates in room three times daily	
	3. Weigh daily prior to breakfast using bed scale	
6-11 N.I.	4. Teach colostomy care	

B-9 TEST YOURSELF
Revision of Incorrectly Written Nursing Interventions: Answers

DATE/INIT	NURSING INTERVENTIONS	REVISED INTERVENTIONS
7/17 P.I.	1. Create a safe environment	Remove obstacles from path of ambulation
10/15 B.A.	2. Ambulates in room three times daily	Assist to ambulate in room tid
	3. Weigh daily prior to breakfast using bed scale	Weigh daily prior to breakfast using bed scale
6-11 N.I.	4. Teach colostomy care	Teach client to apply Bongort pouch on 5/8

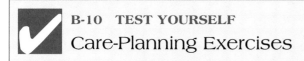

B-10   TEST YOURSELF

Care-Planning Exercises

Read the following case studies. Based on the information provided, identify pertinent cues and develop correctly written diagnoses, outcomes, and nursing interventions. Then, assuming the interventions were implemented, write two evaluative comments reflecting that (1) the outcome has been achieved, and (2) the outcome has not been achieved.

Case 1. Adam Steinman is a 75-year-old gentleman confined to bed as a result of an injury to his spinal column causing some residual weakness of his lower extremities. He is referred to home care by his physician to assist in managing problems with urination. During your visit he voids only 150 ml despite the fact that he has already consumed more than 600 ml of fluid. His bladder is moderately distended. You call his physician and discuss your findings. A decision is made to do a straight urethral catheterization and 350 ml of urine is obtained.

Develop a care plan with **one** nursing diagnosis.

CUES:

NURSING DIAGNOSIS	OUTCOMES	NURSING INTERVENTIONS

EVALUATIVE COMMENT:

(a) *Outcome achieved:*

(b) *Outcome not achieved:*

Continued.

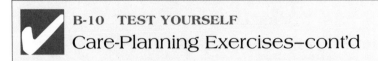

B-10   TEST YOURSELF
Care-Planning Exercises–cont'd

Case 2. Mary Ann LaFleur is a 36-year-old mother of three preschool children. In the sixth month of her last pregnancy, she was found to have a malignant breast tumor for which she had a left modified radical mastectomy. Eighteen months later, she found another mass in her right breast and has been admitted to your unit the morning of the surgery. The client tells you that the physician has explained the anticipated surgical options and has offered her the choice between a lumpectomy followed by radiation and chemotherapy and a second radical mastectomy. The client tells you that she really would prefer the first option but she is very concerned about her ability to handle the difficulties associated with both chemotherapy and radiation. She states, "I know I have to make a decision but neither choice is appealing. If I lose my other breast I will no longer look like a woman."

Develop a care plan with at least **two** nursing diagnoses.

CUES:

NURSING DIAGNOSIS	OUTCOMES	NURSING INTERVENTIONS

EVALUATIVE COMMENT:

(a) *Outcome achieved:*

(b) *Outcome not achieved:*

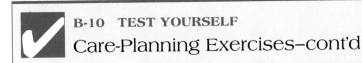

B-10   TEST YOURSELF
Care-Planning Exercises–cont'd

Case 3. Susan Johnson is a 36-year-old housewife who has been diagnosed as having rheumatoid arthritis. As the home health nurse, your initial assessment reveals an alert, oriented woman with joint swelling of the fingers and right knee. During the interview, Susan Johnson grimaces and moans slightly each time she attempts to bend her fingers. She holds her right knee and indicates that she feels best when she lies on her left side with pillows behind her back and between her legs. She states, "I feel so helpless. I'm so stiff in the morning and this pain is really getting me down. My mother has had to come to my house every day to care for my toddlers. I hate when this pain prevents me from performing my responsibilities as a mother."
    Develop a care plan with at least **two** nursing diagnoses.

CUES:

NURSING DIAGNOSIS	OUTCOMES	NURSING INTERVENTIONS

EVALUATIVE COMMENT:
(a) *Outcome achieved:*

(b) *Outcome not achieved:*

Continued.

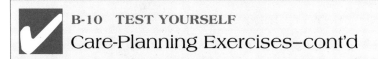

B-10   TEST YOURSELF
Care-Planning Exercises–cont'd

Case 4. Art Herbert is a 75-year-old widower with no nearby relatives. He was recently discharged from the hospital after experiencing a hypertensive crisis. During the course of hospitalization he responded well to the antihypertensive medications. Three days after discharge, the home care nurse finds his B/P is 180/100, his weight is up by 7 lb, and he has edema of the ankles. Art reports that he has not been taking his diuretic as prescribed, because he cannot remember the instructions. He states that he does not want to talk about those pills any more. His real concern is his bowels. He reports he has been constipated for three days, has hard dry stools, and requires straining to accomplish defecation. This is especially distressing because he is accustomed to having a bowel movement daily. Since discharge, Art has been preparing canned soups and small frozen dinners, even though his doctor prescribed a low-salt diet. Prior to hospitalization, his usual diet consisted of home-cooked meals prepared by his neighbor. Art says, "I don't know what is happening to me. Ever since my neighbor left for vacation I have been having all these problems. She cooked for me and reminded me to take my medicine. I can't wait until she comes home."

Develop a care plan with at least **three** nursing diagnoses.

CUES:

NURSING DIAGNOSIS	OUTCOMES	NURSING INTERVENTIONS

EVALUATIVE COMMENT:

(a) *Outcome achieved:*

(b) *Outcome not achieved:*

CASE 1. ADAM STEINMAN

CUES:
Bladder distention
High residual urine
Small frequent voiding

NURSING DIAGNOSIS	OUTCOMES	NURSING INTERVENTIONS

Urinary retention related to diminished sensory/motor impulses	Within one week voids at least ___ ml per void	1. Have client keep record of voiding pattern-time and amounts
		
		2. Assess and document color and consistency of urine
		
		3. Increase oral intake to:
		   100 ml days
		   700 ml evenings
		   300 ml nights
		
		4. Teach client/family to palpate bladder for distention
		
		5. Implement techniques that may encourage voiding: run water in bathroom
		
		6. Consult physician to determine need for further straight catheterizations

EVALUATIVE COMMENT:

(a) *Outcome achieved:*
Reviewed voiding pattern data. Client voiding approximately every three hours. Voiding 200 to 250 ml each time. No evidence of distention at this visit. Has established normal voiding pattern.

(b) *Outcome not achieved:*
Reviewed voiding pattern data. Client voiding approximately every three hours. Voiding only 75 to 100 ml each time. Reports feelings of distention. Has not met outcome.

Continued.

Care-Planning Exercises: Answers–cont'd.

CASE 2. MARY ANN LAFLEUR

Care Plan A

CUES:
Verbalized uncertainty about choices
Verbalized undesired consequences of treatment choices

NURSING DIAGNOSIS	OUTCOMES	NURSING INTERVENTIONS
Decisional conflict (treatment option) related to unknown outcome of choices of therapy	Prior to surgery: verbalizes satisfaction with choice made	1. Encourage client to further verbalize concerns regarding both choices 2. Have client seek input from husband/family 3. Explore her fears regarding chemotherapy and radiation therapy 4. Notify physician that client is still undecided; arrange group conference

EVALUATIVE COMMENT:

(a) *Outcome achieved:*
Client on call to operating room. States that she "thinks that the radical mastectomy is the best thing for me at this time." Identifies that the needs of her family are most important to her at this time.

(b) *Outcome not achieved:*
After group conference with client, husband, physician, nurse, and social worker, client continues to express doubts about decision to have mastectomy.

B-10   TEST YOURSELF
Care-Planning Exercises: Answers–cont'd.

Care Plan B

CUES:
Verbal response to potential change in appearance

NURSING DIAGNOSIS	OUTCOMES	NURSING INTERVENTIONS
Body image disturbance related to feelings of rejection secondary to mastectomies	Verbalizes positive statements about physical appearance prior to discharge	1. Encourage client to discuss negative feelings regarding body 2. Explore feelings regarding effects of surgery and her relationship with her husband 3. Encourage her to discuss fears with her husband 4. Identify personal strengths 5. Assist client to identify other positive aspects of her physical appearance

EVALUATIVE COMMENT:

(a) *Outcome achieved:*
Client dressing in preparation for discharge. Comments that "with my clothes on no one would know that I had surgery." Says that she feels better about herself and knows that she will be able to deal with this. Has improved body image.

(b) *Outcome not achieved:*
Client preparing for discharge. States, "I have nothing to wear after I get home—I'm sure nothing in my closet will do anything to hide my surgery." Body image disturbance not resolved.

Continued.

Care-Planning Exercises: Answers–cont'd.

CASE 3. SUSAN JOHNSON

Care Plan A

CUES:
Grimacing/moaning
Clutching of painful knee
Feelings of helplessness
Reports of pain

NURSING DIAGNOSIS	OUTCOMES	NURSING INTERVENTIONS
Acute pain related to inflammatory process	Verbalizes decreased pain within 30 minutes following initiation of comfort measures	1. Explore pain relief measures that have been helpful in the past 2. Advise client to take hot bath/shower upon arising to reduce stiffness 3. Apply cold as directed by physician 4. Explore with client times of day she can rest with joints in functional position 5. Review knowledge of medication regimen; remind not to miss dose of arthritis medications

B-10   TEST YOURSELF
Care-Planning Exercises: Answers–cont'd.

NURSING DIAGNOSIS	OUTCOMES	NURSING INTERVENTIONS
		6. Explore use of relaxation exercises to reduce stress/anxiety
		7. Consult physical therapy for home physical therapy
		8. Caution against exercising inflamed joints except for ROM exercises

EVALUATIVE COMMENT:

(a) *Outcome achieved:*
Pain regimen is effective. Client reports that she is comfortable when she follows the planned pain regimen.

(b) *Outcome not achieved:*
Pain and comfort measures have not been effective. Client reports that "I am uncomfortable even when I take the medication as planned." She has not been able to get into the bathtub.

Care Plan B

CUES:
States inability to perform role expectations

NURSING DIAGNOSIS	OUTCOMES	NURSING INTERVENTIONS
Altered role performance related to change in health status, effect of acute illness	Demonstrates ability to function within limitations	**1.** Encourage client to verbalize further regarding the effect of the change in health status on her role as wife and mother

Continued.

B-10 TEST YOURSELF
Care-Planning Exercises: Answers–cont'd.

NURSING DIAGNOSIS	OUTCOMES	NURSING INTERVENTIONS
		2. Help client to identify what part of her role she can still perform
		3. Discuss plan for potential change in family member's role function during this acute episode
		4. Discuss need for some temporary child care for children
		5. Explore coping mechanisms that have been successful in the past and explore new options

EVALUATIVE COMMENT:

(a) *Outcome achieved:*
Client has improved perception of her role as mother. Since last week, has arranged for her toddlers to go to child care each day. Mother helps to get the children ready. Says, "This gives me some time to rest without being disturbed." When they come home, she is able to play quietly with them while mother prepares dinner. Says that she feels this is "working well for everyone."

Care Plan B

(b) *Outcome not achieved:*
Role of mother continues to be a problem for client. During visit, Susan cried and stated, "I feel like I'm failing my children—at this point, nothing is working right."

B-10 TEST YOURSELF
Care-Planning Exercises: Answers–cont'd.

CASE 4. ART HERBERT

Care Plan A

CUES:
Inability to meet basic health needs: taking antihypertensive medication (diuretic), following diet

NURSING DIAGNOSIS	OUTCOMES	NURSING INTERVENTIONS
Altered health maintenance related to forgetfulness, lack of support systems	By end of visit: Identifies available resources for maintaining healthy diet, taking medications as ordered	1. Provide and review medication chart, noting purpose and time of medicines 2. Explore client's belief regarding medications/ physician's advice 3. Supply pill sorter and fill on q3 day visit 4. Explore availability of financial resources for homemaker 5. Discuss acceptance of assistance within the home 6. Identify with client other alternative support systems 7. Write all instructions down and place in spot designated by client

Continued.

EVALUATIVE COMMENT:

(a) *Outcome achieved:*

Has identified appropriate strategies to maintain self-care. By the end of visit, client decided to try to have a homemaker come three times a week. He was able to identify a neighbor who could check on him once or twice a day and plans to ask him tomorrow. He agreed that a pill sorter would help him to keep his medications straight. Agreed to try "Meals on Wheels" for two weeks.

(b) *Outcome not achieved:*

By the end of visit, client was still not convinced that he needs someone to help him. Says "I like it the way it is."

Care Plan B

CUES:
Hypertension
Edema of ankles
Weight gain

NURSING DIAGNOSIS	OUTCOMES	NURSING INTERVENTIONS
Fluid volume excess related to:	Within one week:	1. Call physician and notify of client's status
Excessive salt intake	Fluid balance WNL for client	
Noncompliance with medication regimen	Absence of peripheral edema	2. Review with client the interaction of excessive salt on body system
	Return to baseline weight	3. Explore in further detail types of foods he has been eating. Do a refrigerator and pantry review

B-10   TEST YOURSELF
Care-Planning Exercises: Answers–cont'd.

NURSING DIAGNOSIS	OUTCOMES	NURSING INTERVENTIONS
		4. Caution against food with hidden sodium
		5. Instruct client to weigh self on his scale each morning. Start a flow sheet
		6. Review and write down when he should call his doctor: increasing shortness of breath, weight gain, more edema
		7. Explore with physician possibility of antiembolism stockings
		8. Instruct client to elevate feet when sitting
		9. Emphasize importance of adhering to medication regimen

EVALUATIVE COMMENT:

(a) *Outcome achieved:*
Client's fluid volume excess has been resolved. On return visit, Al's weight has returned to baseline of 152 lb. Ankle edema less than 1+. Reports that he has "been eating the food that those people bring." Observed watching TV with feet elevated.

(b) *Outcome not achieved:*
Fluid volume excess continues to be a problem. On return visit, Al has lost only 1 lb and ankles are swollen. States he does not like the food from "Meals on Wheels" and has been eating TV dinners again.

Continued.

B-10   TEST YOURSELF
Care-Planning Exercises: Answers–cont'd.

CUES:
Hard dry stools
Straining
Decreased frequency of bowel movements

NURSING DIAGNOSIS	OUTCOMES	NURSING INTERVENTIONS
Colonic constipation related to changes in dietary intake, change in daily routine	Within two weeks resumes daily bowel movement	1. Evaluate present diet for fiber and fluid content 2. Explore knowledge of role of fluids, fiber, and exercise in management of constipation 3. Investigate possibility of antihypertensive medication contributing to constipation 4. Suggest adding fiber and natural bran to diet 5. Make out fluid intake plan to remind client to drink fluids within his restrictions (1500 ml) 6. Explore temporary use of natural laxatives; instruct on consequences of long-term laxative usage

B-10   TEST YOURSELF

Care-Planning Exercises: Answers–cont'd.

NURSING DIAGNOSIS	OUTCOMES	NURSING INTERVENTIONS
		7. Explore alternatives to providing well balanced meals: Neighbors Meals on Wheels Temporary homemaker
		8. Explore plan for increasing activity level

EVALUATIVE COMMENT:

(a) *Outcome achieved:*
Client's constipation has been relieved. Reports that he has one bowel movement daily without straining.

(b) *Outcome not achieved:*
Client reports that he is "still having problems with his bowel movements." Indicates that he is not straining as much but is only going every other day.

ABBREVIATIONS USED IN TEXT

AIDS	acquired immunodeficiency syndrome
bid	twice a day *(bis in die)*
B/P	blood pressure (expressed in millimeters of mercury [mmHg])
BUN	blood urea nitrogen
CBC	complete blood count
CPR	cardiopulmonary resuscitation
CT	computed tomography
CVA	cerebral vascular accident
CVP	central venous pressure
DX	diagnosis
ED	emergency department
EKG	electrocardiogram
Hct	hematocrit (expressed in grams/deciliter [g/dl])
Hgb	hemoglobin (expressed as vol%)
HIV	human immunodeficiency virus
ICU	intensive care unit
I/O	intake/output
IV	intravenous
IVP	intravenous pyelogram
MI	myocardial infarction
NPO	nothing by mouth *(nil per os)*
OR	operating room
P	pulse rate (expressed in beats/min)
PCA	patient-controlled analgesia
PO	oral *(per os)*
prn	as needed *(pro re nata)*
R	respiration rate (expressed in breaths/min)
RBC	red blood cell
ROM	range of motion
r/t	related to
T	temperature (expressed in degrees Fahrenheit [°F])
tid	three times a day *(ter in die)*
WBC	white blood cell
WNL	within normal limits
2°	secondary to

INDEX

NOTES

NOTES

NOTES

NOTES

NOTES

NOTES

NOTES

NOTES

NOTES

NOTES

NOTES

NOTES

NOTES